Multidrug Resistance: A Global Concern

Editor

Asad U. Khan, Ph.D

*Associate Professor,
Interdisciplinary Biotechnology
Unit, AMU, Aligarh
India*

Co-Editor

Raffaele Zarrilli, M.D. Ph.D.

*Associate Professor in Hygiene and Public Health,
Department of Preventive Medical Sciences,
Federico II University of Naples
Italy*

eBooks End User License Agreement

CONTENTS

Foreword   *i*

Preface   *ii*

List of Contributors   *iii*

CHAPTERS

1. **Role of Multidrug Resistance Associated Proteins in Drug Development**   3
   Shu-Feng Zhou, Jun-Ping Liu, Ming Qian Wei and Wei Duan

2. **Carbapenem-Resistant** *Klebsiella pneumoniae*   36
   Renato Finkelstein

3. **Control of Multi-Drug Resistance**   47
   Spyros Pournaras

4. **Multi-Drug Resistance Among Gram-Negative Bacteria in Thailand**   75
   Pattarachai Kiratisin

5. **Challenges in Management of Tuberculosis in Developing Countries**   90
   Amita Jain and Pratima Dixit

6. **Drug Resistance in Tuberculosis**   100
   UD Gupta and Anuj Kumar Gupta

7. **Extended Spectrum Beta Lactamases: A Critical Update**   115
   Shazi Shakil, Hafiz Muhammad Ali, Raffaele Zarrilli and Asad Ullah Khan

8. **Methicillin Resistant** *Staphylococcus aureus* **(MRSA)**   130
   Esperanza C. Cabrera

9. **Multidrug-Resistant** *Acinetobacter baumannii*: **An Emerging Threat in Health Care Facilities**   142
   Raffaele Zarrilli, Maria Triassi and Asad U. Khan

10. **Prevalence, Mechanisms and Dissemination of Antimicrobial Resistance in Enteric Foodborne Bacteria**   151
    Jing Han, Bashar W. Shaheen, Steven L. Foley and Rajesh Nayak

11. **The Scope of Bacterial Resistance to Antibiotics in Some Countries in the Middle East and North Africa**   176
    Noha Gamal Khalaf and Nancy D. Hanson

12. **Antimicrobial Resistance of Gram-Negative Bacteria in Saudi Arabia**   206
    Jaffar A. Al-Tawfiq and Ziad A. Memish

13. **β-Lactamases as Major Mechanism of Resistance in Gram-Negative Bacteria**   210
    Mariagrazia Perilli, Giuseppe Celenza, Cristina Pellegrini and Gianfranco Amicosante

Index   227

FOREWORD

Once heralded as a miracle drug, penicillin was the first antibiotic in the war against infectious disease. Alexander Fleming recognized the potential for misuse and warned that misuse of antibiotics could result in the development of mutant forms of bacteria that were resistant to those drugs. Fleming's words proved true not just for penicillin but for each antibiotic subsequently developed.

Despite the development of so many antibiotic molecules during the last fifty years, increasing antibiotic resistance worldwide may lead to therapeutic dead-end. In a growing number of cases bacteria are resistant to multiple drugs. This excellent eBook covers many aspects on resistance issues in bacteria. It covers the problem of methicillin resistance in *Staphylococcus aureus* that is observed in hospital and now in the community. The spread of methicillin-resistance in the community in *S. aureus* many complicate significantly its control-antibiotic resistance in tuberculosis which is a growing problem mostly in developing countries. The current situation in this research area is excellently summarized here. By far, its seems that resistance to broad-spectrum antibiotics may significantly hamper the use of those drugs for treating Gram-negative related infections. This is the reason why the parts in this eBook on resistance in Gram-negatives are expanded significantly here. Molecular and biochemical bases of resistance in Gram negatives are given in detail here and all interesting aspects are covered from the most fundamental to the most clinical points of view. The resistance traits often identified first in many developing countries may be spread worldwide at a quite high rate due to globalization and modern travel means. This has been examplified for the carbapenemase NDM-1 that is now identified worldwide. Multidrug resistance in Gram negatives is driven by the emerging carbapenemases and the clavulanic-acid inhibited ESBLs which were among the most important emerging resistance mechanisms in Gram-negatives in 2010. They are associated to other resistance mechanisms (aminoglycosides, fluoroquinolones) explaining the multidrug resistance patterns observed to a large extent. Many excellent chapters here identified those mechanisms and indicated how to control their spread. Control of spread of these multidrug resistant isolated in Gram-negative rods could be possible for a short period of time in hospitals. However, if they will spread in the community their control will be impossible. Treatment of many infections associated to multidrug resistant Gram-negatives infections will need evaluation of clinical efficacy of "old" drugs in combination (colistin, fosfomycin…) or the development of totally novel molecules. We are not sure that such molecules would be available from a clinical point of view within the next five years. Therefore, control of multidrug of those bacteria will be one of the most important issues for the human health.

It shall be kept in mind that many modern techniques in medicine (grafts, heart by-pass…) rely on antibiotics either for a prophylactic usage or for treating possible post-operative infections. Lack of efficient antibiotics may hamper significantly parts of the medicine developed in the last thirty years.

Prof. P. Nordmann
Head Dept. Bacteriology-Virology
Med. School South Paris

PREFACE

Infectious diseases are the world's leading cause of premature deaths, killing almost 50,000 people everyday. An increase in the emergence of health care- and community-associated infections caused by multi drug resistant bacteria is threatening the world population. The presence of antibiotic resistance genes on bacterial plasmids has further helped in the transmission and spread of drug resistance among pathogenic bacteria.

This eBook is composed of wide range of chapters related to multi drug resistance among infectious diseases in different parts of the world. Multiple drug resistance is becoming a big challenge for the physicians and clinicians to treat various infections. It also affects the economy of the country especially pharmaceutical industries where a huge amount of money is going into garbage.

The main focus of this eBook is to understand the different molecular mechanisms responsible for developing resistance against this group of antibiotics. The eBook is composed of 13 chapters describing mechanisms of antimicrobial resistance and their prevalence in various parts of the world. Most of the chapters are covering beta-lactamases and their extended form of enzymes, their variants in infectious diseases as well as in food born pathogens. CTX-M family of enzyme which hydrolyzes third generation of cephalosporins preferably, cefotaxime, belongs to the category of Extended-Spectrum ß-Lactamases (ESBLs) and includes almost 89 variants. These types of enzymes are emerging among Gram-negative bacteria; predominantly *Klebsiella pneumonia*, *Escherichia coli* and other species in different parts of the world. Another important class of beta-lactamases, the bla_{TEM}, and bla_{SHV}, most prevalent among enterobacteriacae in different parts, is also discussed in this eBook. MRSA and VRSA are also analyzed in great detail along with carbapenem resistance in *Acinetobacter baumannii* and *Pseudomonas aeruginosa* in some of the chapters. Drug Resistance in Tuberculosis and its management in developing countries are also analyzed. Finally, several approaches to control the spread of multi-drug resistance organisms are examined.

We are indebted to members of our research group, over a period of 10 years especially for scientific discussions, exchange of ideas and of course experimental data on drug resistance. Dr. Asad is highly thankful to Prof M Saleemuddin for inspiring him to take this task of compiling this information in the form of eBook. We also thank all the authors who kindly agreed to write chapters for the eBook.

We would like to thank Prof. Patrice Nordmann for writing the foreword and Bentham Science Publishers, particularly Mr Mahmood Alam and Ms Salma Siddiqui for their support and efforts.

Asad U. Khan
Biotechnology Unit, AMU, Aligarh
India

Raffaele Zarrilli
Department of Preventive Medical Sciences
Federico II University of Naples
Italy

List of Contributors

Shu-Feng, Zhou Jun-Ping, Liu Ming Qian and Weiwei Duan
RMIT University, Melbourne, Australia.

Renato Finkelstein
Infectious Diseases Unit, Rambam Medical Center, 31096–Bat Galim, Haifa.

Spyros Pournaras
Medical School, University of Thessaly, Uni. Hospital of Larissa, 41110 Larissa, Greece.

Pattarachai Kiratisin
Department of Microbiology, Faculty of Medicine, Siriraj Hospital, Mahidol University, 2 Prannok Rd., Bangkok-Noi, Bangkok 10700, Thailand.

Amita Jain and Pratima Dixit
Department of Microbiology, C.S.M. Medical University, Lucknow, India.

UD Gupta and Anuj Kumar Gupta
National JALMA Institute for Leprosy & Other Mycobacterial Diseases, (ICMR), Tajganj, Agra- 282001, India.

Shazi Shakil, Hafiz Mohammad Ali, Raffaele Zarrilli and Asad Ullah Khan
Interdisciplinary Botechnology Unit, Aligarh Muslim University Aligarh 202002 India.

Esperanza C. Cabrera
Department of Biology, De La Salle University, Manila, Philippines.

Raffaele Zarrilli Maria Triassi and Asad Ullah Khan
Department of Preventive Medical Sciences, Hygiene Section, University of Naples 'Federico II', Naples, Italy.

Jing Han, Bashar Shaheen, Steven L. Foley and Rajesh Nayak
US Food and Drug Administration, National Center for Toxicological Research (HFT-250), Division of Microbiology, 3900 NCTR Road, Jefferson, AK 72079, USA.

Noha Gamal Khalaf and Nancy D. Hanson
Department of Microbioloty and Immunoloty, Faculty of Pharcy, Modern Science and Arts University , Cariro Egypt and Director of Molecular Biology unit at Center for Research in Anti-Infectives and Biotechnology, Department of Medical Microbiology and Immunology, Creighton University School of Medicine, Omaha, NE 68178, USA.

Jaffar A. Al-Tawfiq and Ziad A. Memish
Internal Medicine Services Division, Dhahran Health Center, Saudi Aramco Medical Services Organization, Saudi Aramco, Dhahran, Saudi Arabia.

Mariagrazia Perilli, Giuseppe Celenza, Cristina Pellegrini and Gianfranco Amicosante
Dipartimento di Scienze e Tecnologie Biomediche, Università degli Studi dell'Aquila, Italy.

2

CHAPTER 1

Role of Multidrug Resistance Associated Proteins in Drug Development

Shu-Feng Zhou[1*], Jun-Ping Liu[2], Ming Qian Wei[3] and Wei Duan[4]

[1]*RMIT University, Melbourne, Australia,* [2]*Monash University, Melbourne, Australia and* [3]*Griffith University, Gold Coast, Australia,* [4]*Deakin University, Geelong, Australia*

Abstract: The Multidrug Resistance Associated Proteins ((MRP1, MRP2, MRP3, MRP4, MRP5, MRP6, MRP7, MRP8 and MRP9) belong to the ATP-binding cassette superfamily (ABCC family) of transporters expressed differentially in the liver, kidney, intestine and blood-brain barrier. MRPs transport a structurally diverse array of endo- and xenobiotics and their metabolites (in particular conjugates) and are subject to induction and inhibition by a variety of compounds. An increased efflux of natural product anticancer drugs and other anticancer agents by MRPs in cancer cells is associated with tumor resistance. These transporting proteins play a role in the absorption, distribution and elimination of various compounds in the body. There are increased reports on the clinical impact of genetic mutations of genes encoding MRP1-9. Therefore, MRPs have an important role in drug development, since a better understanding of their function and regulating mechanism can help minimize and avoid drug toxicity, unfavorable drug-drug interactions, and to overcome drug resistance.

Keywords: ATP-binding cassette superfamily, xenobiotics, multidrug resistance, blood-brain barrier, drug toxicity, genetic mutations, tumor resistance, transporting proteins, drug-drug interactions.

INTRODUCTION

The ATP-Binding Cassette (ABC) superfamily of transporters consist of a large number of functionally diverse transmembrane proteins which have been subdivided into seven families designated A through G [1-4]. Members of this transport superfamily display high amino acid similarity of the 200 amino acids surrounding the ATP-binding folds. Approximately 1100 ABC transporters are known at this time. Traffic ATPases and P-glycoproteins (Pgps) are other names used for this family. The family includes bacterial transporters, the cystic fibrosis transmembrane conductance regulator, the *Plasmodium falciparum* drug-resistance gene and genes apparently involved in peptide transport during antigen presentation.

In humans, members of this family serve a variety of physiological roles in transmembrane transport and cell signalling, many of which are associated with disease phenotypes such as multidrug resistance, cystic fibrosis, Tangier disease, adrenoleukodystrophy and Zellwegers' syndrome [1, 2, 4]. The available outline of the human genome contains 48 ABC genes [5]; 16 of these have a known function and 14 are associated with a defined human disease. ABC transporters that pump cytotoxic drugs from the cell are also present in micro-organisms, and this is one of the main mechanisms by which pathogenic species can resist antibiotic treatment. The human family of ABC transporters includes at least 48 members with 7 subfamilies [4]. They facilitate unidirectional translocation of chemically diverse substrates including amino acids, lipids, inorganic ions, peptides, saccharides, metals, drugs, and proteins. Energy derived from the hydrolysis of ATP is used to transport the substrate across the membrane against a concentration gradient [6]. These transporters are present in almost all tissues and cell types in different amounts. A typical ABC transporter is characterized by the presence of three peptide motifs: *Walker* A and B sequences and the so-called ABC-signature sequence ("ALSGGQ") [1, 7]. Most ABC proteins from eukaryotes encode full transporters, consisting of two ATP-binding domains and 12 membrane-spanning regions or half transporters, which are presumed to dimerize [8]. The MRP family contains at least nine members (MRP1-9, ABCC1-6 and ABCC10-12, respectively) with sizes from 1325 to 1545 amino acids. This probably completes the family, as there are no other putative MRP genes among the 52 human ABC transporter genes. ABCC7 (CFTR) is

*Address correspondence to Shu-Feng Zhou: RMIT University, Melbourne, Australia; Tel: +61 3 9925 7794; Fax: +61 3 9925 7178; Email: shufeng.zhou@rmit.edu.au

a chloride channel, and channels are not transporters. ABCC8 and 9 (SUR1 and 2), the sulfonylurea receptors, are the ATP-sensing subunits of a complex potassium channel and are not known to transport any substrates. The MRPs, CFTR, and the SURs are considered to evolve from a common ancestor, and these proteins are now grouped together in the C branch of the ABC transporter family. This paper highlights the pharmacological roles of MRPs and their implications in drug development.

TOPOLOGY OF MRPS

PgP/MDR1 consists of 1276 to 1280 amino acids with a molecular mass of 170 kDa. The commonly accepted model for the topologic structure of PgP has a tandemly duplicated structure, with each half of the molecule contains a Nucleotide-Binding Domain (NBD) and reveals six predicted and highly hydrophobic transmembrane regions [4]. The N- and C-termini, as well as the NBDs, are located intracellularly, and the first extracellular loop is *N*-glycosylated. Both NBDs are essential for proper functioning of the protein. Each consists of two core consensus motifs referred to as the *Walker A* and *B* motifs and a S signature of ABC transporters [9]. These motifs generally are found in a wide range of ATPases, and they are involved directly in the binding and hydrolysis of nucleotides. Structures of bacterial ABC transporter proteins suggest that the two NBDs form a common binding site where the energy of ATP is harvested to promote efflux through a pore that is delineated by the transmembrane helice [10]. The two half molecules are separated by a highly charged "linker region" which is phosphorylated at several sites by protein kinase C. Different topologic orientations of PgP have been reported, and several studies have indicated that conformational changes in the structure of PgP are involved in the mechanism of substrate efflux [11].

Like PgP, MRPs belong to ABC transporter superfamily. All MRP members have 2 hydrophobic transmembrane domains (TMD1 & TMD2) and 2 cytoplasmic NBDs [12]. The NBDs are responsible for the ATP binding/hydrolysis that drives drug transport, and their structure is conserved independently of the degree of primary- sequence homology [13]. The TMDs contain the drug-binding sites that are likely located in a flexible internal chamber that is sufficiently large to accommodate different drugs. MRPs can be categorized according to the presence or absence of a third (NH_2-terminal) membrane-spanning domain (TMD_0) in their structure (Fig. **1**) [14-16]. This topological feature can be found in MRP1, MRP2, MRP3, MRP6, and MRP7, while it is not possessed by MRP4, MRP5, MRP8, and MRP9 [17-20]. TMD_0 is not essential for catalytic function or intracellular routing; the function of this domain is unknown [21]. MRPs with this structural feature have the ability to transport conjugates, while MRPs without it are able to transport cyclic nucleotides. Long MRPs share an L_0 segment with a highly conserved sequence near its N-terminus. This sequence is also present near the N terminus of the short MRPs. It is essential for function and appears to associate with the membrane.

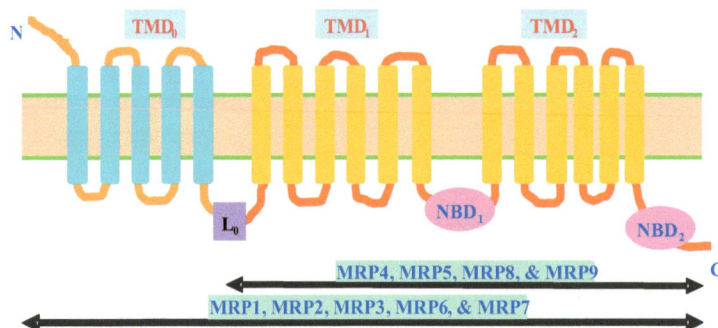

Figure 1: Predicted topological structure of MRP1-9 (ABCC1-6 & 10-12). All MRP members have two hydrophobic transmembrane domains (TMD1 and TMD2) and two cytoplasmic Nucleotide Binding Domains (NBDs) responsible for the ATP binding and hydrolysis that drives drug transport. MRPs can be categorized according to the presence or absence of a third (NH_2-terminal) membrane-spanning domain (TMD_0) in their structure. This topological feature can be found in MRP1, MRP2, MRP3, MRP6, and MRP7, while it is not possessed by MRP4, MRP5, MRP8, and MRP9. TMD_0 is not essential for catalytic function or intracellular routing; the function of this domain is unknown. Long MRPs share an L_0 segment with a highly conserved sequence near its N terminus. This sequence is also present near the N terminus of the short MRPs. It is essential for function and appears to associate with the membrane.

SUBSTRATE SPECIFICITY, RESISTANCE PROFILES AND INHIBITOR SELECTIVITY OF MRPS

The first member of MRP family, MRP1 (ABCC1), was found in 1992 in lung cancer cell line conferring resistance to doxorubicin which was not related to PgP [22]. The genes encoding MRP1 and PgP are evolutionarily very distant, and the primary structure of the two proteins is quite dissimilar, sharing only 15 percent amino acid identity [22]. Most of the sequence similarity between MRP1 and PgP is found within the nucleotide-binding domains that generally are conserved among members of the ABC superfamily [23]. MRP1 is larger than other full-length ABC proteins, containing approximately 250 additional amino acids in its NH_2 terminal. Thus, in addition to the 12 transmembrane segments characterizing PgP, MRP1 has five transmembrane domains. MRP1 is nearly present in all major tissues and in all peripheral blood cell types [24, 25]. The expression levels of MRP1 are different in various organs and cell lines [26-29]. Natural product drugs such as vincristine, etoposide and doxorubicin are substrates for MRP1 [30]. Although MRP1 and PgP have some identical substrates, they show difference in the substrate specificity. PgP can transport drugs in original form, while MRP1 can transport glutathione (GSH), oxidized GSH (GSSG), as well as a number of GSH, glucuronate and sulfate conjugates of drugs (Fig. **2**) [30-32]. Additionally, MRP1 has several physiologic substrates, such as 17-β-D-estradiol-glucuronide ($E_2$17βG), the GSH-conjugated cysteinyl leukotriene C_4 (LTC_4), sulfated bile acids, prostaglandin (PG) A GSH conjugates, and unconjugated bilirubin [33-38]. The high affinity for LTC_4 is a specific feature of MRP1, which may contribute to the distinguished role of MRP1 in immune responses associated with cellular excretion of LTC_4 [39, 40]. In contrast, PgP shows poor resistance to these conjugated organic anions [31]. Moreover, significant species difference in the substrate specificity of MRP1 has been noted.

Substrates of MRP1 also include neutral and basic cytotoxic compounds without conjugation with GSH or other anionic drugs [41, 42]. However, intracellular GSH is needed when MRP1 transports these chemicals [43, 44]. GSH concentrations increase in some organs of *mrp* knockout mice [45], and decrease in cells overexpressing MRP1 [31, 46]. MRP1 may reduce the harm of xenobiotics to cells by co-transporting the xenobiotics and GSH out [45]. Overexpression of MRP1 is associated with an increased transport activity of compounds conjugated with GSH, glucuronide, or sulfate, which is known as glutathione conjugate pumps [35, 47, 48]. GSH not only can enhance MRP1-mediated transport of hydrophobic xenobiotics, but also certain hydrophilic conjugated endobiotics [29]. However, MRP1 has low affinity to GSH [49, 50]. Drugs including verapamil and apigenin have been demonstrated to increase the affinity of MRP1 to GSH [51, 52]. Vincristine uptake is inhibited by vinblastine but not daunorubicin or doxorubicin. Although GSH or vincristine alone has little effect on the MRP1-mediated transport of LTC_4, the combination of them becomes the potent inhibitor of MRP1-mediated transport of LTC_4 [49].

Human MRP1 confers resistance to anthracycline drugs, while Mrp1 from other species do not [53, 54]. Unlike PgP, however, MRP1 appears to cause resistance to some heavy metal ions, including arsenite and antimonials [55, 56], which is consistent with the extensive homology of *MRP1* with the *Leishmania* arsenite transporter-encoding gene (*ltpgpA*) and the yeast cadmium factor gene (*ycf1*). In addition to alkaloid cytotoxic drugs, MRP1 is resistant to methotrexate (MTX), ZD1694 and GW1843 [57, 58]. The topoisomerase I inhibitors, camptothecin derivative, CPT-11 (irinotecan), and its active metabolite, SN-38 in unconjugated and conjugated forms are also actively effluxed out of cells by MRP1 [59]. MRP1 confers resistance to doxorubicin, vincristine, etoposide, and mitoxantrone [60, 61]. MRP1 substrates also include conjugates of thiotepa, cyclophosphamide, chlorambucil, and melphalan [60, 62, 63]. The resistance capability of MRP1 to melphalan can be increased by co-upregulation of glutathione S-transferases or the GSH biosynthetic enzyme, γ-glutamylcysteine synthetase [62, 63].

MRP1 also confers resistance to arsenic in association with GSH [55]. The ability of MRP1 to cause arsenite resistance in transfected or selected cellsand the overexpression of MRP1 in cells selected for arsenite [55] has raised the question of whether MRP1 might be responsible for the arsenite resistance of patients treated with arsenite for acute promyelocytic leukemia. However, that the $Mrp1^{-/-}$ mouse is not hypersensitive to arsenite [64], which suggests that MRP1 is not a critical factor in the cellular defense against arsenite. This could be due to the rapid excretion of the complexes of arsenite and methylarsenite with GSH into bile [65].

MRP1 transports the protease inhibitors, ritonavir and saquinavir [66-68], the antiandrogen drug flutamide and its metabolite hydroxyflutamide [69], and the GSH conjugates of ethacrynic acid (a diuretic) [70]. In addition, the radiopharmaceuticals [99mTc]-Sestamibi, [99mTc]-Tetrofosmin, and the gadolinium chelate B22956/1 are substrates of MRP1 [71-73]. Such compounds are used in clinical functional imaging studies and recently they may be used for *in vivo* imaging of hepatobiliary transport function.

A number of chemical toxicants and their metabolites are known to be the substrates for MRP1. Aflatoxin B1 and several *S* and *R* GSH conjugate stereoisomers of aflatoxin B1 [74], the GSH conjugates of herbicide metolachlor [75], and the GSH conjugates of the model toxicants 1-chloro-2,4-dinitrobenzene [76] and 4-nitroquinoline 1-oxide [77] have been identified as MRP1 substrates. However, a recent study indicated that carcinogen aflatoxin B1 induced a similar number of lung and liver tumors in both *mrp1*-null and wide type mice [78]. This may be due to the redundancy of transmembrane export pumps, other pumps may effectively vicariate for MRP1-mediated transport of aflatoxin B1 and its glutathione conjugates. In addition, the 3β-*O*-glucuronide conjugate of the tobacco metabolite 4-(methylnitrosamino)-1-(3-pyridyl)-1-butanol (NNAL) is also a substrate of MRP1 [52]. Notably, the NNAL-*O*-glucuronide transport by MRP1 requires physiological concentrations of GSH [52]. NNAL is a lung cancer inducer.

MRP1 and murine Mrp1 are normally located in intracellular vesicles of undefined nature and in the basolateral membrane of epithelial membranes. Hence, MRP1 secretes drugs into the body, rather than moving them out of the body as PgP or MRP2 do. This makes MRP1 a system of cellular defense rather than one of total organism defense like Mdr1 Pgp and MRP2, which eliminate drugs from the body. The importance of this cellular function is highlighted by the fact that mice lacking Mrp1 are hypersensitive to etoposide [64, 79], whereas an increased sensitivity to vincristine is uncovered in the TKO mice (triple knockout mice in which the disrupted *Mrp1* alleles are combined with disruptions of the two drug-transporting Pgp (ABCB1) genes, *Mdr1a* and *Mdr1b*) [79]. In mice, loss of Mrp1 is associated only with increased sensitivity to epipodophyllotoxins (*e.g.* etoposide) and *Vinca* alkaloids (*e.g.* vincristine), the drugs also most affected by the absence of Mrp1 in *Mrp1* (−/−) embryonic stem cells [64]. Knockout mice without *mrp1* have a decreased response to inflammatory stimuli, increased levels of GSH, and increased sensitivity to etoposide but are otherwise healthy and fertile [40, 64].

Table 1. Tissue distribution, substrates and inhibitors of MRPs.

Name	Symbol	Tissue Location	Expression Levels	Major Drug Substrates	Physiologic Substrates	Inhibitors
MRP1	ABCC1	All major tissues	Differ in various organs and cell lines	Doxorubicin, vincristine, etoposide, MTX, camptothecin, CPT-11, SN-38, cyclophosphamide, conjugates	Glutathione, LTC4, E$_2$17βG, sulfated bile acids, bilirubin, PGA GSH conjugate, GSH, GSSG	Probenecid, sulfinpyrazone, indomethacin, verapamil, quercetin, genistein, cyclosporine, PAK-104P, steroid analogs, MK571, ONO-1078, sulphonylurea, glibenclamide
MRP2	ABCC2, cMOAT	Liver, kidney, intestine, brain		Conjugates, cisplatin, etoposide, vinca alkaloids, anthracyclines, Camptothecins, MTX, lopinavir, olmesartan	LTC4, GSH, GSSG, bilirubin conjugates, LTD4, LTE4,	MK571, furosemide,
MRP3	ABCC3	Small intestine, pancreas, colon, placenta, adrenal gland	Low level in liver, brain, kidney and prostate	Etoposide, teniposide, dinitrophenyl S-glutathione, acetaminophen glucuronide, vincristine, MTX	LTC4, E$_2$17βG, cholate, glycocholate, taurocholate	Etoposide, MTX
MRP4	ABCC4	Kidneys	Low levels in other tissues	MTX, 6-thioguanine, PMEA, 6-mercaptopurine, topotecan	cGMP, cAMP, DHEAS, E$_2$17βG, PGE$_1$, PGE$_2$	MK571, celecoxib, rofecoxib, diclofenac
MRP5	ABCC5	Most tissues	Low levels	6-Mercaptopurine, 6-thioguanine, PMEA, heavy metals, *S*-(2,4-dinitrophenyl)glutathione	cGMP, cAMP	Probenecid, sulfinpyrazone, benzbromarone, MK571
MRP6	ABCC6	Liver, kidney	Low levels in other tissues	LTC4, N-ethylmaleimide S-glutathione, dinitrophenol glutathione, etoposide, doxorubicin, cisplatin, daunorubicin	?	Indomethacin, probenecid, benzbromarone
MRP7	ABCC10	Most tissues	Very low levels	?	E$_2$17βG	?
MRP8	ABCC11	Normal breast, testis	Low levels in liver, brain, and placenta	5-FU, ddC, PMEA, MTX, bile acids	cGMP, cAMP, LTC4, DHEAS,	?
MRP9	ABCC12	Breast cancer, normal breast, testis, brain, skeletal muscle, ovary	Low levels	?	?	?

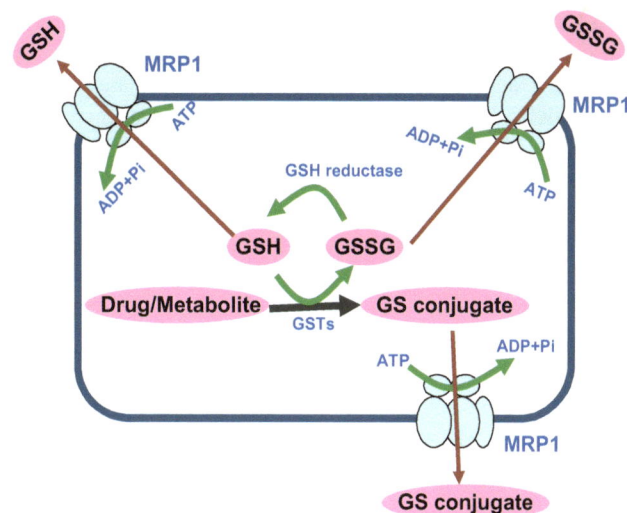

Figure 2: Glutathione (GSH)-dependent transport of drugs and their GSH conjugates by MRP1. P-glycoprotein can transport drugs in original form, while MRP1 can transport GSH, oxidized GSH (GSSG), as well as a number of GSH, glucuronate and sulfate conjugates of drugs. However, MRP1 has low affinity to GSH and GSSH. GSH not only enhances MRP1-mediated transport of hydrophobic xenobiotics, but also certain hydrophilic conjugated endobiotics, which represents a major detoxifying pathway.

A variety of inhibitors of MRP1 have been identified, but their specificity as yes to be determined. Some general inhibitors of organic anion transport including probenecid, sulfinpyrazone and indomethacin are able to inhibit MRP1 [80-82]. The inhibitors of PgP such as verapamil, quercetin, genistein and cyclosporine can also suppress the transport activity of MRP1 [83-87]. Other PgP and MRP1 dual inhibitors include the dihydropyridine PAK-104P [88], the polyhydroxylated sterol acetate agosterol A [89], steroid analogs [90, 91], and imidazothiazole derivatives [92]. The MRP1 inhibiting bioflavonoids, such as genistein, quercetin, biochanin A, and kaempferol, can also decrease the intracellular GSH levels [84-87]. The non-nucleoside reverse transcriptase inhibitors (delavirdine, efavirenz, and nevirapine), nucleoside reverse transcriptase inhibitors (abacavir, emtricitabine, and lamivudine), and tenofovir as a nonnucleotide reverse transcriptase inhibitor also inhibited MRP1 *in vitro* [93].

There are some inhibitors specific to MRP family members. For example, the LTD4 receptor antagonist, MK571, is a GSH conjugate inhibiting both MRP1 and MRP2 [94]. Different to MK571 in structure, the peptide leukotriene receptor antagonist ONO-1078, has also been demonstrated to reduce LTC$_4$-efflux in lung tumor cells by blocking MRP1 function [95]. The sulphonylurea, glibenclamide also shows inhibitory activity to both MRP1 and MRP2 [96]. In addition, several highly specific ad potent MRP1 inhibitors have been identified. These include tricyclic isoxazole derivatives such as LY475776 and LY402913 [97-99]. It has been reported that some antisense oligonucleotides are also able to inhibit MRP1 activity by reducing MRP1 mRNA levels and the protein synthesis [100-102]. For instance, some antisense oligonucleotides reduce the expression level of the MRP1 protein by 46% and its mRNA level by 76% [102]. ISIS 7597, an antisense oligonucleotide, is able to quickly decrease intracellular MRP1 mRNA levels by up to 90% at a low concentration (0.5 μM) [100].

MRP2 (ABCC2) is also known as the Canalicular Multispecific Organic Anion Transporter (cMOAT). The amino acids of MRP2 have 49% identity with MRP1 [103]. Human *MRP2* maps to chromosome 10q23-24 and consists of 32 exons spanning 65 kb [104]. The location of MRP2 is unique, as it is present on the apical plasma membranes of polarized cells such as hepatocytes, pneumocytes, kidney proximal tubules, and specialized cells in the intestine and brain [105, 106], while other MRPs are all located on basolateral membrane of polarized cells. Based on its localization and substrate specificity, it is proposed that the primary physiological function of MRP2 is to export amphiphilic organic anions and xenobiotics into bile and into the lumen of excretory organs [107].

Like MRP1, MRP2 transfected cells are resistant to etoposide, vinca alkaloids, anthracyclines, camptothecins, CPT-11 and MTX [58, 108-110]. The substrates of MPR1 and MRP2 have similarity with regard to the transport of GSH and glucuronate, and sulfate conjugates, but there are some important differences. The affinity of MRP2 to GSH conjugates is less than that of MRP1 [111, 112]. For instance, the affinity to MRP2 for both LTC_4 and N-ethylmaleimide glutathione is found to be significantly lower than that of MRP1 [82], whereas bilirubin mono- and bis-glucuronides have higher affinity for MRP2 [105, 113]. MRP2 is distinct from MRP1 with the ability to confer resistance to cisplatin [108-110], probably in the presence of GSH [47]. Cisplatin resistance in MRP2-overexpressing cells is thus abrogated by MRP2 antisense cDNA. GSH itself appears to be a relatively low affinity substrate for MRP2 [114], but the co-transport of GSH with MRP2 substrate is similar to that observed for MRP1 [112, 115].

MRP2 transports an array of conjugated endogenous metabolites. In addition to LTC_4, GSH, GSSG, and bilirubin conjugates, MRP2 is able to transport LTD_4, LTE_4, and the glucuronide conjugates of estrodiol and triiodo-L-thyronine [111]. The substrates of MRP2 also include the glucuronide conjugates of grepafloxacin, diclofenac and acetaminophen [111, 116, 117]. Moreover, sulfated MRP2 substrates include taurolithocholate sulfate and taurochenodeoxycholate sulfate, but not estrone 3-sulfate [118, 119].

MRP2 also transport ampicillin, ceftriaxone, pravastatin, temocaprilat, grepafloxacin and BQ-123 [118, 120]. Olmesartan, a novel angiotensin II blocker, is a substrate of MRP2 [121]. A previous study reported that the biliary excretion of olmesartan is mediated by Mrp2 based on low biliary excretion in Eisai Hyperbilirubinemic Rats (EHBR), which are inherited mrp2-deficient rats, compared with Sprague-Dawley Rats [122]. Moreover, the HIV protease inhibitors saquinavir, lopinavir, ritonavir and indinavir are MRP2 substrates [123, 124]. Similar to MRP1, MRP2 can transport ^{99m}Tc-labeled compounds used in functional imaging studies [125].

Interestingly, MRP2 shows its ability to transport certain carcinogens and other toxicants as conjugates or as unconjugated organic anions. For example, MRP2 can transport the tobacco carcinogen NNAL, and in contrast to MRP1, GSH is not needed [52]. MRP2 is also capable of transporting the GSH conjugate of (+)-anti-benzo[a]pyrene-7,8-diol-9,10-epoxide, the active metabolite of benzo[a]pyrene [126]. Other toxicants as substrates of MRP2 include arsenite, cadmium and α-naphthylisothiocyanate with the need of GSH [127, 128]. This suggests a role of MRP2 in chemoprotection n the body.

Many inhibitors of MRP2 have been established, and most of which do not have high selectivity to MRP2. For instance, MK571 can also inhibit MRP1 and MRP3. The organic anions have different inhibitory effects on MRP2. For example, probenecid and furosemide inhibit, whereas under certain conditions, sulfinpyrazone, penicillin G, and indomethacin considerably stimulated MRP2 transport activity [82]. However, all these compounds inhibit MRP1-ATPase capability. MRP1 may be a more potent transporter of GSH conjugates and free GSH than MRP2, but several anions are preferred substrates for MRP2. This may indicate different modulation selectivity on MRP1 or MRP2 in drug resistant cancer cells [82]. The MPR2-mediated transport of known substrate $E_2 17\beta G$ can be blocked by bile acids and certain amphipathic anions [129, 130]. The antisense cDNA expression is also used to block the drug resistance capability of MRP2 [131]. The non-nucleoside reverse transcriptase inhibitors (delavirdine, efavirenz, and nevirapine), nucleoside reverse transcriptase inhibitors (abacavir, emtricitabine, and lamivudine), and tenofovir as a nonnucleotide reverse transcriptase inhibitor also inhibited MRP2 *in vitro* [93].

Among the MRP family, MRP3 has the highest amino acid sequence resemblance (58%) with MRP1 [132]. Less is known about this protein than either MRP1 or MRP2. Although most closely related to MRP1 and MRP2, MRP3 has its own particular pattern of tissue localisation and substrate specificity. MRP3 mRNA is mainly detected in small intestine, pancreas, colon, placenta, and adrenal gland, while lower levels are found in liver, brain, kidney and prostate [133-135]. MRP3 is mainly localized in the basolateral membrane of polarized cells such as cholangiocytes, hepatocytes an enterocytes [129].

MRP3 confers resistance to a much narrower spectrum of anticancer drugs compared to MRP1 and MRP2, and the drugs are limited to vincristine, methotrexate, epipodophyllotins (etoposide and teniposide) [136,

137]. MRP3-mediated transport of etoposide is inhibited by some organic anion transport inhibitors, but is not influenced by the reduction of intracellular GSH level. MRP3 is also involved in the transport of $E_2$17βG, LTC4, dinitrophenyl S-glutathione, acetaminophen glucuronide, but not GSH and etoposide glucuronide [138, 139]. Both etoposide and MTX can block the MRP3-mediated transport of $E_2$17βG [140]. Unlike MRP1 and MRP2, MRP3 has a higher affinity to glucuronate conjugates than to GSH conjugates [141]. Furthermore, the resistance capacity of MRP3 to etoposide and vincristine is much lower than that of MRP1. However, MRP3 shows poor resistance to some natural product drugs, such as anthracyclines and Taxol [137]. MRP3 is present in cancer cell lines from many tissues, but initial studies on MRP3 in a panel of drug-resistant cancer cell lines did not turn up any association between MRP3 levels and drug resistance [142]. However, there was a strong correlation between MRP3 and doxorubicin resistance in lung cancer lines [143].

In contrast to MRP1 and MRP2, MRP3 has a greater capacity to transport glucuronate conjugates than GSH conjugates, and it can not increase GSH efflux in transfected cells [144]. MRP3 also transports monovalent bile salts such as cholate, glycocholate and taurocholate which are not substrates for MRP1 and MRP2 [137, 145]. Conversely, the conjugated cholate 3-O-glucronide, taurochenodeoxycholate 3-sulfae and taurolithocholate-3-sulfte are substrates for all three MRP proteins [138]. Thus, MRP3 may have a role in entero-hepatic circulation of bile salts and it is considered to function as a backup detoxifying pathway for hepatocytes when normal canalicular route is damaged by cholestatic diseases and the function of MRP1 and MRP2 is impaired [146-148]. The non-nucleoside reverse transcriptase inhibitors (delavirdine, efavirenz, and nevirapine), nucleoside reverse transcriptase inhibitors (emtricitabine, and lamivudine), and tenofovir as a nonnucleotide reverse transcriptase inhibitor also inhibited MRP3 *in vitro* [93].

MRP4 (ABCC4) has particular tissue expression profile, drug resistance selectivity, and substrate and inhibitor specificity, in comparison with other MRPs. Although MRP4 mRNA is present in most organs, MRP4 protein is mainly detected in the kidneys [133]. MRP4 is a lipophilic anion pump capable of transporting some physiological and endogenous compounds. These include cyclic adenosine monophosphate (cAMP) and cyclic guanosine monophosphate (cGMP), GSH [149], and folate [150-152]. MRP4 is also able to mediate the uptake of PGE_1 and PGE_2, while MRP1, MRP2, MRP3, and MPR5 can not transport PGE_1 and PGE_2 [153, 154].

MRP4 is able to transport several endogenous organic anions and steroid conjugates, including $E_2$17βG [34, 35, 138], and dehydroepiandrosterone-3-sulfate (DHEAS) which is the major circulating steroid made in the adrenal gland in humans [155]. The affinity of MRP4 for $E_2$17βG is similar to that of MRP3, while lower than that of MRP1 and MRP2 [34, 35, 138]. No transport of DHEAS by MRP2 or MRP3 is found [155]. MRP4 mediates ATP-dependent co-transport of GSH or S-methyl-glutathione together with cholyltaurine, cholylglycine, or cholate [156]. A recent study has identified conjugated bile acids, especially sulfated derivatives, as substrates of MRP4 [155]. Bile acids, like the steroid $E_2$17βG, contain a cholesterol backbone structure and may thus represent physiological substrates of MRP4. GSH plays an important role in the function of MRP4, as MRP4 transports many of its substrates in a GSH-dependent manner and depletion of intracellular GSH by the GSH synthesis inhibitor, DL-buthionine-(S,R)-sulphoximine, blocks the MRP4-mediated export of cAMP and abolishes resistance to nucleoside analogues [149]. MRP4 participates in the hepatic basolateral excretion of sulfate conjugates [157].

A variety of nucleoside (purine and pyrimidine) analogues are found to be substrates for MRP4. These include ganciclovir [158], azidothymidine monophosphate [159], 9-(2-phosphonylmethoxyethyl)adenine (PMEA) [159, 160], bis(pivaloxymethyl)-9-(2-phosphonylmethoxyethyl)adenine, a lipophilic ester prodrug) [161], 6-mercaptopurine and 6-thioguanine [162]. ATP-dependent uptake of the acyclic nucleotide phosphonates, adefovir and tenofovir but not cidofovir, was observed only in the membrane vesicles expressing MRP4 [163]. The kidney accumulation of adefovir and tenofovir was significantly greater in Mrp4 knockout mice (130 *vs* 66 and 191 *vs* 87 pmol/g tissue, respectively); thus, the renal luminal efflux clearance was estimated to be 37 and 46%, respectively, of the control [163]. There was no change in the kinetic parameters of cidofovir in Mrp4 knockout mice. There was no difference in the fraction of mono- and diphosphorylated forms of adefovir in the kidney between wild-type and Mrp4 knockout mice [163]. These findings indicate that MRP4 is involved in the renal luminal efflux of both adefovir and tenofovir, but it makes only a limited contribution to the urinary excretion of cidofovir. MRP4 is also an efflux pump for urate, the purine end metabolite [164] and thioxanthosine monophosphate and thioinosine monophosphate (both thiopurine metabolites) [165]. Moreover, MRP4 transports the anticancer agents topotecan [166], leucovorin [151], and MTX [136, 151, 160]. Topotecan is a semi-synthetic, water-soluble derivative of camptothecin, a cytotoxic plant alkaloid isolated from the Chinese tree *Camptotheca acuminata* [167]. It is used as a second-line treatment for patients with ovarian carcinoma. Moreover, MRP4 can mediate the efflux of the glutathione conjugate of monochlorobimane, a bimane that forms fluorescent adduct with thiols [168].

A variety of inhibitors for MRP4 have been identified. Like MRP1 and MRP2, MRP4 is also inhibited by the leukotriene antagonist MK571 [152, 169]. The cellular efflux of cGMP by both MRP4 and MRP5 is inhibited by PGA1 and PGE1, the steroid progesterone and the anticancer drug estramustine (a combination of estrogen and mechlorethamine) [170]. PGA1 inhibited the ATP-dependent efflux of MTX, another MRP4 substrate [151, 171]. PGF1α, PGF2α, PGA1, and thromboxane B2 are high-affinity inhibitors (therefore presumably substrates) of MRP4-mediated transport of PGE1 and PGE2 [172]. The MRP4-mediated transport of PGE1 and PGE2 is also inhibited by rofecoxib and celecoxib (both COX-2-specific inhibitors), and diclofenac [172]. Sulfinpyrazone is a potent inhibitor (IC_{50} = 420 μM) of PMEA efflux in MRP4-overexpressing HEK293 cells [172]. MTX can inhibit the MRP4-mediated transport of $E_2 17\beta G$ [162]. Glucuronide and glutathione conjugates can also inhibit MRP4-mediated transport of MTX [151, 152]. The MRP4-mediated transport of $E_2 17\beta G$ is blocked in the presence of estradiol 3,17-disulphate, taurolithocholate 3-sulphate [155], or topotecan [166]. The MRP4-mediated transport of bimane-glutathione is totally inhibited in the presence of carbonylcyanide *m*-chlorophenylhydrasone (an uncoupler of oxidative phosphorylation) and significant inhibition is also observed with known inhibitors of MRP transporters including benzbromarone, verapamil, indomethacin, MTX, and 6-TG [168]. Such transport is also inhibited by 1-chloro-2,4-dinitrobenzene (CDNB) which is metabolized to the glutathione conjugate after entry into cells.

MRP4 may be regulated at transcriptional, translational and posttranslational level. Its expression is substantially increased in livers of mice with disruption of the farnesyl/bile acid nuclear receptor, which have increased levels of serum and hepatocellular bile acids, and MRP4 can be further upregulated by cholic acid feeding [173]. The constitutively active nuclear receptor (CAR) is required to coordinately upregulate hepatic expression of MRP4 and an enzyme known to sulfate hydroxy-bile acids and steroids (Sult2a1) [174]. CAR activators increased MRP4 and Sult2a1 expression in primary human hepatocytes and HepG2, a human liver cell line. Sult2a1 was down-regulated in MRP4-null mice, further indicating an inter-relation between MRP4 and Sult2a1 gene expression. Based on the hydrophilic nature of sulfated bile acids and MRP4's capability to transport sulfated steroids, these findings suggest that MRP4 and Sult2a1 participate in an integrated pathway mediating elimination of sulfated steroid and bile-acid metabolites from the liver. In addition, a recent study in infected human macrophages indicates that azidiothymidine treatment induces MRP4 mRNA [175].

Analysis of tissue RNA suggests that MRP5 is ubiquitously expressed. The highest levels are found in skeletal muscle and brain [142]. In comparison with MRP1-3, MRP5 (ABCC5) has its particular drug resistance selectivity and shows no resistance to natural anticancer compounds or MTX. MRP5 and MRP4 share only 36% amino acids identity, and their substrate specificity is similar. Both MRP4 and MRP5 are able to mediate the Mg^{++}/ATP-dependent transport of cGMP and cAMP. MRP4 has a higher affinity for cAMP than that of MRP5, while MRP5 has a higher affinity for cGMP that of MRP4 [162]. Like MRP4, MRP5 is capable to transporting purine derivatives including PMEA and 6-mercaptopurine [176, 177]. However, MRP4 is also able to transport some substrates of MRP1-3, such as $E_2 17\beta G$ and MTX [136]. MRP5 is able to transport *S*-(2,4-dinitrophenyl)glutathione which is inhibited by typical organic anion transport inhibitors, including sulfinpyrazone and benzbromarone [176]. However, most glutathione and glucuronate conjugates are not substrates of MRP5. Notably, MRP5 shows resistance to heavy metals including cadmium chloride and potassium antimonyl tartrate [177]. MRP5 can be modulated by general organic anion transport inhibitors, including probenecid, sulfinpyrazone, benzbromarone, and MK571 [172]. Like MRP4, there are no specific inhibitors of MRP5.

The physiological functions and possible role in drug resistance of MRP4 and 5 remain to be defined. Obviously, the discovery that these pumps can transport cyclic nucleotides, notably cGMP, has raised the question of whether MRP4/5 can affect the signal transduction role of cGMP by removing it from the cell, which would supplement the degradation by phosphodiesterases. There is also evidence for an extracellular signaling role for cGMP in kidney and several other tissues, and MRP4/5 might be involved. No human disease has been associated with alterations in MRP5, and the Mrp5 KO mouse, generated by Wijnholds *et al.* [176], has no obvious phenotype. It is possible, however, that the overlapping substrate specificities of MRP5 and MRP4 (and possibly MRP8 and 9) may hide the physiological function of Mrp5, *e.g.*, in cyclic nucleotide transport, and that the breeding of mice lacking all these transporters may lead to an understanding of the physiological function of each of them.

Human MRP6 is most closely related to MRP1 and MRP2 with 45% and 43% amino acid identity, respectively. The highest levels of MRP6 mRNA and protein expression are detected in kidney and liver while low levels are found in most other tissues such as skin and retina [178-180]. MRP6 is located on the basolateral membranes in hepatocytes and kidney proximal tubules [181]. Overexpression of MRP6 does lead to weak resistance to chemotherapeutic drugs [182]. Rat Mrp6 transported the cyclic cyclopentapeptide endothelin-1 receptor antagonist BQ123, although endothelin-1 itself is not a substrate of Mrp6 [183]. However, rat Mrp6 did not transport glucuronide, sulfate and GSH conjugates, hydrophobic drugs, PG s or aminophospholipids [183]. More recently, MRP6 was found to transport glutathione conjugates, such as LTC_4, N-ethylmaleimide S-glutathione and dinitrophenol glutathione, while $E_2 17\beta G$ appears a poor MRP6 substrate [182, 184]. Effective inhibitors of MRP1 and MRP2, including indomethacin, probenecid, and benzbromarone, can block the MRP6-mediated transport [184]. MRP6 also exhibited low-level resistant activity to a variety of natural product anticancer drugs, such as etoposide, teniposide, doxorubicin, cisplatin, and daunorubicin and dactinomycin [182]. These findings suggest that MRP6 may transport conjugated organic anions and probably confers resistance to anticancer drugs to a less effective extent than MRP1-3.

MRP7 (ABCC10) has the lowest amino acid sequence identity (33-36%) with other MRP family members [17]. Although MRP7 mRNA can be detected in most tissues, but the expression levels are usually very low [17]. MRP7 is able to transport $E_2 17\beta G$ with a high K_m (58 μM) [185]. This suggests that MRP7 may be a lipophilic anion transporter. In contrast, MRP7 did not transport other typical MRP substrates, such as cyclic nucleotides, MTX, or bile acids [185, 186]. Interestingly, MRP7 is as closely related to the SUR K_i channel regulators, but the functional implication is yet to be determined.

MRP8 (ABCC11) has 40% amino acids identity with MRP5, and has been characterized as an amphipathic anion transporter. MRP8 is mainly present in normal breast and testis, while little is present in liver, brain, and placenta [18]. With the ability to efflux cAMP and cGMP, MRP8 confers resistance to purine and pyrimidine nucleotide derivatives, including anticancer fluoropyrimidines, and several antiviral agents. Similar to the case for other MRPs that possess only two membrane spanning domains (MRP4 and MRP5), MRP8 is a cyclic nucleotide efflux pump that is able to confer resistance to nucleoside-based agents, such as PMEA and 5-FU [187]. In contrast, little resistance is found for some natural product anticancer drugs [188]. Recently, MRP8 is found to transport a variety of physiological and synthetic lipophilic anions, including the LTC_4, steroid sulfates such as dehydroepiandrosterone (DHEAS) and estrone 3-sulfate, $E_2 17\beta G$, leukotriene C4 and dinitrophenyl-S-glutathione, the monoanionic bile acids glycocholate and taurocholate, and MTX [189-192].

Both MRP8 and MRP9 genes are identified using a functional genomic approach and bioinformatics tools. Both MRP8 and MRP9 (ABCC12) have the highest degree of similarity with MRP5. One major difference between MRP8 and MRP9 is that MRP9 has only one ATP-binding domain but two transmembrane domains each with four membrane-spanning regions. The MRP9 gene is unusual because it encodes two transcripts of different sizes [193]. The larger 4.5-kb RNA is found in breast cancer, normal breast, and testis and encodes an MRP-like protein that lacks transmembrane domains 3, 4, 11, and 12 and the second nucleotide-binding domain. The smaller 1.3-kb RNA is detected in brain, skeletal muscle, and ovary and seems to encode the second nucleotide-binding domain. There is a lack of information on the substrate specificity of MRP9. It is speculated that MRP9 may have a different function from other family members. Because both MRP8 and MRP9 are membrane proteins with very restricted expression in essential tissues [20], they may represent potential molecular targets for targeted therapy with antibodies, antibody conjugates, and immunotoxins.

Various MRPs show considerable differences in their tissue distribution, substrate specificities, and proposed physiological and pharmacological functions. The tissue distribution, substrates and inhibitors of MRPs are listed in Table 1 MRPs are capable of transporting a structurally diverse array of endo- and xenobiotics including many therapeutic drugs and their metabolites across cell membranes. They play an important role in the absorption, disposition and elimination of many therapeutic agents in the body.

INDUCTION OF MRPS

Regulation of ABC transporter gene expression involves participation of numerous nuclear receptors [194-196]. Nuclear receptors constitute a family of transcription factors that act as heterodimers, which bind to promoter elements and induce gene expression. Transporter genes are regulated at several levels, including membrane retrieval and reinsertion, translation, and transcription. Nuclear receptors relevant for the expression of ABC transporters are Liver X Receptor (LXR), Farnesoid Receptor (FXR), Pregnane X Receptor (PXR), and peroxisome proliferator-activated receptors α and γ (PPARα and PPARγ) [4]. The induction of *CYP3A4* and *CYP2B6* genes by numerous xenobiotics is well known to be mediated through activation of PXR [197]. PXR is activated by a diverse number of compounds, including rifampicin, phenobarbital, and mifepristone in humans. PXR mediates the expression of rodent Oatp1a4 [195], Oatp2 [198, 199], human MDR1 [200], mouse MRP1 [201], Mrp2 [201] and Mrp3 [202]. Furthermore, CAR activation induces Mrp2-7 mRNA in mouse liver [203] and is involved in the regulation of Mrp4 and sulfotransferase2a1 [174]. The PPARα agonist clofibrate induces gene and protein expression of Mrp3 and Mrp4 efflux transporters in a PPARα-dependent manner while having little effect on mRNA expression of Ntcp, Oatp1a1, Oatp1a4, and Oatp1b2 uptake transporters in mouse liver [204].

In primary cultures of human hepatocytes, MRP1 was increased by rifampin [205]. In mouse liver, carbon tetrachloride induced Mrp1 [206]. MRP1 is up-regulated when exposed to rifampin [207, 208] or mitoxantrone in tumor cells [209]. The expression of MRP1 in human colorectal cancer cell lines was induced by sulindac [210]. The promoter regions of the human *MRP2* and the rat *Mrp2* gene contain a number of putative consensus binding sites for AP1, SP1, HNF1, and HNF3β [211]. The -431 to -258 region also contains important elements that control expression in HepG2 cells, particularly the CCAAT-enhancer binding protein β. AhR ligands (2,3,7,8-tetrachlorodibenzo-p-dioxin, polychlorinated biphenyl 126, and β-naphthoflavone), the CAR activator 1,4-bis[2-(3,5-dichloropyridyloxy)]benzene, and nuclear factor-E2-related factor 2 (Nrf2) activators (butylated hydroxyanisole, oltipraz, and ethoxyquin) increased Mrp2 expression in mouse liver, suggesting that AhR, CAR, and Nrf2 may be important for modulating Mrp2 expression by chemicals [203]. Induction of rat Mrp2 has been observed with numerous chemicals, such as pregnenolone-16α-carbonitrile, spironolactone, and dexamethasone (all PXR ligands), phenobarbital (CAR ligand), and oltipraz (Nrf2 activator) [212, 213]. Similar induction of Mrp2 with indole-3-carbinol and β-naphthoflavone, both AhR ligands, has also been observed in rat liver [214]. Ligands for FXR, PXR, and CAR all induced Mrp2 mRNA in primary cultures of rat hepatocytes and characterized a putative ER-8 at -401 to -376 of the rat Mrp2 promoter that bound the corresponding FXR/RXR, PXR/RXR, and CAR/RXR heterodimers [215]. Treatment with the chemical carcinogen 2-acetylaminofluorene, cisplatin, and the protein-synthesis inhibitor cycloheximide increased expression of Mrp2 in rat liver [216]. *Trans*-Stilbene oxide also induced rat Mrp2 expression *via* CAR-independent manner [217].

The inducibility of *Mrp2* gene expression in primate liver was investigated in rhesus monkeys treated with tamoxifen or rifampin [218]. Both tamoxifen and rifampin strongly induced Mrp2 mRNA in two male and two female rhesus; tamoxifen induced Mrp2 protein in both male and female rhesus, whereas rifampin showed some inducing effect in a female but was inactive in a male monkey. Carotenoids and retinol also induced MRP2 through PXR activation [219]. Human Mrp2 is similarly up-regulated by the PXR activators rifampicin and tamoxifen, which differ from known rodent ligands for PXR [220]. Similarly, Mrp2 is induced by phenobarbital [221] and by *tert*-butyl hydroquinone in HepG2 cells [201], which suggests that CAR and Nrf2, respectively, may regulate expression of the human *MRP2* gene. These results suggest that the gene for *Mrp*2 may be similarly up-regulated by PXR agonists in human and rat, but mouse Mrp2 may not be as sensitive to PXR ligands. In clinical studies, expression of MRP2 mRNA and protein was decreased in patients with obstructive cholestasis who were poorly drained by percutaneous transhepatic biliary drainage [222]. In another clinical study, rifampin treatment of normal human subjects increased MRP2 mRNA and protein in the duodenum [223]. Additionally, induction of chronic renal failure in rats increased Mrp2 mRNA and protein levels in both the kidney and the liver [224]. This may represent a compensatory mechanism during renal failure, although the human response has not yet been documented.

The expression of MRP3 in rat and human liver is low under normal conditions but is induced during cholestasis and in the absence of MRP2 or Bile Salt Export Pump (BSEP) [173, 225]. Bile acids, in particular lithocholic acid, have been demonstrated to activate PXR likely as a mechanism to control their production and metabolism to prevent their accumulation to toxic levels [226]. In rats, mice, and humans, Mrp3 has been shown to be regulated by phenobarbital, diallyl sulfide, and polychlorinated biphenyl 99 [227], compounds that induce Cyp2B1/2 and are known or hypothesized CAR activators. *trans*-Stilbene oxide also induced rat Mrp3 expression *via* CAR-independent manner [217]. Similar to Mrp2, Mrp3 is highly up-regulated by oltipraz [203], suggesting that Nrf2 might be an important transcription factor that regulates Mrp3 [227]. In humans, induction by β-naphthoflavone and rifampicin suggests that Mrp3 might be regulated *via* AhR or PXR, respectively [221]. Using a large collection of human liver tissues, it was found that omeprazole was an inducer of MRP3 expression, probably through a AhR-dependent pathway [228]. This effect could be reproduced with HepG2 hepatoma cells, which showed a concentration-dependent induction of MRP3 expression by omeprazole. Overall, Mrp3 seems to be regulated similarly in rats, mice, and humans, with potential transcriptional regulation by AhR, PXR, CAR, PPARα, and Nrf2.

The CAR activator 1,4-bis[2-(3,5-dichloropyridyloxy)]benzene and Nrf2 activators (butylated hydroxyanisole, oltipraz, and ethoxyquin) induced Mrp4 in mouse liver [203], indicating potential roles for CAR and Nrf2 in the regulation of mouse Mrp4. In rats, Mrp4 is induced in liver by the Nrf2 activators oltipraz, and ethoxyquin [229]. *trans*-Stilbene oxide also induced rat Mrp4 expression *via* CAR-independent manner [217]. Little data exists on induction of Mrp4 in humans. However, studies in CAR-null mice have definitively shown that induction of Mrp4 by 1,4-bis[2-(3,5-dichloropyridyloxy)]benzene and phenobarbital is *via* CAR [174]. Taken together, the most likely means of induction of Mrp4 is by transcriptional activation by CAR and Nrf2.

Few chemicals have been observed to modulate expression of MRP6 in rats or humans. However, AhR, CAR, and Nrf2 activators induced expression of Mrp6 in mouse liver [203]. A recent study found that the expression of this gene in cells of hepatic origin is significantly upregulated by retinoids, acting as agonists of the Retinoid X Receptor (RXR) rather than the Retinoid A Receptor (RAR) [230].

One of the patterns of Mrp expression of note is that AhR and Nrf2 activators often induce the same transporter (*i.e.*, Mrp2, 3, 5, and 6). Several genes known to be regulated by Nrf2 are also regulated in a similar manner compared with these Mrps. Rat UDP-glucuronosyltransferase 1A6 is induced by oltipraz, a classical Nrf2 activator, and oltipraz induction of UDP-glucuronosyltransferase 1A6 is dependent on the binding of AhR to the xenobiotic response element [231]. Furthermore, one of the known target genes of Nrf2 activation, Nqo1, can be induced by the classical AhR ligand 2,3,7,8-tetrachlorodibenzo-*p*-dioxin, and that induction was Nrf2-dependent [232]. Although the mechanism of this cross-activation is not well defined, MRPs may share a similar pattern of inducibility to the phase I and II enzymes known to be regulated by these two receptors. Thus, it is unclear whether the induction of MRPs by some of the microsomal enzyme inducers is mediated through direct mechanisms (transcription factor binding to its cognate response element) or indirect mechanisms that involve some sort of "cross talk" (activation of multiple receptors by a chemical and/or transcriptional up-regulation of another gene or transcription factor that acts on the gene of interest.

MRPS AND INTESTINAL ABSORPTION OF DRUGS

Many orally administered drugs must overcome several barriers before reaching their target site [233]. The first major obstacle to cross is the intestinal epithelium. MRP2 and MRP4, together with Pgp/MDR1 (ABCB1) and BCRP/MXR (ABCG2), have been shown to localize at the apical/lumenal membrane of enterocytes, and thus are thought to form a barrier to intestinal absorption of substrate drugs (Fig. **3**) [233]. Their expression level varies between different segments of the intestine. In general, BCRP/MXR (ABCG2), MRP2 (ABCC2) and Pgp/MDR1 (ABCB1) are expressed at high level in the small intestine [233], considered by many in the field as the rate limiting barrier to oral drug absorption.

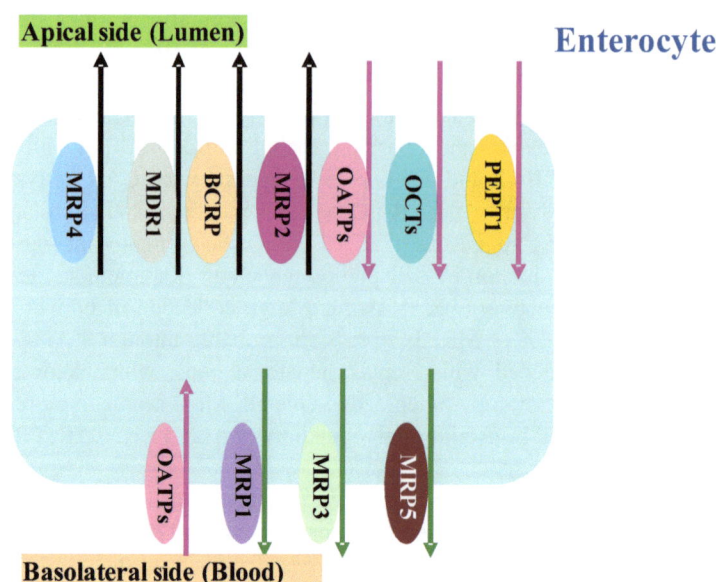

Figure 3: MRP2 and MRP4, together with **Pgp/MDR1 (ABCB1)** and **BCRP/MXR (ABCG2),** are localize at the apical/lumenal membrane of enterocytes, and thus are thought to form a physical barrier to intestinal absorption of a number of substrate drugs. OATPs, OCTs and PEPT1 are also located at this side. Their expression level varies between different segments of the intestine. **In general, BCRP/MXR (ABCG2), MRP2 (ABCC2) and Pgp/MDR1 (ABCB1) are expressed at high level in the small intestine, considered by many in the field as the rate limiting barrier to oral drug absorption.** MRP1, 3, & 5 and OATPs are expressed at the basolateral membrane of enterocytes.

Regarding their role in limiting intestinal absorption, MDR1 is the most thoroughly characterized and well accepted. Although the expression levels of both the MRP2 and MXR are higher in the small intestine than the expression of MDR1, there are much fewer data available on their role in drug absorption [233]. MRP2 has been shown to limit absorption of a phenylimidazo [4, 5-b] pyridine (PhIP) derivative, a food-derived carcinogen, and MXR has been shown to limit absorption of topotecan.

MRPS AND BILIARY EXCRETION OF DRUGS

Hepatic transporters are involved in the regulation of bile formation and disposition of xenobiotics. The hepatocyte has a polarized plasma membrane with basolateral and apical domains, enabling vectorial movement of endogenous and exogenous compounds from blood into bile. Drugs that reach the blood are then passed to the liver, where they are metabolized and subject to biliary excretion, often by MRPs and other important ABC transporters (Fig. **4**) [4, 233, 234]. Canalicular secretion of bile components represents the rate-limiting step in bile formation. Bile acids, glutathione conjugates, and xenobiotics are removed from hepatocytes and concentrated into the bile by canalicular efflux transporters in an ATP-dependent manner.

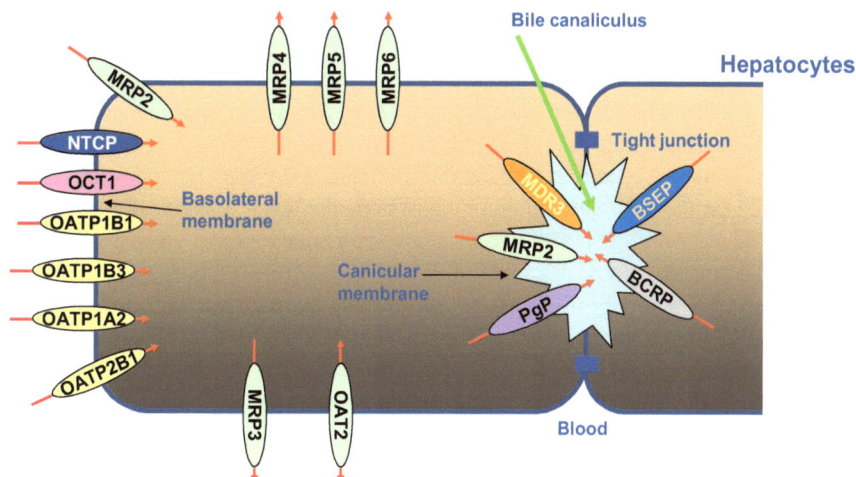

Figure 4: Localization of MRP transporters in hepatocytes. MRP2, localized on the basolateral (sinusoidal) membrane of hepatocytes, plays a critical role in the hepatic excretion of drugs and their metabolites (mainly conjugates). MRP3-6 facilitate the efflux of non-membrane-permeable molecules out of the hepatic cells. Human **NTCP** (Na$^+$-taurocholate co-transporting polypeptide) is a Na$^+$-dependent taurocholate uptake transporter located on the basolateral (sinusoidal) membrane of hepatocytes. NTCP mediates the Na$^+$-coupled uptake of bile salts from the space of Disse. The conjugated bile salts are then secreted into bile by the canalicular Bile Salt Export Pump (BSEP). Phosphatidylcholine (lecithin) is transported to the outer leaflet of the canalicular membrane by the phospholipid flippase, MDR3, from where it is stripped into bile by secreted bile salts. Uptake of organic cations is mediated by a family of Organic Cation Transporters (OCTs). Uptake or organic anions is mediated by families of Organic Anion Transporting Polypeptides (OATPs) and Organic Anion Transporters (OATs). Human **OATPs,** located on the basolateral membrane of hepatocytes, are responsible for the uptake of bile salts, organic anions, hormones, cholates along with their metabolites and conjugates. After conjugation, the organic anions, as well as glutathione, are then secreted into bile by MRP2. A wide variety of amphipathic compounds (including many drugs and organic cations) are exported from the hepatocytes into bile by apical MDR1.

Four MRP transporters (MRP2, 3, 4, and 6) are expressed to an appreciable extent in liver. In liver, MRP2 is the only MRP localized to the canalicular membrane and participates in excretion of chemicals into bile. Alternatively, MRP3 and MRP4 are localized to the basolateral membrane and efflux chemicals from hepatocytes into blood. Mrp6 is thought to be localized to the basolateral membrane as well, but a high-affinity substrate for this transporter has not been identified. The Mrps play an important role in the hepatic elimination of metabolites, and modulation of Mrp expression in liver can alter drug disposition.

Both organic cations and anions are taken up into the hepatocyte by groups of transport proteins (OCTs & OATPs respectively) with overlapping specificity. None of the known OATPs import unconjugated bilirubin. Organic anions (including bilirubin and glutathione) are transported across the hepatocyte into bile, usually after being modified by covalent conjugation in the microsomes. These conjugates are secreted into bile by MRP2. After uptake, some compounds may reflux back into the plasma, either by passive diffusion, by MRPs and export by the newly discovered, dimeric organic solute tranporter (OSTα,β) [235]; these are expressed at the basolateral membrane of the hepatocyte and show considerable overlap of substrate specificity. MRP1 exports both unconjugated and conjugated bilirubins, whereas MRP3&4 and OSTα,β best export conjugated bile salts [235]. All of them have low expression in the normal liver, but are upregulated in cholestasis [234, 236].

Some MRPs (*e.g.* MRP2) play a critical role in the hepatic excretion of drugs and their metabolites [234]. Decreased MRP function can thus impair hepatic capacity to excrete drugs and their metabolites. For example, altered MRP2 function can change the clearance of many clinically important drugs, including cancer chemotherapeutics (irinotecan, methotrexate, and vinblastine), antibiotics (ampicillin, ceftriaxone, and rifampin), antihyperlipidemics, and angiotensin-converting enzyme inhibitors, as well as many toxins and their conjugates [237].

MRP3-6 facilitates the efflux of non-membrane-permeable molecules out of the hepatic cells. Human **NTCP** (Na$^+$-taurocholate co-transporting polypeptide) is a Na$^+$-dependent taurocholate uptake transporter located on the basolateral (sinusoidal) membrane of hepatocytes. The conjugated bile salts are then secreted into bile by the canalicular Bile Salt Export Pump (BSEP/ABCB11) [234]. Phosphatidylcholine (lecithin) is transported to the outer leaflet of the canalicular membrane by the phospholipid flippase [238], MDR3, from where it is stripped into bile by secreted bile salts [239]. Uptake of organic cations is mediated by a family of Organic Cation Transporters (OCTs). Uptake or organic anions is mediated by families of Organic Anion Transporting Polypeptides (OATPs) and Organic Anion Transporters (OATs) [234, 236]. Human **OATPs,** located on the basolateral membrane of hepatocytes, are responsible for the uptake of bile salts, organic anions, hormones, cholates along with their metabolites and conjugates [236]. After conjugation, the organic anions, as well as glutathione, are then secreted into bile by MRP2. A wide variety of amphipathic compounds (including many drugs and organic cations) are exported from the hepatocytes into bile by apical MDR1 [240]. With regard to the transporters involved in biliary excretion, it is known that PgP (MDR1/ABCB1), MRP2 (ABCC2), the bile salt export protein (BSEP/ABCB11), and BCRP/ABCG2 are predominantly expressed on canalicular membrane [233].

MRPS AND RENAL DRUG EXCRETION

Pgp/MDR1 (ABCB1), MRP2 (ABCC2), MRP4 (ABCC4) primarily localize to the apical (luminal) membrane of renal epithelial cells, while **MRP1 (ABCC1)** and MRP6 have been shown to be expressed on the basolateral membrane (Fig. **5**) [103, 241-244]. Substrates of MRP2 and MRP4 have been shown to have altered renal clearance in animals lacking transporter function [242]. These transporters export compounds from the cytoplasm of renal tubular cells to the urine, therefore, substrates of these transporters are expected to have higher renal elimination than it is expected by glomerular filtration. Tenofovir, an anti-HIV agent, is actively excreted from the proximal tubule cells by MRP2 and MRP4 [245]. Further studies are needed to the detailed role of these transporters in pharamacokinetics.

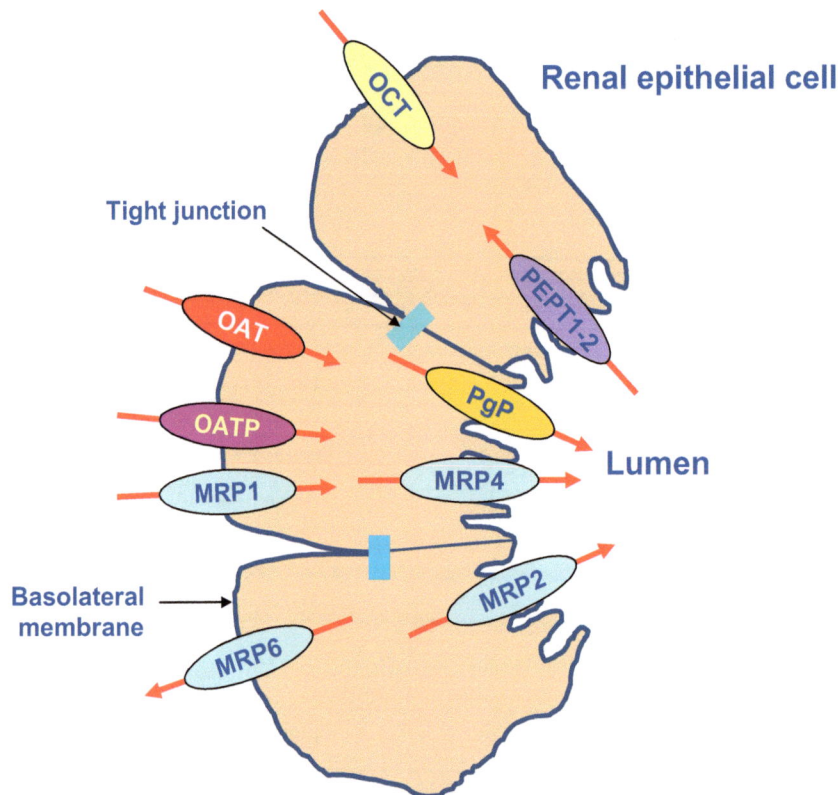

Figure 5: MRP2 (ABCC2) and **MRP4 (ABCC4)** are primarily localized to the apical (luminal) membrane of renal epithelial cells, while **MRP1 (ABCC1)** and MRP6 are expressed on the basolateral membrane of proximal tubule cells. **Pgp/MDR1 (ABCB1) is also located** to the apical membrane of renal epithelial cells. Moreover, **OATP, OCT** (OCT1-3) and **OAT** (OAT1, 3, & 4) transporters have been identified in the basolateral membrane of proximal tubule cells.

Additionally, members of the **OATP, OCT** (OCT1-3) and **OAT** (OAT1, 3, 4) transporter families have been identified in the basolateral membrane of proximal tubule cells [242, 246-248]. OAT3 has shown to be responsible for the renal elimination of pravastatin [249]. Substrates of OCTs have been shown to have greatly reduced renal clearance and increased plasma concentration in mice lacking OCT1 and OCT2 [250]. On the other hand, the two peptide transporters **PEPT1** and **PEPT2** are present on the luminal membrane of proximal tubule cells and were shown to be responsible for the tubular re-absorption of peptide-like drugs such as β-lactam antibiotics across the brush-border membranes [251]. The reabsorbtion process results in lower renal clearance than it is expected by glomerular filtration. Furthermore, the uptake process might result in increased concentration of drugs in the cytoplasm of proximal tubular cells, leading to toxic effects in the kidney. The nephorotoxic effect of the antibiotic cephaloridine was linked to OAT3 function [252, 253], while OCT2 was identified as the major determinant of the nephrotoxicity of the anti-cancer drug cisplatin [254].

MRP2 inhibition by tenofovir may contribute to the known interaction between tenofovir and didanosine. Coadministration of these two antiretroviral drugs leads to an increase of the area under the didanosine concentration-time curve (AUC) by 44 to 60% [255]. This may occur through tenofovir-induced inhibition of the active uptake of didanosine into the proximal tubule cells by the human organic anion transporter 1 [256] or by inhibition of purine nucleoside phosphorylase, an enzyme involved in the degradation of didanosine [245, 257]. However, assuming that the MRP2 inhibitor didanosine is also an MRP2 substrate, the increase in didanosine AUC could also be achieved by inhibition of MRP2-mediated efflux in the tubular brush-border membrane or in other tissues. Inhibition of several MRP could also have contributed to the life-threatening toxicity (*e.g.* neutropenia) of the MRP substrate vinblastine in a patient with HIV-associated multicentric Castleman's disease who was maintained on lamivudine, abacavir, and nevirapine [258]. Another patient with HIV-associated Hodgkin's disease also experienced life-threatening neutropenia when treated with ABVD (doxorubicine, bleomycine, vinblastine, dacarbazine) chemotherapy and lopinavir-ritonavir based antiretroviral therapy [259]. Vinblastine and lopinavir-ritonavir interaction was managed with lopinavir-ritonavir interruption around chemotherapy administration, with complete remission and immunovirological success after six cycles.

MRPS AND THE BLOOD-BRAIN BARRIER (BBB)

The BBB is formed by the tight junctions that connect the brain endothelial cells, thus restricting the entry of compounds from the circulating blood to the brain *via* paracellular and transcellular routes [260-265]. The BBB acts as an anatomical and transporter barrier notably due to the presence of tight junctions and a multitude of ABC transporters such as PgP, BCRP, and MRP1, 2, 4, and 5 (Fig. **6**) [4, 261, 262, 265-267]. As such, the BBB contributes to brain homeostasis by protecting the brain from potentially harmful endogenous and exogenous substances [268]. It is well established that the **Pgp/MDR1 (ABCB1) and BCRP/MXR (ABCG2)** localized in the apical/luminal membrane of the brain capillary endothelial cells are a major barrier of brain penetration of drugs.

Functional studies have assigned a role for human **MRP2 (ABCC2)** in the blood-brain barrier. **MRP1 (ABCC1)** is also implicated in protecting the brain tissue against xenobiotics (*e.g.* somatostatin analogs). MRP1 is localized in the basolateral membrane of the choroid epithelial cells and prevents the penetration of drugs and toxicants into the cephalo-spinal fluid. Similarity between the localization of MRP2, MXR (BCRP) and MDR1 in the brain microvessel endothelial cells and in the enteral epithelial cells suggests that these transporters function together to serve as physiological barriers against xenobiotics at the intestinal brush-border membrane and at the blood-brain barrier. MRP4 and MRP5 have been located in the brain capillary endothelial cells forming the blood-brain barrier. MRP1, MRP4, and MRP5 are clearly localized to the luminal side of brain capillary endothelial cells.

Despite advances in brain research, Central Nervous System (CNS) disorders remain very difficult to treat because the majority of drugs do not cross the BBB. The BBB blocks delivery of more than 98% of CNS acting drugs [263, 269]. Successful brain penetration is a prerequisite for the design of chemical lead substances for CNS acting drugs. To restrict CNS adverse effects, brain penetration properties are also important for the development of non-CNS acting drugs. Therefore, for both drug classes their BBB penetration is useful to be tested in advance. PgP and other ABC transporters can limit the penetration of drugs into the brain and thus modulate effectiveness and central nervous system toxicity of numerous drugs [263, 270, 271]. The drug delivery challenge posed by the BBB is compelling, particularly as the population ages and the incidence of neurodegenerative diseases such as stroke, Alzheimer's disease, and Parkinson's disease increase in prevalence. Despite advances in brain research, central nervous system disorders remain very difficult to treat because the majority of drugs do not cross the BBB. The BBB limits the ability of many drugs to penetrate brain tissue by restricting paracellular and transcellular transport [263]. To circumvent the limited access of drugs into the brain, different approaches have been investigated, including drug delivery systems such as liposomes, nanoparticles, peptide-vector strategy, MDR1 modulators, modulators of endothelial tight junctions, or osmotic pressure modification [272].

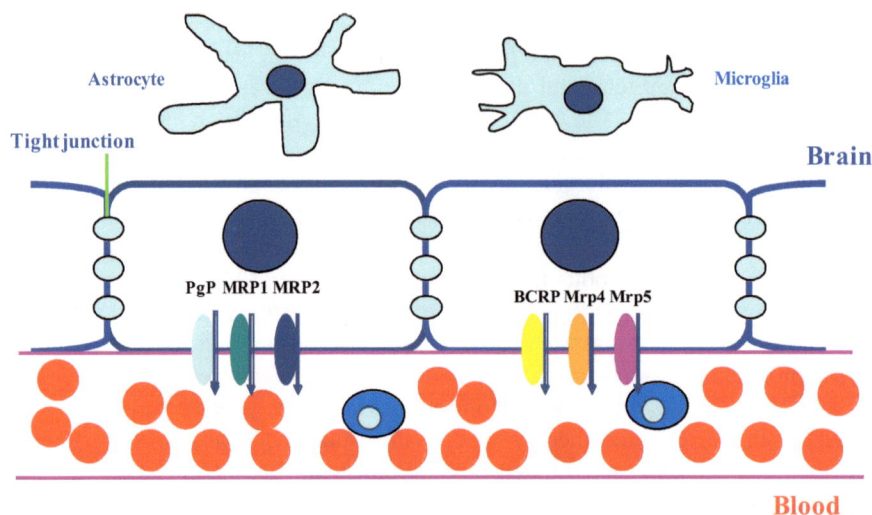

Figure 6: MRP1, MRP2, MRP4, and MRP5 are clearly localized to the luminal (apical) side of brain capillary endothelial cells of the blood-brain barriers. It is well established that the **Pgp/MDR1 (ABCB1) and BCRP** protein localized in the apical/luminal membrane of the brain capillary endothelial cells are a major barrier of brain penetration of drugs. These transporters are also expressed in astrocytes and microglias.

MRP alterations may also affect the distribution of their substrates, thus altering therapeutics or toxicology. For example, MRP4-deficient mice had enhanced accumulation of topotecan in brain tissue and cerebrospinal fluid [166]. On the other hand, modulation of MRPs in blood-brain barrier may facilitate the management of diseases of the central nervous system by enhancing penetration of drugs into the brain. Such MRP-based barrier may be circumvented by targeted site-specific drug delivery systems, such as immunoliposome and nanoparticulate systems [273]. Moreover, development of novel approaches for bypassing the impact of these drug transporters and for the design of effective drugs that are not substrates and the development of selective and potent inhibitors for the MRP transporters becomes a high imperative for the pharmaceutical industry [270].

MRPs enhanced the ability of tumor cells to efflux chemotherapy drugs out of cells to reduce the cellular drug concentration leading to resistance to anticancer drugs. Increased expression of these drug transporters in tumor cells is associated with resistance to a number of important chemotherapeutic agents. With the accumulation of information on drug resistance profile and physiological function of MRP family, the relationship between drug selectivity and specific transporter level will be more and more significant and helpful in clinical cancer treatment and development of novel anticancer agents.

MRPs can be regulated at the level of transcription, translation and post-translation. Like PgP, MRPs are also subject to induction and inhibition by a number of compounds. Not surprisingly, the induction and inhibition of MRPs by various agents are of pharmacokinetic and pharmacodynamic importance. The identification of induces and inhibitors for each MRP may also allow the prediction of potential drug-drug interactions.

MRPS AND DRUG TOXICITY

MRPs can efflux the GSH conjugated xenobiotics and endobiotics from the intracellular compartment into extracellular medium. This can protect cells from the toxic effects of xenobiotics and endobiotics. Therefore, screening the substrates and inhibitors of MRPs could point out the physiological function for each member of MRPs. Also, this could give information on toxicity and efficacy of individual drug. Modulation of MRPs activity seems to be significant to find new mechanism of drug-drug interaction and optimize drug bioavailability.

In addition to playing an important role in drug excretion through the bile, MRPs serve as protective shields by preventing uptake or facilitating clearance of toxic substances in the liver. Anti-toxic effects of MRP1-3 have been studied in more details. **MRP2 (ABCC2)** is involved in hepato-biliary excretion of GSH conjugates of inorganic arsenic and its chemical derivatives. In addition, some food-derived carcinogens and pre-carcinogens and their glucuronide conjugates are also transported by **MRP2 (ABCC2), MRP1 (ABCC1)** and **MRP3 (ABCC3)** may also contribute to the toxicological defense function by eliminating a number of toxic agents and their conjugates from epithelial tissues. It has been observed, that **MRP3 (ABCC3)** expression is strongly upregulated in the liver of the **MRP2 (ABCC2)** deficient patients and animals implying that basolateral MRP1 and MRP3-mediated efflux of toxicants may become of pivotal importance when administering MRP2-interacting drugs. ABC pumps play important function in the homeostasis of their own endogenous substrates. At pharmacological blockade of the transport, endogenous substrates may cause toxicity and adverse effects. **MRP2 (ABCC2)**, which transports sulfated bile salts as well as bilirubin conjugates, and **MDR3 (ABCB4),** the phosphatidyl choline flippase, in particular carry important functions, therefore full or partial blockade of these proteins may evoke toxicity and adverse effects.

PHARMACOGENETICS OF MRPS

In vitro site-directed mutagenesis studies indicate that mutants of MRPs may exhibit an altered substrate specificity, plasma membrane trafficking, ATP binding and transport activity [11, 274-276]. The replacement of Glu^{1089} with a neutral or positive charged amino acid reduced or completely eliminated the anthracycline resistance of MRP1 without influencing transport of LTC_4 and $E_217\beta G$ [11]. Substitution of the aromatic residue (Trp^{653} in NBD1 and Tyr^{1302} in NBD2) with a polar cysteine residue, such as W653C or Y1302C, decreased the affinity for ATP, resulting in greatly increased K_d values for ATP binding or K_m values for ATP in ATP-dependent LTC4 transport [274]. In addition, the mutation N597A near transmembrane helix increased and decreased resistance to vincristine and VP-16, respectively, while S605A decreased resistance to vincristine, VP-16 and doxorubicin and S604A selectively increased $E_217\beta G$ transport [275].

A number of mutations in MRP1 have been found in different ethnic populations, but these are not associated with any known genetic diseases. Nevertheless, some of these *MRP1* mutations may be associated with altered drug disposition. Substitution of Arg^{433} with Ser predicted to be close to TM8 of MRP1 caused by the low frequency G1299T polymorphism in exon 10 leads to a substrate selective change in organic anion transport activity and drug resistance using MRP1-expressing HeLa cells [277] or human leukemia CEM-7A cells [278]. The 128C *MRP1* polymorphism in exon 2 resulting in Cys43Ser substitution disrupted plasma membrane trafficking and reduced resistance to doxorubicin, vincristine and arsenite in HeLa cells expressing this MRP1 mutant while the transport of conjugated organic anion remained comparable to wild type MRP1 [279, 280]. Further studies are needed to explore the pharmacological role of *MRP1* polymorphism in humans.

Spontaneous mutant strains of hyperbilirubinemic rat, the Groningen yellow/transport deficient Wistar rat and the Eisai hyperbilirubinemic Sprague-Dawley rat are deficient in biliary excretion of bilirubin glucuronides and glucuronide and glutathione conjugates of xenobiotics due to mutations of *Mrp2* gene

[281-283]. Such mutations in the *Mrp2* gene cause premature termination codons. Cloning of *mrp2* has made possible an understanding of its structure-function relationships, localization and regulation of expression, and characterization of the defect in patients with the Dubin-Johnson Syndrome (DJS). Mutations of MRP2 are responsible for DJS, which is characterized with impairment of hepatobiliary elimination of organic anions such as conjugated hyperbilirubinaemia, increased urinary coproporphyrin I fraction (>80%), and deposition of melanin-like pigment in the liver [104, 283, 284]. Patients with DJS may also have a decreased biliary clearance of bromosulfophthalein and some degree of jaundice [104]. The absence of functional MRP2 is the molecular basis of transport defect of DJS [284]. Many single nucleotide polymorphisms in DJS patients have been reported (Table **2**) [117, 285-289]. These include C-24T (promoter), G1249A (exon 10), G2026C (exon 16), T2125C (exon 17), C2302T (exon 18), C2366 (exon 18), A3517T (exon 25), G3449 (exon 25), C3972T (exon 28) and G4348A (Exon 31). Many of these mutations are localized to NBD1 or NBD2. For instance, G4348A may affect MRP2 function because it is located in the Walker C motif within the carboxyl terminal NBD region of MRP2 [117]. S789F and A1450T which are less frequently than V417I substitution may be more relevant to the *in vivo* function of MRP2 than V417I [287]. Homozygous mutations lead to classic Dubin-Johnson syndrome, whereas heterozygous mutants have moderately elevated urinary coproporphyrin 1 fraction (~40%) with normal total and direct bilirubin [104]. Unlike other mutations, R1150H mutants of the MRP2 protein mature and are properly localized, but transport activity is impaired [289]. In addition, a significant allelic association between the 1249G>A SNP in *MRP2* gene and tenofovir-induced tenofovir-induced proximal tubulopathy [290]. Future studies are needed to identify any polymorphisms and their impact on MRP2 function.

Lang *et al.* [291] have reported the *MRP3* gene polymorphisms in 103 Caucasians. A total of 51 mutations were identified and 15 SNPs were located in the coding exons of MRP3, six of which are nonsynonymous mutations. The SNPs G39GC (allele frequency = 0.5%, in exon 1), C202T (1.6%, exon 2), C1037T (0.5%, exon 9), C1537A (0.5%, exon 12), G3890A (5.2%, exon 27) and G4267A (0.6%, exon 29) led to Lys13Asn, His68Tyr, Ser346Phe, Gln513Lys, Arg1297His and Gly1423Arg amino acid substitutions, respectively. A splice site mutation (G1339-1T) was found at the intron 10-exon 11 boundary. There was a significant correlation of C-211T with *MRP3* mRNA expression, with individuals homozygous and heterozygous for the C-211T promoter polymorphism having significantly lower *MRP3* transcript levels compared to wild-type individuals.

Pseudoxanthoma elasticum (PXE) is an autosomally inherited disorder characterized by accumulation of mineralized and fragmented elastic fibers in the skin, Bruch's membrane in the retina, and vessel walls with abnormalities of collagen and matrix constituents in the soft connective tissues [292-294]. The ophthalmic and dermatologic expression of PXE and its vascular complications are heterogeneous, with considerable variation in phenotype, progression, and mode of inheritance. Clinical manifestations mainly include coalesced papules and laxity in the flexural areas of skin, retinal angioid streaks and recurrent hemorrhage and vessel alterations similar to those in atherosclerosis [295]. Lower expression of MRP6 was found in tissues affected by PXE, including skin, retina, and vessel walls. PXE is considered to be caused by mutations in *MRP6*. Small peptides transported by MRP6 in humans may be essential for extracellular matrix deposition or turnover of connective tissue at specific sites in the body.

Mutant alleles of *MRP6* occurred in homozygous, compound heterozygous and heterozygous forms. The great majority of mutations were located from exon 24 to 30, with exon 24 being the most affected [296-299]. Among the others, exons 2, 9 and 12 were particularly involved [296, 300]. Almost all mutations were located in the intracellular site of MRP6.

A physiological function has only been established for MRP8, for which a single nucleotide polymorphism determines wet *vs* dry earwax type [190]. However, the constituent of earwax that is susceptible to transport by MRP8 has not been identified. The functional characteristics and its genetic mutations of MRP9 are currently unknown.

Since MRPs are able to transport a wide range of drugs with various structures, the analysis of polymorphisms of these drug transporters may provide a potent tool for improving the risk assessment, prevention, early diagnosis and treatment of diseases. Naturally occurring mutations in MRP/ABCC-related drug transporters have been reported, some of which are non-synonymous single nucleotide polymorphisms [276]. The consequences of the resulting amino acid changes can sometimes be predicted from *in vitro* site-directed mutagenesis studies or from knowledge of mutations of analogous (conserved) residues in ABCC proteins that cause DJS, PXE (ABCC6), cystic fibrosis (CFTR/ABCC7) or persistent hyperinsulinemic hypoglycemia of infancy (SUR1/ABCC8) [276]. Polymorphisms of MRPs could be recognized as an important source of interindividual variability of pharmacokinetics and pharmacodynamics of many drugs. Also, this could help to establish a more powerful patient orientated drug therapy against severe adverse effects and for better therapeutic outcome. Eventually, this may provide a powerful tool for drug development, particularly for those with a narrow therapeutic window, such as anticancer drugs.

MRPS AS POTENTIAL THERAPEUTIC TARGETS IN MULTIDRUG RESISTANCE

PgP-mediated or classic multidrug resistance (MDR), which was identified in the 1970s, is a well-characterized experimental phenomenon. Classic MDR is characterized by: a) cross-resistance between a series of chemically unrelated drugs, b) decreased drug accumulation in cancer cells, c) increased expression of PgP, and d) reversal of the phenotype by a variety of different compounds [301]. The drugs most often involved in PgP-mediated MDR are of fungal or plant origin, including the anthracyclines (*e.g.* primarily daunorubicin and doxorubicin) and vinca alkaloids. Apart from drugs within these groups, a number of other, nonrelated compounds are able to induce PgP-mediated MDR (*e.g.*, epipodophyllotoxins, actinomycin D, colchicine, the taxanes, and the anthracenedione derivatives [301]. All these drugs are hydrophobic, and most are weak bases.

MRP members play an important role in cancer chemotherapy. The differences in substrate selectivity, organ distribution, and membrane localization of these pumps play major function in related cancer drug transports. The knowledge about the mechanism of drug resistance may be useful in predicting the human response of chemotherapy. The overlapping substrates range of MRPs may have significant contributions for the clinical use of modulators aimed to block the resistant activity of pumps and increase the intracellular drug levels.

Most compounds that efficiently block PgP have only low affinity for MRP1, MRP2 and other MRPs. Despite that there are only a few effective and specific MRP inhibitors available, drug targeting of these transporters may play a role in cancer chemotherapy and in the pharmacokinetics of substrate drugs [302]. The perfect reversing agent is efficient, lacks unrelated pharmacological effects, shows no pharmacokinetic interactions with other drugs, tackles specific mechanisms of resistance with high potency and is readily administered to patients. Selective down-regulation of resistance genes in cancer cells by antisense or interfering RNA is an emerging approach in therapeutics. Because there is sufficient evidence to implicate several MRPs as negative prognostic markers during cancer chemotherapy, the pharmacological reversal of MRP1 function becomes a possible approach for overcoming tumor resistance. Disulfiram, a drug approved for use in treating alcoholism, reverses either MDR1- or MRP1-mediated efflux of fluorescent drug substrates *via* inhibiting ATP hydrolysis and the binding of [α-32P]8-azidoATP to P-glycoprotein and MRP1 [303].

Design of novel anticancer agents that evade transporter-mediated efflux is a potential approach to avoid multidrug resistance. Epothilones are novel microtubule-targeting agents with a paclitaxel-like mechanism of action that are not recognized by PgP, providing proof of the concept that new classes of anticancer agents that do not interact with the multidrug transporters can be developed to improve response to therapy. As most anticancer agents subject to efflux are currently irreplaceable in chemotherapy regimens, an attractive solution would be to chemically modify their susceptibility to being transported while retaining antineoplastic activity. Although such modifications frequently decrease the bioavailability or efficacy of drugs, some novel agents have been developed using this approach [304]. The intracellular concentration of drugs can also be elevated by increasing the rate of influx by improving the formulation. Encapsulation of doxorubicin in polyethylene glycol-coated liposomes might be safer and occasionally more effective than conventional doxorubicin [305]. Overexpression of ABC transporters, particularly PgP, BCRP and MRPs, has consistently been implicated as a cause for MDR both *in vitro* and *in vivo*.

New and effective strategies are needed to engage, evade or exploit these transporters to improve cancer therapy.

CONCLUSIONS AND FUTURE DIRECTIONS

MRPs which belong to the ABC transporter family are able to transport a remarkable array of diverse endo- and xenobiotics and their metabolites. MRP1, MRP2 and MRP3 are lipophilic anion transporters with similar substrate ranges and confer resistance to some natural compounds and methotrexate. MRP4, MRP5, and MRP8 are cyclic nucleotide transporters. Each member of MRP family has its own specified substrates. Notably, the 190 kDa MRP and PgP only have 15% the same amino acid and differ greatly in many aspects. Substrates for PgP are mainly neutral or mildly positive lipophilic compounds, while MRP is able to pump conjugated organic anions and neutral organic compounds.

Differences in substrate range, subcellular localization, expression profiles and kinetic parameters of transport dictate distinct physiological functions for MRPs [4]. For example, MRP1 is distinguished from MRP2 and MRP3 by its higher affinity for LTC_4, a feature that is reflected in the specific role that MRP1 plays in mediating immune responses involving cellular export of this cystinyl leukotriene [40]. By contrast with MRP1, MRP2 is primarily expressed at canalicular (apical) surfaces of hepatocytes where it functions in the extrusion of endogenous organic anions such as bilirubin glucuronide and certain anticancer agents and in the provision of the biliary fluid constituent glutathione. In addition to the transport of glutathione and glucuronate conjugates, MRP3 has the additional capability of mediating the transport of monoanionic bile acids. The latter feature, in combination with its induction at basolateral surfaces of hepatocytes and cholangiocytes under cholestatic conditions, support the notion that it functions as a compensatory backup mechanism to eliminate from these cells potentially toxic compounds that are ordinarily excreted into the bile. With regard to drug-resistance capabilities, MRP1, MRP2, and MRP3 are able to confer cellular resistance to natural product agents to varying extents, and all three pumps are potent methotrexate resistance factors [8]. Recent investigations of MRP4 and MRP5 indicate that they have the facility for mediating the transport of cyclic nucleotides, a property that has implicated the two pumps in the regulation of intracellular levels of these second messengers as well as in the cellular extrusion of cAMP involved in intercellular signalling [4]. In accord with their capacity to transport cyclic nucleotides, MRP4 and MRP5 have the facility for conferring resistance to certain antiviral and anticancer nucleotide analogs but do not seem to be capable of effluxing natural product agents [8]. MRP6, whose hereditary deficiency results in PXE, a disease that affects elastic tissues in the skin, eyes, and cardiovascular system, has recently been determined to be competent in the transport of glutathione conjugates and the cyclic pentapeptide BQ123 [183]. MRP7 was able to catalyze the MgATP-energized transport of the glucuronide $E_2 17\beta G$. By comparison with $E_2 17\beta G$, only modest transport was observed for LTC_4, and transport of a range of other compounds that are established substrates of other MRP family members was not detected to any extent [185]. Further studies are needed to elucidate the clinical, pharmacological and toxicological relevance of all these MRPs.

Interindividual differences of drug response are an important cause of treatment failures and adverse drug reactions. The identification of polymorphisms explaining distinct phenotypes of drug metabolizing enzymes contributed in part to the understanding of individual variations of drug plasma levels. However, bioavailability also depends on a major extent from the expression and activity of drug transport across cellular membranes. In particular, the ABC family such as PgP/ABCB1, MRPs and BCRP/ABCG2 have been identified as major determinants of chemoresistance in tumor cells. They are expressed in the apical membranes of many barrier tissues such as the intestine, liver, blood-brain barrier, kidney, placenta, testis and in lymphocytes, thus contributing to plasma, liquor, but also intracellular drug disposition [306]. Since expression and function exhibit a broad variability, it was hypothesized that hereditary variances in the genes of ABC transporters could explain at least in part interindividual differences of pharmacokinetics and clinical outcome of a variety of drugs [276, 306]. The pharmacogenetic studies on MRPs including the single nucleotide polymorphism may provide powerful tools for drug development. Studies on the functions of MRPs may give more information on drug toxicity and drug-drug interaction. Continual updating of databases of sequence variants and haplotype analysis, together with *in vitro* biochemical validation assays and pharmacological studies in knockout animals, should make it possible to determine how genetic variation in the MRP-related transporters contributes to the range of responses to drugs and chemicals observed in different human populations. However, the mechanisms of MRPs activity and the substrates of some members of MRP family are unclear. In the future, we need to do more molecular, proteomic and genetic studies on MRPs to identify the regulation mechanism for individual MRPs.

The ability of transport proteins including MDR1, BCRP and MRPs to reduce oral bioavailability and alter tissue distribution has obvious implications for drug design [307]. Indeed, the identification of transporters that influence the disposition and safety of drugs has become a new challenge for drug discovery programmes. It is essential to know, first, whether drugs can freely cross pharmacological barriers or whether their passage is restricted by ABC transporters; and, second, whether drugs can influence the passage of other compounds through the inhibition of ABC transporters. Consequently, the evaluation of transport susceptibility of drug candidates has become an important step in the development of novel therapeutics, and the pharmaceutical industry has adopted routine evaluation of PgP susceptibility in the drug discovery process. In the early stages of drug development, it is important to identify drugs as substrates, inducers, inhibitors, or modulators for MRPs, as this may help to avoid drug toxicity, drug resistance and drug-drug interactions and to optimize cancer chemotherapy. The identification always involves the application of proper models and probes, such as *in vitro* (*e.g.* purified MRP protein or MRP-overexpressing cells) and *in vivo* models.

REFERENCES

[1]   Locher KP. Structure and mechanism of ABC transporters. Curr Opin Struct Biol 2004; 14: 426-31.

[2]   Tian Q, Zhang J, Chan E, *et al.* Multidrug resistance proteins (MRPs) and implication in drug development. Drug Dev Res 2005; 51: 1-18.

[3]   Piddock LJ. Multidrug-resistance efflux pumps - not just for resistance. Nat Rev Microbiol 2006; 4: 629-36.

[4]   Borst P, Elferink RO. Mammalian ABC transporters in health and disease. Annu Rev Biochem 2002; 71: 537-92.

[5]   Dean M, Rzhetsky A, Allikmets R. The human ATP-binding cassette (ABC) transporter superfamily. Genome Res 2001; 11: 1156-66.

[6]   Jones PM, George AM. The ABC transporter structure and mechanism: perspectives on recent research. Cell Mol Life Sci 2004; 61: 682-99.

[7]   Klein I, Sarkadi B, Varadi A. An inventory of the human ABC proteins. Biochim Biophys Acta 1999; 1461: 237-62.

[8]   Borst P, Evers R, Kool M *et al.* A family of drug transporters: the multidrug resistance-associated proteins. J Natl Cancer Inst 2000; 92: 1295-302.

[9]   Walker JE, Saraste M, Runswick MJ, *et al.* Distantly related sequences in the a- and b-subunits of ATP synthase, myosin, kinases and other ATP-requiring enzymes and a common nucleotide binding fold. Embo J 1982; 1: 945-51.

[10]   Chang G, Roth CB. Structure of MsbA from *E. coli*: a homolog of the multidrug resistance ATP binding cassette (ABC) transporters. Science 2001; 293: 1793-800.

[11]   Zhang DW, Cole SP, Deeley RG. Identification of a nonconserved amino acid residue in multidrug resistance protein 1 important for determining substrate specificity: evidence for functional interaction between transmembrane helices 14 and 17. J Biol Chem 2001; 276: 34966-74.

[12]   Higgins C. ABC transporters: from microorganisms to man. Annu Rev Cell Biol 1992; 8: 67-113.

[13]   Altenberg GA. Structure of multidrug-resistance proteins of the ATP-binding cassette (ABC) superfamily. Curr Med Chem Anti-Canc Agents 2004; 4: 53-62.

[14]   Kruh GD, Belinsky MG. The MRP family of drug efflux pumps. Oncogene 2003; 22: 7537-52.

[15]   Dean M RA, Allikmets R. The human ATP-binding cassette (ABC) transporter superfamily. Genome Res 2001; 11: 1156-66.

[16]   Belinsky MG, Bain LJ, Balsara BB, *et al.* Characterization of MOAT-C and MOAT-D, new members of the MRP/cMOAT subfamily of transporter proteins. J Natl Cancer Inst 1998; 90: 1735-41.

[17]   Hopper E, Belinsky MG, Zeng H, *et al.* Analysis of the structure and expression pattern of MRP7 (ABCC10), a new member of the MRP subfamily. Cancer Lett 2001; 162: 181-91.

[18]   Bera TK, Lee S, Salvatore G *et al.* MRP8, a new member of ABC transporter superfamily, identified by EST database mining and gene prediction program, is highly expressed in breast cancer. Mol Med 2001; 7: 509-16.

[19]   Tammur J PC, Arnould I, Rzhetsky A, *et al.* Two new genes from the human ATP-binding cassette transporter superfamily, ABCC11 and ABCC12, tandemly duplicated on chromosome 16q12. Gene 2001; 273: 89-96 2001;273:89-96.

[20]   Yabuuchi H SH, Takayanagi S, Ishikawa T. Multiple splicing variants of two new human ATP-binding cassette transporters, ABCC11 and ABCC12. Biochem Biophys Res Commun 2001; 288: 933-9.

[21]   Bakos E, Evers R, Szakacs G, *et al.* Functional multidrug resistance protein (MRP1) lacking the *N*-terminal transmembrane domain. J Biol Chem 1998; 273: 32167-75.

[22]   Cole SP, Bhardwaj G, Gerlach JH, *et al.* Overexpression of a transporter gene in a multidrug-resistant human lung cancer cell line. Science 1992; 258: 1650-4.

[23]   Cole SP, Deeley RG. Multidrug resistance mediated by the ATP-binding cassette transporter protein MRP. Bioessays 1998; 20: 931-40.

[24]   Zaman GJ, Versantvoort CH, Smit JJ, *et al.* Analysis of the expression of MRP, the gene for a new putative transmembrane drug transporter, in human multidrug resistant lung cancer cell lines. Cancer Res 1993; 53: 1747-50.

[25]   Burger H, Nooter K, Zaman GJ, *et al.* Expression of the multidrug resistance-associated protein (MRP) in acute and chronic leukemias. Leukemia 1994; 8: 990-97.

[26]   Stride BD, Valdimarsson G, Gerlach JH, *et al.* Structure and expression of the messenger RNA encoding the murine multidrug resistance protein, an ATP-binding cassette transporter. Mol Pharmacol 1996; 49: 962-71.

[27]   Flens MJ, Zaman GJ, van der Valk P, *et al.* Tissue distribution of the multidrug resistance protein. Am J Pathol 1996; 148: 1237-47.

[28]   Wijnholds J, Scheffer GL, van der Valk M, *et al.* Multidrug resistance protein 1 protects the oropharyngeal mucosal layer and the testicular tubules against drug-induced damage. J Exp Med 1998; 188: 797-808.

[29]   Qian YM, Song WC, Cui H, *et al.* Glutathione stimulates sulfated estrogen transport by multidrug resistance protein 1. J Biol Chem 2001; 276: 6404-11.

[30]   Leslie EM, Deeley RG, Cole SP. Toxicological relevance of the multidrug resistance protein 1, MRP1 (ABCC1) and related transporters. Toxicology 2001; 167: 3-23.

[31]   Lautier D, Canitrot Y, Deeley RG, *et al.* Multidrug resistance mediated by the multidrug resistance protein (MRP) gene. Biochem Pharmacol 1996; 52: 967-77.

[32]   Hammond CL, Marchan R, Krance SM, *et al.* Glutathione export during apoptosis requires functional multidrug resistance-associated proteins. J Biol Chem 2007; 282: 14337-47.

[33]   Leier I, Jedlitschky G, Buchholz U, *et al.* ATP-dependent glutathione disulphide transport mediated by the MRP gene-encoded conjugate export pump. Biochem J 1996; 314 (Pt 2): 433-7.

[34]   Loe DW, Almquist KC, Cole SP, *et al.* ATP-dependent 17β-estradiol 17-(β-D-glucuronide) transport by multidrug resistance protein (MRP). Inhibition by cholestatic steroids. J Biol Chem 1996; 271: 9683-9.

[35]   Jedlitschky G, Leier I, Buchholz U, *et al.* Transport of glutathione, glucuronate, and sulfate conjugates by the MRP gene-encoded conjugate export pump. Cancer Res 1996; 56: 988-94.

[36]   Rigato I, Pascolo L, Fernetti C, *et al.* The human multidrug-resistance-associated protein MRP1 mediates ATP-dependent transport of unconjugated bilirubin. Biochem J 2004; 383: 335-41.

[37]   Evers R, Cnubben NH, Wijnholds J, *et al.* Transport of glutathione prostaglandin A conjugates by the multidrug resistance protein 1. FEBS Lett 1997; 419: 112-6.

[38]   Akimaru K, Kuo MT, Furuta K, *et al.* Induction of MRP/GS-X pump and cellular resistance to anticancer prostaglandins. Cytotechnology 1996; 19: 221-7.

[39]   Robbiani DF, Finch RA, Jager D, *et al.* The leukotriene C₄ transporter MRP1 regulates CCL19 (MIP-3β, ELC)-dependent mobilization of dendritic cells to lymph nodes. Cell 2000; 103: 757-68.

[40]   Wijnholds J, Evers R, van Leusden MR, *et al.* Increased sensitivity to anticancer drugs and decreased inflammatory response in mice lacking the multidrug resistance-associated protein. Nat Med 1997; 3: 1275-9.

[41]   Cole SP, Sparks KE, Fraser K, *et al.* Pharmacological characterization of multidrug resistant MRP-transfected human tumor cells. Cancer Res 1994; 54: 5902-10.

[42]   Zaman GJ, Flens MJ, van Leusden MR, *et al.* The human multidrug resistance-associated protein MRP is a plasma membrane drug-efflux pump. Proc Natl Acad Sci U S A 1994; 91: 8822-6.

[43]   Versantvoort CH, Broxterman HJ, Bagrij T, *et al.* Regulation by glutathione of drug transport in multidrug-resistant human lung tumour cell lines overexpressing multidrug resistance-associated protein. Br J Cancer 1995; 72: 82-9.

[44]   Zaman GJ, Lankelma J, van Tellingen O, *et al.* Role of glutathione in the export of compounds from cells by the multidrug-resistance-associated protein. Proc Natl Acad Sci U S A 1995; 92: 7690-4.

[45]　Rappa G, Lorico A, Flavell RA, *et al.* Evidence that the multidrug resistance protein (MRP) functions as a co-transporter of glutathione and natural product toxins. Cancer Res 1997; 57: 5232-7.

[46]　Cole SP, Downes HF, Mirski SE, *et al.* Alterations in glutathione and glutathione-related enzymes in a multidrug-resistant small cell lung cancer cell line. Mol Pharmacol 1990; 37: 192-7.

[47]　Leier I, Jedlitschky G, Buchholz U, *et al.* The MRP gene encodes an ATP-dependent export pump for leukotriene C4 and structurally related conjugates. J Biol Chem 1994; 269: 27807-10.

[48]　Muller M, Meijer C, Zaman GJ, *et al.* Overexpression of the gene encoding the multidrug resistance-associated protein results in increased ATPdependent glutathione *S*-conjugate transport. Proc Natl Acad Sci USA 1994; 91: 8822-6.

[49]　Loe DW, Deeley RG, Cole SP. Characterization of vincristine transport by the M(r) 190,000 multidrug resistance protein (MRP): evidence for cotransport with reduced glutathione. Cancer Res 1998; 58: 5130-6.

[50]　Salerno M, Garnier-Suillerot A. Kinetics of glutathione and daunorubicin efflux from multidrug resistance protein overexpressing small-cell lung cancer cells. Eur J Pharmacol 2001; 421: 1-9.

[51]　Leslie EM, Deeley RG, Cole SP. Bioflavonoid stimulation of glutathione transport by the 190-kDa multidrug resistance protein 1 (MRP1). Drug Metab Dispos 2003;31:11-5.

[52]　Leslie EM, Ito K, Upadhyaya P, *et al.* Transport of the β-*O*-glucuronide conjugate of the tobacco-specific carcinogen 4-(methylnitrosamino)-1-(3-pyridyl)-1-butanol (NNAL) by the multidrug resistance protein 1 (MRP1). Requirement for glutathione or a non-sulfur-containing analog. J Biol Chem 2001; 276: 27846-54.

[53]　Yang Z, Horn M, Wang J, *et al.* Development and characterization of a recombinant Madin-Darby canine kidney cell line that expresses rat multidrug resistance-associated protein 1 (rMRP1). AAPS PharmSci 2004; 6: E8.

[54]　Nunoya K, Grant CE, Zhang D, *et al.* Molecular cloning and pharmacological characterization of rat multidrug resistance protein 1 (mrp1). Drug Metab Dispos 2003; 31: 1016-26.

[55]　Leslie EM, Haimeur A, Waalkes MP. Arsenic transport by the human multidrug resistance protein 1 (MRP1/ABCC1). Evidence that a tri-glutathione conjugate is required. J Biol Chem 2004; 279: 32700-8.

[56]　Ito K, Olsen SL, Qiu W, *et al.* Mutation of a single conserved tryptophan in multidrug resistance protein 1 (MRP1/ABCC1) results in loss of drug resistance and selective loss of organic anion transport. J Biol Chem 2001; 276: 15616-24.

[57]　Zeng H, Chen ZS, Belinsky MG, *et al.* Transport of methotrexate (MTX) and folates by multidrug resistance protein (MRP) 3 and MRP1: effect of polyglutamylation on MTX transport. Cancer Res 2001; 61: 7225-32.

[58]　Hooijberg JH, Broxterman HJ, Kool M, *et al.* Antifolate resistance mediated by the multidrug resistance proteins MRP1 and MRP2. Cancer Res 1999; 59: 2532-5.

[59]　Chu XY, Suzuki H, Ueda K, *et al.* Active efflux of CPT-11 and its metabolites in human KB-derived cell lines. J Pharmacol Exp Ther 1999; 288: 735-41.

[60]　Morrow CS, Smitherman PK, Diah SK, *et al.* Coordinated action of glutathione S-transferases (GSTs) and multidrug resistance protein 1 (MRP1) in antineoplastic drug detoxification. Mechanism of GST A1-1- and MRP1-associated resistance to chlorambucil in MCF7 breast carcinoma cells. J Biol Chem 1998; 273: 20114-20.

[61]　Morrow CS, Peklak-Scott C, Bishwokarma B, *et al.* Multidrug resistance protein 1 (MRP1, ABCC1) mediates resistance to mitoxantrone *via* glutathione-dependent drug efflux. Mol Pharmacol 2006; 69: 1499-505.

[62]　Paumi CM, Ledford BG, Smitherman PK, *et al.* Role of multidrug resistance protein 1 (MRP1) and glutathione *S*-transferase A1-1 in alkylating agent resistance. Kinetics of glutathione conjugate formation and efflux govern differential cellular sensitivity to chlorambucil *vs* melphalan toxicity. J Biol Chem 2001; 276: 7952-6.

[63]　Barnouin K, Leier I, Jedlitschky G, *et al.* Multidrug resistance protein-mediated transport of chlorambucil and melphalan conjugated to glutathione. Br J Cancer 1998; 77: 201-9.

[64]　Lorico A, Rappa G, Finch RA, *et al.* Disruption of the murine MRP (multidrug resistance protein) gene leads to increased sensitivity to etoposide (VP-16) and increased levels of glutathione. Cancer Res 1997; 57: 5238-42.

[65]　Paulusma CC, van Geer MA, Evers R, *et al.* Canalicular multispecific organic anion transporter/multidrug resistance protein 2 mediates low-affinity transport of reduced glutathione. Biochem J 1999; 338: 393-401.

[66]　Meaden ER, Hoggard PG, Newton P, *et al.* P-glycoprotein and MRP1 expression and reduced ritonavir and saquinavir accumulation in HIV-infected individuals. J Antimicrob Chemother 2002; 50: 583-8.

[67]　Williams GC, Liu A, Knipp G, *et al.* Direct evidence that saquinavir is transported by multidrug resistance-associated protein (MRP1) and canalicular multispecific organic anion transporter (MRP2). Antimicrob Agents Chemother 2002; 46: 3456-62.

[68]　Dallas S, Ronaldson PT, Bendayan M, *et al.* Multidrug resistance protein 1-mediated transport of saquinavir by microglia. Neuroreport 2004; 15: 1183-6.

[69] Grzywacz MJ, Yang JM, Hait WN. Effect of the multidrug resistance protein on the transport of the antiandrogen flutamide. Cancer Res 2003; 63: 2492-8.

[70] Zaman GJ, Cnubben NH, van Bladeren PJ, *et al.* Transport of the glutathione conjugate of ethacrynic acid by the human multidrug resistance protein MRP. FEBS Lett 1996; 391: 126-30.

[71] Hendrikse NH, Kuipers F, Meijer C, *et al.* *In vivo* imaging of hepatobiliary transport function mediated by multidrug resistance associated protein and P-glycoprotein. Cancer Chemother Pharmacol 2004; 54: 131-8.

[72] Chen WS, Luker KE, Dahlheimer JL, *et al.* Effects of MDR1 and MDR3 P-glycoproteins, MRP1, and BCRP/MXR/ABCP on the transport of (99m)Tc-tetrofosmin. Biochem Pharmacol 2000; 60: 413-26.

[73] Lorusso V, Pascolo L, Fernetti C, *et al.* *In vitro* and *in vivo* hepatic transport of the magnetic resonance imaging contrast agent B22956/1: role of MRP proteins. Biochem Biophys Res Commun 2002; 293: 100-5.

[74] Loe DW, Stewart RK, Massey TE, *et al.* ATP-dependent transport of aflatoxin B_1 and its glutathione conjugates by the product of the multidrug resistance protein (MRP) gene. Mol Pharmacol 1997; 51: 1034-41.

[75] Geisler M, Girin M, Brandt S, *et al.* Arabidopsis immunophilin-like TWD1 functionally interacts with vacuolar ABC transporters. Mol Biol Cell 2004; 15: 3393-405.

[76] Diah SK, Smitherman PK, Townsend AJ, *et al.* Detoxification of 1-chloro-2,4-dinitrobenzene in MCF7 breast cancer cells expressing glutathione *S*-transferase P1-1 and/or multidrug resistance protein 1. Toxicol Appl Pharmacol 1999; 157: 85-93.

[77] Morrow CS, Diah S, Smitherman PK, *et al.* Multidrug resistance protein and glutathione *S*-transferase P1-1 act in synergy to confer protection from 4-nitroquinoline 1-oxide toxicity. Carcinogenesis 1998; 19: 109-15.

[78] Lorico A, Nesland J, Emilsen E, *et al.* Role of the multidrug resistance protein 1 gene in the carcinogenicity of aflatoxin B_1: investigations using mrp1-null mice. Toxicology 2002; 171: 201-5.

[79] Johnson DR, Finch RA, Lin ZP, et al. The pharmacological phenotype of combined multidrug-resistance mdr1a/1b- and mrp1-deficient mice. Cancer Res 2001; 61: 1469-76.

[80] Gollapudi S, Kim CH, Tran BN, *et al.* Probenecid reverses multidrug resistance in multidrug resistance-associated protein-overexpressing HL60/AR and H69/AR cells but not in P-glycoprotein-overexpressing HL60/Tax and P388/ADR cells. Cancer Chemother Pharmacol 1997; 40: 150-8.

[81] Draper MP, Martell RL, Levy SB. Indomethacin-mediated reversal of multidrug resistance and drug efflux in human and murine cell lines overexpressing MRP, but not P-glycoprotein. Br J Cancer 1997; 75: 810-5.

[82] Bakos E, Evers R, Sinko E, *et al.* Interactions of the human multidrug resistance proteins MRP1 and MRP2 with organic anions. Mol Pharmacol 2000; 57: 760-8.

[83] Barrand MA, Rhodes T, Center MS, *et al.* Chemosensitisation and drug accumulation effects of cyclosporin A, PSC-833 and verapamil in human MDR large cell lung cancer cells expressing a 190k membrane protein distinct from P-glycoprotein. Eur J Cancer 1993; 29A: 408-15.

[84] Hooijberg JH, Broxterman HJ, Heijn M, *et al.* Modulation by (iso)flavonoids of the ATPase activity of the multidrug resistance protein. FEBS Lett 1997; 413: 344-8.

[85] Hooijberg JH, Broxterman HJ, Scheffer GL, *et al.* Potent interaction of flavopiridol with MRP1. Br J Cancer 1999; 81: 269-76.

[86] Versantvoort CH, Broxterman HJ, Lankelma J, *et al.* Competitive inhibition by genistein and ATP dependence of daunorubicin transport in intact MRP overexpressing human small cell lung cancer cells. Biochem Pharmacol 1994; 48: 1129-36.

[87] Nguyen H, Zhang S, Morris ME. Effect of flavonoids on MRP1-mediated transport in Panc-1 cells. J Pharm Sci 2003; 92: 250-7.

[88] Marbeuf-Gueye C, Salerno M, Quidu P, *et al.* Inhibition of the P-glycoprotein- and multidrug resistance protein-mediated efflux of anthracyclines and calceinacetoxymethyl ester by PAK-104P. Eur J Pharmacol 2000; 391: 207-16.

[89] Aoki S, Chen ZS, Higasiyama K, *et al.* Reversing effect of agosterol A, a spongean sterol acetate, on multidrug resistance in human carcinoma cells. Jpn J Cancer Res 2001; 92: 886-95.

[90] Bandi N, Kompella UB. Budesonide reduces multidrug resistance-associated protein 1 expression in an airway epithelial cell line (Calu-1). Eur J Pharmacol 2002; 437: 9-17.

[91] Payen L, Delugin L, Courtois A, *et al.* Reversal of MRP-mediated multidrug resistance in human lung cancer cells by the antiprogestatin drug RU486. Biochem Biophys Res Commun 1999; 258: 513-8.

[92] Naito S, Koike K, Ono M, *et al.* Development of novel reversal agents, imidazothiazole derivatives, targeting MDR1- and MRP-mediated multidrug resistance. Oncol Res 1998; 10: 123-32.

[93] Weiss J, Theile D, Ketabi-Kiyanvash N, *et al.* Inhibition of MRP1/ABCC1, MRP2/ABCC2, and MRP3/ABCC3 by nucleoside, nucleotide, and non-nucleoside reverse transcriptase inhibitors. Drug Metab Dispos 2007; 35: 340-4.

[94]   Gekeler V, Ise W, Sanders KH, *et al.* The leukotriene LTD$_4$ receptor antagonist MK571 specifically modulates MRP associated multidrug resistance. Biochem Biophys Res Commun 1995; 208: 345-52.

[95]   Nakano R, Oka M, Nakamura T, *et al.* A leukotriene receptor antagonist, ONO-1078, modulates drug sensitivity and leukotriene C$_4$ efflux in lung cancer cells expressing multidrug resistance protein. Biochem Biophys Res Commun 1998; 251: 307-12.

[96]   Payen L, Delugin L, Courtois A, *et al.* The sulphonylurea glibenclamide inhibits multidrug resistance protein (MRP1) activity in human lung cancer cells. Br J Pharmacol 2001; 132: 778-84.

[97]   Mao Q, Qiu W, Weigl KE, *et al.* GSH-dependent photolabeling of multidrug resistance protein MRP1 (ABCC1) by [^{125}I]LY475776. Evidence of a major binding site in the COOH-proximal membrane spanning domain. J Biol Chem 2002; 277: 28690-9.

[98]   Norman BH, Dantzig AH, Kroin JS, *et al.* Reversal of resistance in multidrug resistance protein (MRP1)-overexpressing cells by LY329146. Bioorg Med Chem Lett 1999; 9: 3381-6.

[99]   Qian YM, Grant CE, Westlake CJ, *et al.* Photolabeling of human and murine multidrug resistance protein 1 with the high affinity inhibitor [^{125}I]LY475776 and azidophenacyl-[35S]glutathione. J Biol Chem 2002; 277: 35225-31.

[100] Stewart AJ, Canitrot Y, Baracchini E, *et al.* Reduction of expression of the multidrug resistance protein (MRP) in human tumor cells by antisense phosphorothioate oligonucleotides. Biochem Pharmacol 1996; 51: 461-9.

[101] Peaston AE, Gardaneh M, Franco AV, *et al.* MRP1 gene expression level regulates the death and differentiation response of neuroblastoma cells. Br J Cancer 2001; 85: 1564-71.

[102] Niewiarowski W, Gendaszewska E, Rebowski G, *et al.* Multidrug resistance-associated protein--reduction of expression in human leukaemia cells by antisense phosphorothioate olignucleotides. Acta Biochim Pol 2000; 47: 1183-8.

[103] Evers R, Kool M, van Deemter L, *et al.* Drug export activity of the human canalicular multispecific organic anion transporter in polarized kidney MDCK cells expressing cMOAT (MRP2) cDNA. J Clin Invest 1998; 101: 1310-9.

[104] Toh S, Wada M, Uchiumi T, *et al.* Genomic structure of the canalicular multispecific organic anion-transporter gene (MRP2/cMOAT) and mutations in the ATP-binding-cassette region in Dubin-Johnson syndrome. Am J Human Genet 1999; 64: 739-46.

[105] Keppler D, Leier I, Jedlitschky G. Transport of glutathione conjugates and glucuronides by the multidrug resistance proteins MRP1 and MRP2. Biol Chem 1997; 378: 787-91.

[106] Masuda M IiY, Yamazaki M, Nishigaki R, *et al.* Methotrexate is excreted into the bile by canalicular multispecific organic anion transporter in rats. Cancer Res 1997; 57: 3506-10.

[107] Keppler D, and Kartenbeck, J. The canalicular conjugate export pump encoded by the cmrp/cmoat gene. Prog Liver Dis 1996; 14: 55-67.

[108] Cui Y, Konig J, Buchholz JK, *et al.* Drug resistance and ATP-dependent conjugate transport mediated by the apical multidrug resistance protein, MRP2, permanently expressed in human and canine cells. Mol Pharmacol 1999; 55: 929-37.

[109] Kawabe T CZ, Wada M, Uchiumi T, *et al.* Enhanced transport of anticancer agents and leukotriene C4 by the human canalicular multispecific organic anion transporter (cMOAT/MRP2). FEBS Lett 1999; 456: 327-31.

[110] Koike K KT, Tanaka T, Toh S, *et al.* A canalicular multispecific organic anion transporter (cMOAT) antisense cDNA enhances drug sensitivity in human hepatic cancer cells. Cancer Res 1997; 57: 5475-9.

[111] Xiong H, Turner KC, Ward ES, *et al.* Altered hepatobiliary disposition of acetaminophen glucuronide in isolated perfused livers from multidrug resistance-associated protein 2-deficient TR⁻ rats. J Pharmacol Exp Ther 2000; 295: 512-8.

[112] Evers R, de Haas M, Sparidans R, *et al.* Vinblastine and sulfinpyrazone export by the multidrug resistance protein MRP2 is associated with glutathione export. Br J Cancer 2000; 83: 375-83.

[113] Konno T, Ebihara T, Hisaeda K, *et al.* Identification of domains participating in the substrate specificity and subcellular localization of the multidrug resistance proteins MRP1 and MRP2. J Biol Chem 2003; 278: 22908-17.

[114] Rebbeor JF, Connolly GC, Henson JH, *et al.* ATP-dependent GSH and glutathione *S*-conjugate transport in skate liver: role of an Mrp functional homologue. Am J Physiol Gastrointest Liver Physiol 2000; 279: G417-25.

[115] Paulusma CC, van Geer MA, Evers R, *et al.* Canalicular multispecific organic anion transporter/multidrug resistance protein 2 mediates low-affinity transport of reduced glutathione. Biochem J 1999; 338 (Pt 2):393-401.

[116] Xiong H, Suzuki H, Sugiyama Y, *et al.* Mechanisms of impaired biliary excretion of acetaminophen glucuronide after acute phenobarbital treatment or phenobarbital pretreatment. Drug Metab Dispos 2002; 30: 962-9.

[117] Suzuki H, Sugiyama Y. Single nucleotide polymorphisms in multidrug resistance associated protein 2 (MRP2/ABCC2): its impact on drug disposition. Adv Drug Deliv Rev 2002; 54: 1311-31.

[118] Sasaki M, Suzuki H, Ito K, *et al.* Transcellular transport of organic anions across a double-transfected Madin-Darby canine kidney II cell monolayer expressing both human organic anion-transporting polypeptide (OATP2/SLC21A6) and Multidrug resistance-associated protein 2 (MRP2/ABCC2). J Biol Chem 2002; 277: 6497-503.

[119] Akita H, Suzuki H, Ito K, *et al.* Characterization of bile acid transport mediated by multidrug resistance associated protein 2 and bile salt export pump. Biochim Biophys Acta 2001;1511:7-16.

[120] Kobayashi N, Tani T, Hisaka A, *et al.* Hepatobiliary transport of a nonpeptidic endothelin antagonist, (+)-(5*S*,6*R*,7*R*)-2-butyl-7-[2((2*S*)-2-carboxypropyl)-4-methoxyphenyl]-5-(3,4-methylenedioxyphenyl) cyclopentenol[1,2-b]pyridine-6-carboxylic acid: uptake by isolated rat hepatocytes and canalicular membrane vesicles. Pharm Res 2003; 20: 89-95.

[121] Nakagomi-Hagihara R, Nakai D, Kawai K, *et al.* OATP1B1, OATP1B3, and MRP2 are involved in hepatobiliary transport of olmesartan, a novel angiotensin II blocker. Drug Metab Dispos 2006; 34: 862-9.

[122] Takayanagi M, Sano N, Takikawa H. Biliary excretion of olmesartan, an anigotensin II receptor antagonist, in the rat. J Gastroenterol Hepatol 2005; 20: 784-8.

[123] Huisman MT, Smit JW, Crommentuyn KM, *et al.* Multidrug resistance protein 2 (MRP2) transports HIV protease inhibitors, and transport can be enhanced by other drugs. Aids 2002; 16: 2295-301.

[124] Agarwal S, Pal D, Mitra AK. Both P-gp and MRP2 mediate transport of Lopinavir, a protease inhibitor. Int J Pharm 2007.

[125] Hendrikse NH, Franssen EJ, van der Graaf WT, *et al.* Visualization of multidrug resistance *in vivo*. Eur J Nucl Med 1999; 26: 283-93.

[126] Srivastava SK, Watkins SC, Schuetz E, *et al.* Role of glutathione conjugate efflux in cellular protection against benzo[*a*]pyrene-7,8-diol-9,10-epoxide-induced DNA damage. Mol Carcinog 2002; 33: 156-62.

[127] Terlouw SA, Graeff C, Smeets PH, *et al.* Short- and long-term influences of heavy metals on anionic drug efflux from renal proximal tubule. J Pharmacol Exp Ther 2002; 301: 578-85.

[128] Dietrich CG, Ottenhoff R, de Waart DR, *et al.* Role of MRP2 and GSH in intrahepatic cycling of toxins. Toxicology 2001;167:73-81.

[129] Bodo A, Bakos E, Szeri F, *et al.* Differential modulation of the human liver conjugate transporters MRP2 and MRP3 by bile acids and organic anions. J Biol Chem 2003; 278: 23529-37.

[130] Zelcer N, Huisman MT, Reid G, *et al.* Evidence for two interacting ligand binding sites in human multidrug resistance protein 2 (ATP binding cassette C2). J Biol Chem 2003; 278: 23538-44.

[131] Koike K, Kawabe T, Tanaka T, *et al.* A canalicular multispecific organic anion transporter (cMOAT) antisense cDNA enhances drug sensitivity in human hepatic cancer cells. Cancer Res 1997; 57: 5475-9.

[132] Kiuchi Y SH, Hirohashi T, Tyson CA, *et al.* cDNA cloning and inducible expression of human multidrug resistance associated protein 3 (MRP3). FEBS Lett 1998;433:149-52.

[133] Kool M, de Haas M, Scheffer GL, *et al.* Analysis of expression of cMOAT (MRP2), MRP3, MRP4, and MRP5, homologues of the multidrug resistance-associated protein gene (MRP1), in human cancer cell lines. Cancer Res 1997;57:3537-47.

[134] Zimmermann C, Gutmann H, Hruz P, *et al.* Mapping of MDR1 and MRP1-5 mRNA expression along the human intestinal tract. Drug Metab Dispos 2004.

[135] Nies AT, Jedlitschky G, Konig J, *et al.* Expression and immunolocalization of the multidrug resistance proteins, MRP1-MRP6 (ABCC1-ABCC6), in human brain. Neuroscience 2004;129:349-60.

[136] Kool M, van der Linden M, de Haas M, *et al.* MRP3, an organic anion transporter able to transport anti-cancer drugs. Proc Natl Acad Sci U S A 1999; 96: 6914-9.

[137] Zeng H, Bain LJ, Belinsky MG, *et al.* Expression of multidrug resistance protein-3 (multispecific organic anion transporter-D) in human embryonic kidney 293 cells confers resistance to anticancer agents. Cancer Res 1999; 59: 5964-7.

[138] Zeng H, Liu G, Rea PA, *et al.* Transport of amphipathic anions by human multidrug resistance protein 3. Cancer Res 2000; 60: 4779-84.

[139] Chu XY, Huskey SE, Braun MP, *et al.* Transport of ethinylestradiol glucuronide and ethinylestradiol sulfate by the multidrug resistance proteins MRP1, MRP2, and MRP3. J Pharmacol Exp Ther 2004; 309: 156-64.

[140] Zelcer N, Saeki T, Reid G, *et al.* Characterization of drug transport by the human multidrug resistance protein 3 (ABCC3). J Biol Chem 2001; 276: 46400-7.

[141] Hirohashi T, Suzuki H, Sugiyama Y. Characterization of the transport properties of cloned rat multidrug resistance-associated protein 3 (MRP3). J Biol Chem 1999; 274: 15181-5.

[142] Kool M, de Haas M, Scheffer GL, *et al.* Analysis of expression of cMOAT (MRP2), MRP3, MRP4, and MRP5, homologues of the multidrug resistance-associated protein gene (MRP1), in human cancer cell lines. Cancer Res 1997; 57: 3537-47.

[143] Young LC, Campling BG, Voskoglou-Nomikos T, *et al.* Expression of multidrug resistance protein-related genes in lung cancer: correlation with drug response. Clin Cancer Res 1999; 5: 673-80.

[144] Ishikawa T. The ATP-dependent glutathione S-conjugate export pump. Trends Biochem Sci 1992; 17: 463-8.

[145] Hirohashi T SH, Takikawa H, Sugiyama Y. ATP-dependent transport of bile salts by rat multidrug resistance-associated protein 3 (Mrp3). J Biol Chem 2000; 275: 2905-10.

[146] Kullak-Ublick GA, Stieger B, Meier PJ. Enterohepatic bile salt transporters in normal physiology and liver disease. Gastroenterology 2004; 126: 322-42.

[147] Ros JE, Libbrecht L, Geuken M, *et al.* High expression of MDR1, MRP1, and MRP3 in the hepatic progenitor cell compartment and hepatocytes in severe human liver disease. J Pathol 2003; 200: 553-60.

[148] Zollner G, Fickert P, Silbert D, *et al.* Adaptive changes in hepatobiliary transporter expression in primary biliary cirrhosis. J Hepatol 2003; 38: 717-27.

[149] Lai L, Tan TM. Role of glutathione in the multidrug resistance protein 4 (MRP4/ABCC4)-mediated efflux of cAMP and resistance to purine analogues. Biochem J 2002;361:497-503.

[150] Chen ZS, Lee K, Kruh GD. Transport of cyclic nucleotides and estradiol 17-b-D-glucuronide by multidrug resistance protein 4. Resistance to 6-mercaptopurine and 6-thioguanine. J Biol Chem 2001; 276: 33747-54.

[151] Chen ZS, Lee K, Walther S, *et al.* Analysis of methotrexate and folate transport by multidrug resistance protein 4 (ABCC4): MRP4 is a component of the methotrexate efflux system. Cancer Res 2002; 62: 3144-50.

[152] van Aubel RA, Smeets PH, Peters JG, *et al.* The MRP4/ABCC4 gene encodes a novel apical organic anion transporter in human kidney proximal tubules: putative efflux pump for urinary cAMP and cGMP. J Am Soc Nephrol 2002; 13: 595-603.

[153] Reid G, Wielinga P, Zelcer N, *et al.* The human multidrug resistance protein MRP4 functions as a prostaglandin efflux transporter and is inhibited by nonsteroidal antiinflammatory drugs. Proc Natl Acad Sci U S A 2003; 100: 9244-9.

[154] Rius M, Thon WF, Keppler D, *et al.* Prostanoid transport by multidrug resistance protein 4 (MRP4/ABCC4) localized in tissues of the human urogenital tract. J Urol 2005; 174: 2409-14.

[155] Zelcer N, Reid G, Wielinga P, *et al.* Steroid and bile acid conjugates are substrates of human multidrug-resistance protein (MRP) 4 (ATP-binding cassette C_4). Biochem J 2003; 371: 361-7.

[156] Rius M, Nies AT, Hummel-Eisenbeiss J, *et al.* Cotransport of reduced glutathione with bile salts by MRP4 (ABCC4) localized to the basolateral hepatocyte membrane. Hepatology 2003; 38: 374-84.

[157] Zamek-Gliszczynski MJ, Nezasa K, Tian X, *et al.* Evaluation of the role of multidrug resistance-associated protein (MRP) 3 and MRP4 in hepatic basolateral excretion of sulfate and glucuronide metabolites of acetaminophen, 4-methylumbelliferone, and harmol in $ABCC3^{-/-}$ and $ABCC4^{-/-}$ mice. J Pharmacol Exp Ther 2006; 319: 1485-91.

[158] Adachi M, Sampath J, Lan LB, *et al.* Expression of MRP4 confers resistance to ganciclovir and compromises bystander cell killing. J Biol Chem 2002; 277: 38998-9004.

[159] Sampath J, Adachi M, Hatse S, *et al.* Role of MRP4 and MRP5 in biology and chemotherapy. AAPS PharmSci 2002; 4: E14.

[160] Lee K, Klein-Szanto AJ, Kruh GD. Analysis of the MRP4 drug resistance profile in transfected NIH3T3 cells. J Natl Cancer Inst 2000; 92: 1934-40.

[161] Dallas S, Schlichter L, Bendayan R. Multidrug resistance protein (MRP) 4- and MRP 5-mediated efflux of 9-(2-phosphonylmethoxyethyl)adenine by microglia. J Pharmacol Exp Ther 2004; 309: 1221-9.

[162] Chen ZS, Lee K, Kruh GD. Transport of cyclic nucleotides and estradiol 17-beta-D-glucuronide by multidrug resistance protein 4. Resistance to 6-mercaptopurine and 6-thioguanine. J Biol Chem 2001; 276: 33747-54.

[163] Imaoka T, Kusuhara H, Adachi M, *et al.* Functional involvement of multidrug resistance-associated protein 4 (MRP4/ABCC4) in the renal elimination of the antiviral drugs adefovir and tenofovir. Mol Pharmacol 2007; 71: 619-27.

[164] van Aubel RA, Smeets PH, Van Den Heuvel JJ, *et al.* Human organic anion transporter MRP4 (ABCC4) is an efflux pump for the purine end metabolite urate with multiple allosteric substrate binding sites. Am J Physiol Renal Physiol 2004.

[165] Wielinga PR, Reid G, Challa EE, *et al.* Thiopurine metabolism and identification of the thiopurine metabolites transported by MRP4 and MRP5 overexpressed in human embryonic kidney cells. Mol Pharmacol 2002; 62:1321-31.

[166] Leggas M, Adachi M, Scheffer GL, *et al.* Mrp4 confers resistance to topotecan and protects the brain from chemotherapy. Mol Cell Biol 2004; 24: 7612-21.

[167] Wall M, Wani MC, Cook CE, *et al.* Plant antitumor agents: 1, the isolation and structure of camptothecin, anovel alkaloidal leukemia and tumor inhibitor from *Camptotheca acuminata*. J Am Chem Soc 1966; 88: 3888-90.

[168] Bai J, Lai L, Yeo HC, *et al.* Multidrug resistance protein 4 (MRP4/ABCC4) mediates efflux of bimane-glutathione. Int J Biochem Cell Biol 2004; 36: 247-57.

[169] Chen ZS, Lee K, Kruh GD. Transport of cyclic nucleotides and estradiol 17-β-D-glucuronide by multidrug resistance protein 4: Resistance to 6-mercaptopurine and 6-thioguanine. J Biol Chem 2001; 276:33747-54.

[170] Wielinga PR, van der Heijden I, Reid G, *et al.* Characterization of the MRP4- and MRP5-mediated transport of cyclic nucleotides from intact cells. J Biol Chem 2003; 278: 17664-71.

[171] Assaraf YG, Sierra EE, Babani S, *et al.* Inhibitory effects of prostaglandin A$_1$ on membrane transport of folates mediated by both the reduced folate carrier and ATP-driven exporters. Biochem Pharmacol 1999; 58: 1321-7.

[172] Reid G, Wielinga P, Zelcer N, *et al.* Characterization of the transport of nucleoside analog drugs by the human multidrug resistance proteins MRP4 and MRP5. Mol Pharmacol 2003; 63: 1094-103.

[173] Schuetz EG, Strom S, Yasuda K, *et al.* Disrupted bile acid homeostasis reveals an unexpected interaction among nuclear hormone receptors, transporters, and cytochrome P450. J Biol Chem 2001; 276: 39411-8.

[174] Assem M, Schuetz EG, Leggas M, *et al.* Interactions between hepatic Mrp4 and Sult2a as revealed by the constitutive androstane receptor and Mrp4 knockout mice. J Biol Chem 2004; 279: 22250-7.

[175] Jorajuria S, Dereuddre-Bosquet N, Becher F, *et al.* ATP binding cassette multidrug transporters limit the anti-HIV activity of zidovudine and indinavir in infected human macrophages. Antivir Ther 2004; 9: 519-28.

[176] Wijnholds J, Mol CA, van Deemter L, *et al.* Multidrug-resistance protein 5 is a multispecific organic anion transporter able to transport nucleotide analogs. Proc Natl Acad Sci U S A 2000; 97: 7476-81.

[177] McAleer MA, Breen MA, White NL, *et al.* pABC11 (also known as MOAT-C and MRP5), a member of the ABC family of proteins, has anion transporter activity but does not confer multidrug resistance when overexpressed in human embryonic kidney 293 cells. J Biol Chem 1999; 274: 23541-8.

[178] Kool M, van der Linden M, de Haas M, *et al.* Expression of human MRP6, a homologue of the multidrug resistance protein gene MRP1, in tissues and cancer cells. Cancer Res 1999; 59: 175-82.

[179] Scheffer GL, Hu X, Pijnenborg AC, *et al.* MRP6 (ABCC6) detection in normal human tissues and tumors. Lab Invest 2002; 82: 515-8.

[180] Boraldi F, Quaglino D, Croce MA, *et al.* Multidrug resistance protein-6 (MRP6) in human dermal fibroblasts. Comparison between cells from normal subjects and from Pseudoxanthoma elasticum patients. Matrix Biol 2003; 22: 491-500.

[181] Sinko E, Ilias A, Ujhelly O, *et al.* Subcellular localization and *N*-glycosylation of human ABCC6, expressed in MDCKII cells. Biochem Biophys Res Commun 2003; 308: 263-9.

[182] Belinsky MG, Chen ZS, Shchaveleva I, *et al.* Characterization of the drug resistance and transport properties of multidrug resistance protein 6 (MRP6, ABCC6). Cancer Res 2002; 62: 6172-7.

[183] Madon J, Hagenbuch B, Landmann L, *et al.* Transport function and hepatocellular localization of mrp6 in rat liver. Mol Pharmacol 2000; 57: 634-41.

[184] Ilias A UZ, Seidl TL, Le Saux O, *et al.* Loss of ATP-dependent transport activity in pseudoxanthoma elasticum-associated mutants of human ABCC6 (MRP6). J Biol Chem 2002; 277: 16860-7.

[185] Chen ZS, Hopper-Borge E, Belinsky MG, *et al.* Characterization of the transport properties of human multidrug resistance protein 7 (MRP7, ABCC10). Mol Pharmacol 2003; 63: 351-8.

[186] Hopper-Borge E, Chen ZS, Shchaveleva I, *et al.* Analysis of the drug resistance profile of multidrug resistance protein 7 (ABCC10): resistance to docetaxel. Cancer Res 2004; 64: 4927-30.

[187] Oguri T, Bessho Y, Achiwa H, *et al.* MRP8/ABCC11 directly confers resistance to 5-fluorouracil. Mol Cancer Ther 2007; 6: 122-7.

[188] Guo Y, Kotova E, Chen ZS, *et al.* MRP8, ATP-binding cassette C11 (ABCC11), is a cyclic nucleotide efflux pump and a resistance factor for fluoropyrimidines 2',3'-dideoxycytidine and 9'-(2'-phosphonylmethoxyethyl)adenine. J Biol Chem 2003; 278: 29509-14.

[189] Chen LM, Wu XP, Ruan JW, *et al.* Screening novel, potent multidrug-resistant modulators from imidazole derivatives. Oncol Res 2004; 14: 355-62.

[190] Kruh GD, Guo Y, Hopper-Borge E, *et al.* ABCC10, ABCC11, and ABCC12. Pflugers Arch 2007; 453: 675-84.

[191] Bortfeld M, Rius M, Konig J, *et al.* Human multidrug resistance protein 8 (MRP8/ABCC11), an apical efflux pump for steroid sulfates, is an axonal protein of the CNS and peripheral nervous system. Neuroscience 2006; 137: 1247-57.

[192] Chen ZS, Guo Y, Belinsky MG, *et al.* Transport of bile acids, sulfated steroids, estradiol 17b-D-glucuronide, and leukotriene C$_4$ by human multidrug resistance protein 8 (ABCC11). Mol Pharmacol 2005; 67: 545-57.

[193] Bera TK IC, Kumar V, Lee S, *et al.* MRP9, an unusual truncated member of the ABC transporter superfamily, is highly expressed in breast cancer. Proc Natl Acad Sci U S A 2002; 99: 6997-7002.

[194] Urquhart BL, Tirona RG, Kim RB. Nuclear receptors and the regulation of drug-metabolizing enzymes and drug transporters: implications for interindividual variability in response to drugs. J Clin Pharmacol 2007; 47: 566-78.

[195] Staudinger JL, Madan A, Carol KM, *et al.* Regulation of drug transporter gene expression by nuclear receptors. Drug Metab Dispos 2003;31:523-7.

[196] Klaassen CD, Slitt AL. Regulation of hepatic transporters by xenobiotic receptors. Curr Drug Metab 2005; 6: 309-28.

[197] Bertilsson G, Heidrich J, Svensson K, *et al.* Identification of a human nuclear receptor defines a new signaling pathway for CYP3A induction. Proc Natl Acad Sci U S A 1998; 95: 12208-13.

[198] Kliewer SA, Willson TM. Regulation of xenobiotic and bile acid metabolism by the nuclear pregnane X receptor. J Lipid Res 2002; 43: 359-64.

[199] Staudinger JL, Goodwin B, Jones SA, *et al.* The nuclear receptor PXR is a lithocholic acid sensor that protects against liver toxicity. Proc Natl Acad Sci U S A 2001; 98: 3369-74.

[200] Geick A, Eichelbaum M, Burk O. Nuclear receptor response elements mediate induction of intestinal MDR1 by rifampin. J Biol Chem 2001; 276: 14581-7.

[201] Kauffmann HM, Pfannschmidt S, Zoller H, *et al.* Influence of redox-active compounds and PXR-activators on human *MRP1* and *MRP2* gene expression. Toxicology 2002; 171: 137-46.

[202] Teng S, Jekerle V, Piquette-Miller M. Induction of ABCC3 (MRP3) by pregnane X receptor activators. Drug Metab Dispos 2003; 31: 1296-9.

[203] Maher JM, Cheng X, Slitt AL, *et al.* Induction of the multidrug resistance-associated protein family of transporters by chemical activators of receptor-mediated pathways in mouse liver. Drug Metab Dispos 2005; 33: 956-62.

[204] Moffit JS, Aleksunes LM, Maher JM, *et al.* Induction of hepatic transporters multidrug resistance-associated proteins (MRP) 3 and 4 by clofibrate is regulated by peroxisome proliferator-activated receptor a. J Pharmacol Exp Ther 2006; 317: 537-45.

[205] Nishimura M, Koeda A, Suzuki E, *et al.* Regulation of mRNA expression of MDR1, MRP1, MRP2 and MRP3 by prototypical microsomal enzyme inducers in primary cultures of human and rat hepatocytes. Drug Metab Pharmacokinet 2006; 21: 297-307.

[206] Aleksunes LM, Scheffer GL, Jakowski AB, *et al.* Coordinated expression of multidrug resistance-associated proteins (MRPs) in mouse liver during toxicant-induced injury. Toxicol Sci 2006; 89: 370-9.

[207] Magnarin M, Morelli M, Rosati A, *et al.* Induction of proteins involved in multidrug resistance (P-glycoprotein, MRP1, MRP2, LRP) and of CYP 3A4 by rifampicin in LLC-PK1 cells. Eur J Pharmacol 2004; 483: 19-28.

[208] Pfrunder A, Gutmann H, Beglinger C, et al. Gene expression of CYP3A4, ABC-transporters (MDR1 and MRP1-MRP5) and hPXR in three different human colon carcinoma cell lines. J Pharm Pharmacol 2003; 55: 59-66.

[209] Nieth C, Lage H. Induction of the ABC-transporters Mdr1/P-gp (Abcb1), mrpl (Abcc1), and bcrp (Abcg2) during establishment of multidrug resistance following exposure to mitoxantrone. J Chemother 2005; 17: 215-23.

[210] Tatebe S, Sinicrope FA, Kuo MT. Induction of multidrug resistance proteins MRP1 and MRP3 and g-glutamylcysteine synthetase gene expression by nonsteroidal anti-inflammatory drugs in human colon cancer cells. Biochem Biophys Res Commun 2002; 290: 1427-33.

[211] Kauffmann HM, Schrenk D. Sequence analysis and functional characterization of the 5'-flanking region of the rat multidrug resistance protein 2 (*mrp2*) gene. Biochem Biophys Res Commun 1998; 245: 325-31.

[212] Johnson DR, Klaassen CD. Regulation of rat multidrug resistance protein 2 by classes of prototypical microsomal enzyme inducers that activate distinct transcription pathways. Toxicol Sci 2002; 67: 182-9.

[213] Courtois A, Payen L, Le Ferrec E, *et al.* Differential regulation of multidrug resistance-associated protein 2 (MRP2) and cytochrornes P4502B1/2 and 3A1/2 in phenobarbital-treated hepatocytes. Biochem Pharmacol 2002; 63: 333-41.

[214] Cherrington NJ, Hartley DP, Li N, *et al.* Organ distribution of multidrug resistance proteins 1, 2, and 3 (Mrp1, 2 and 3) mRNA and hepatic induction of Mrp3 by constitutive androstane receptor activators in rats. J Pharmacol Exp Ther 2002; 300: 97-104.

[215] Kast HR, Goodwin B, Tarr PT, *et al.* Regulation of multidrug resistance-associated protein 2 (ABCC2) by the nuclear receptors pregnane X receptor, farnesoid X-activated receptor, and constitutive androstane receptor. J Biol Chem 2002; 277: 2908-15.

[216] Kauffmann HM, Keppler D, Kartenbeck J, *et al.* Induction of cMrp/cMOAT gene expression by cisplatin, 2-acetylaminofluorene, or cycloheximide in rat hepatocytes. Hepatology 1997; 26: 980-5.

[217] Slitt AL, Cherrington NJ, Fisher CD, *et al.* Induction of genes for metabolism and transport by trans-stilbene oxide in livers of Sprague-Dawley and Wistar-Kyoto rats. Drug Metab Dispos 2006; 34: 1190-7.

[218] Kauffmann HM, Keppler D, Gant TW, *et al.* Induction of hepatic MRP2 (cMRP/cMOAT) gene expression in nonhuman primates treated with rifampicin or tamoxifen. Arch Toxicol 1998; 72: 763-8.

[219] Ruhl R, Sczech R, Landes N, *et al.* Carotenoids and their metabolites are naturally occurring activators of gene expression *via* the pregnane X receptor. Eur J Nutr 2004;43:336-43.

[220] Jones SA, Moore LB, Shenk JL, *et al.* The pregnane x receptor: a promiscuous xenobiotic receptor that has diverged during evolution. Mol Endocrinol 2000;14:27-39.

[221] Schrenk D, Baus PR, Ermel N, *et al.* Up-regulation of transporters of the MRP family by drugs and toxins. Toxicol Lett 2001;120:51-7.

[222] Shoda J, Kano M, Oda K, *et al.* The expression levels of plasma membrane transporters in the cholestatic liver of patients undergoing biliary drainage and their association with the impairment of biliary secretory function. Am J Gastroenterol 2001; 96: 3368-78.

[223] Fromm MF, Kauffmann HM, Fritz P, *et al.* The effect of rifampin treatment on intestinal expression of human MRP transporters. Am J Pathol 2000; 157: 1575-80.

[224] Laouari D, Yang R, Veau C, *et al.* Two apical multidrug transporters, P-gp and MRP2, are differently altered in chronic renal failure. Am J Physiol Renal Physiol 2001; 280: F636-45.

[225] Konig J, Rost D, Cui Y, *et al.* Characterization of the human multidrug resistance protein isoform MRP3 localized to the basolateral hepatocyte membrane. Hepatology 1999; 29: 1156-63.

[226] Xie W, Radominska-Pandya A, Shi Y, *et al.* An essential role for nuclear receptors SXR/PXR in detoxification of cholestatic bile acids. Proc Natl Acad Sci U S A 2001; 98: 3375-80.

[227] Cherrington NJ, Slitt AL, Maher JM, *et al.* Induction of multidrug resistance protein 3 (mrp3) *in vivo* is independent of constitutive androstane receptor. Drug Metab Dispos 2003; 31: 1315-9.

[228] Hitzl M, Klein K, Zanger UM, *et al.* Influence of omeprazole on multidrug resistance protein 3 expression in human liver. J Pharmacol Exp Ther 2003; 304: 524-30.

[229] Chen C, Klaassen CD. Rat multidrug resistance protein 4 (Mrp4, Abcc4): molecular cloning, organ distribution, postnatal renal expression, and chemical inducibility. Biochem Biophys Res Commun 2004; 317: 46-53.

[230] Ratajewski M, Bartosz G, Pulaski L. Expression of the human *ABCC6* gene is induced by retinoids through the retinoid X receptor. Biochem Biophys Res Commun 2006; 350: 1082-7.

[231] Auyeung DJ, Kessler FK, Ritter JK. Mechanism of rat UDP-glucuronosyltransferase 1A6 induction by oltipraz: evidence for a contribution of the Aryl hydrocarbon receptor pathway. Mol Pharmacol 2003; 63: 119-27.

[232] Ma Q, Kinneer K, Bi Y, *et al.* Induction of murine NAD(P)H:quinone oxidoreductase by 2,3,7,8-tetrachlorodibenzo-p-dioxin requires the CNC (cap 'n' collar) basic leucine zipper transcription factor Nrf2 (nuclear factor erythroid 2-related factor 2): cross-interaction between AhR (aryl hydrocarbon receptor) and Nrf2 signal transduction. Biochem J 2004; 377: 205-13.

[233] Chan LM, Lowes S, Hirst BH. The ABCs of drug transport in intestine and liver: efflux proteins limiting drug absorption and bioavailability. Eur J Pharm Sci 2004; 21: 25-51.

[234] Alrefai WA, Gill RK. Bile Acid Transporters: Structure, Function, Regulation and Pathophysiological Implications. Pharm Res 2007.

[235] Ballatori N, Christian WV, Lee JY, *et al.* OSTa-OSTb: a major basolateral bile acid and steroid transporter in human intestinal, renal, and biliary epithelia. Hepatology 2005; 42: 1270-9.

[236] Geier A, Wagner M, Dietrich CG, *et al.* Principles of hepatic organic anion transporter regulation during cholestasis, inflammation and liver regeneration. Biochim Biophys Acta 2007; 1773: 283-308.

[237] Gerk PM, Vore M. Regulation of expression of the multidrug resistance-associated protein 2 (MRP2) and its role in drug disposition. J Pharmacol Exp Ther 2002; 302: 407-15.

[238] Zachowski A, Henry JP, Devaux PF. Control of transmembrane lipid asymmetry in chromaffin granules by an ATP-dependent protein. Nature 1989; 340: 75-6.

[239] Smith AJ, Timmermans-Hereijgers JL, Roelofsen B, *et al.* The human MDR3 P-glycoprotein promotes translocation of phosphatidylcholine through the plasma membrane of fibroblasts from transgenic mice. FEBS Lett 1994; 354: 263-6.

[240] Smit JW, Weert B, Schinkel AH, *et al.* Heterologous expression of various P-glycoproteins in polarized epithelial cells induces directional transport of small (Type 1) and bulky (Type 2) cationic drugs. J Pharmacol Exp Ther 1998; 286: 321-7.

[241] Matsuzaki Y, Nakano A, Jiang QJ, *et al.* Tissue-specific expression of the ABCC6 gene. J Invest Dermatol 2005; 125: 900-5.

[242] van de Water FM, Masereeuw R, Russel FG. Function and regulation of multidrug resistance proteins (MRPs) in the renal elimination of organic anions. Drug Metab Rev 2005; 37: 443-71.

[243] Kim WJ, Kakehi Y, Kinoshita H, *et al.* Expression patterns of multidrug-resistance (MDR1), multidrug resistance-associated protein (MRP),glutathione-S-transferase-pi (GST-pi) and DNA topoisomerase II (Topo II) genes in renal cell carcinomas and normal kidney. J Urol 1996; 156: 506-11.

[244] Inui KI, Masuda S, Saito H. Cellular and molecular aspects of drug transport in the kidney. Kidney Int 2000; 58: 944-58.

[245] Ray AS, Cihlar T, Robinson KL, *et al.* Mechanism of active renal tubular efflux of tenofovir. Antimicrob Agents Chemother 2006; 50: 3297-304.

[246] Sekine T, Miyazaki H, Endou H. Molecular physiology of renal organic anion transporters. Am J Physiol Renal Physiol 2006; 290: F251-61.

[247] Launay-Vacher V, Izzedine H, Karie S, *et al.* Renal tubular drug transporters. Nephron Physiol 2006; 103: 97-106.

[248] Terada T, Inui K. Peptide transporters: structure, function, regulation and application for drug delivery. Curr Drug Metab 2004; 5: 85-94.

[249] Nishizato Y, Ieiri I, Suzuki H, *et al.* Polymorphisms of *OATP-C* (SLC21A6) and *OAT3* (SLC22A8) genes: consequences for pravastatin pharmacokinetics. Clin Pharmacol Ther 2003; 73: 554-65.

[250] Jonker JW, Wagenaar E, Van Eijl S, *et al.* Deficiency in the organic cation transporters 1 and 2 (OCT1/OCT2 [Slc22a1/Slc22a2]) in mice abolishes renal secretion of organic cations. Mol Cell Biol 2003; 23: 7902-8.

[251] Ganapathy ME, Brandsch M, Prasad PD, *et al.* Differential recognition of b -lactam antibiotics by intestinal and renal peptide transporters, PEPT 1 and PEPT 2. J Biol Chem 1995; 270: 25672-7.

[252] Jung KY, Takeda M, Shimoda M, *et al.* Involvement of rat organic anion transporter 3 (rOAT3) in cephaloridine-induced nephrotoxicity: in comparison with rOAT1. Life Sci 2002; 70: 1861-74.

[253] Deguchi T, Kusuhara H, Takadate A, *et al.* Characterization of uremic toxin transport by organic anion transporters in the kidney. Kidney Int 2004; 65: 162-74.

[254] Yonezawa A, Masuda S, Nishihara K, *et al.* Association between tubular toxicity of cisplatin and expression of organic cation transporter rOCT2 (Slc22a2) in the rat. Biochem Pharmacol 2005;70:1823-31.

[255] Kearney BP, Sayre JR, Flaherty JF, *et al.* Drug-drug and drug-food interactions between tenofovir disoproxil fumarate and didanosine. J Clin Pharmacol 2005;45:1360-7.

[256] Kearney BP, Flaherty JF, Shah J. Tenofovir disoproxil fumarate: clinical pharmacology and pharmacokinetics. Clin Pharmacokinet 2004;43:595-612.

[257] Ray AS, Olson L, Fridland A. Role of purine nucleoside phosphorylase in interactions between 2',3'-dideoxyinosine and allopurinol, ganciclovir, or tenofovir. Antimicrob Agents Chemother 2004;48:1089-95.

[258] Kotb R, Vincent I, Dulioust A, *et al.* Life-threatening interaction between antiretroviral therapy and vinblastine in HIV-associated multicentric Castleman's disease. Eur J Haematol 2006;76:269-71.

[259] Makinson A, Martelli N, Peyriere H, *et al.* Profound neutropenia resulting from interaction between antiretroviral therapy and vinblastine in a patient with HIV-associated Hodgkin's disease. Eur J Haematol 2007;78:358-60.

[260] Banks WA. Physiology and pathology of the blood-brain barrier: implications for microbial pathogenesis, drug delivery and neurodegenerative disorders. J Neurovirol 1999;5:538-55.

[261] Loscher W, Potschka H. Blood-brain barrier active efflux transporters: ATP-binding cassette gene family. NeuroRx 2005;2:86-98.

[262] Couture L, Nash JA, Turgeon J. The ATP-binding cassette transporters and their implication in drug disposition: a special look at the heart. Pharmacol Rev 2006;58:244-58.

[263] Girardin F. Membrane transporter proteins: a challenge for CNS drug development. Dialogues Clin Neurosci 2006;8:311-21.

[264] de Boer AG, Gaillard PJ. Drug targeting to the brain. Annu Rev Pharmacol Toxicol 2007;47:323-55.

[265] Dallas S, Miller DS, Bendayan R. Multidrug resistance-associated proteins: expression and function in the central nervous system. Pharmacol Rev 2006;58:140-61.

[266] de Boer AG, van der Sandt IC, Gaillard PJ. The role of drug transporters at the blood-brain barrier. Annu Rev Pharmacol Toxicol 2003;43:629-56.

[267] Hawkins BT, Davis TP. The blood-brain barrier/neurovascular unit in health and disease. Pharmacol Rev 2005;57:173-85.

[268] Terasaki T, Ohtsuki S. Brain-to-blood transporters for endogenous substrates and xenobiotics at the blood-brain barrier: an overview of biology and methodology. NeuroRx 2005;2:63-72.

[269] Taylor EM. The impact of efflux transporters in the brain on the development of drugs for CNS disorders. Clin Pharmacokinet 2002;41:81-92.

[270] Begley DJ. ABC transporters and the blood-brain barrier. Curr Pharm Des 2004;10:1295-312.

[271] Deeley RG, Westlake C, Cole SP. Transmembrane transport of endo- and xenobiotics by mammalian ATP-binding cassette multidrug resistance proteins. Physiol Rev 2006;86:849-99.

[272] Siegal T, Zylber-Katz E. Strategies for increasing drug delivery to the brain: focus on brain lymphoma. Clin Pharmacokinet 2002;41:171-86.

[273] Fricker G, Miller DS. Modulation of drug transporters at the blood-brain barrier. Pharmacology 2004;70:169-76.

[274] Zhao Q, Chang XB. Mutation of the aromatic amino acid interacting with adenine moiety of ATP to a polar residue alters the properties of multidrug resistance protein 1. J Biol Chem 2004;279:48505-12.

[275] Zhang DW, Nunoya K, Vasa M, et al. Transmembrane helix 11 of multidrug resistance protein 1 (MRP1/ABCC1): identification of polar amino acids important for substrate specificity and binding of ATP at nucleotide binding domain 1. Biochemistry 2004;43:9413-25.

[276] Conseil G, Deeley RG, Cole SP. Polymorphisms of MRP1 (ABCC1) and related ATP-dependent drug transporters. Pharmacogenet Genomics 2005;15:523-33.

[277] Conrad S, Kauffmann HM, Ito K, et al. A naturally occurring mutation in MRP1 results in a selective decrease in organic anion transport and in increased doxorubicin resistance. Pharmacogenetics 2002;12:321-30.

[278] Assaraf YG, Rothem L, Hooijberg JH, et al. Loss of multidrug resistance protein 1 expression and folate efflux activity results in a highly concentrative folate transport in human leukemia cells. J Biol Chem 2003;278:6680-6.

[279] Leslie EM, Letourneau IJ, Deeley RG, et al. Functional and structural consequences of cysteine substitutions in the NH2 proximal region of the human multidrug resistance protein 1 (MRP1/ABCC1). Biochemistry 2003;42:5214-24.

[280] Ito K, Oleschuk CJ, Westlake C, et al. Mutation of Trp1254 in the multispecific organic anion transporter, multidrug resistance protein 2 (MRP2) (ABCC2), alters substrate specificity and results in loss of methotrexate transport activity. J Biol Chem 2001;276:38108-14.

[281] Buchler M, Konig J, Brom M, et al. cDNA cloning of the hepatocyte canalicular isoform of the multidrug resistance protein, cMRP, reveals a novel conjungate export pump deficient in hyperbilirubinemic rats. J Biol Chem 1996;271:15091-8.

[282] Ito K, Suzuki H, Hirohashi T, et al. Molecular cloning of canalicular multispecific organic anion transporter defective in EHBR. Am J Physiol 1997;272:G16-G22.

[283] Paulusma CC, Bosma PJ, Zaman GJ, et al. Congenital jaundice in rats with a mutation in a multidrug resistance-associated protein gene. Science 1996;271:1126-8.

[284] Kartenbeck J, Leuschner U, Mayer R, et al. Absence of the canalicular isoform of the MRP gene-encoded conjugate export pump from the hepatocytes in Dubin-Johnson syndrome. Hepatology 1996;23:1061-6.

[285] Machida I, Inagaki Y, Suzuki S, et al. Mutation analysis of the multidrug resistance protein 2 (MRP2) gene in a Japanese patient with Dubin-Johnson syndrome. Hepatol Res 2004;30:86-90.

[286] Wakusawa S, Machida I, Suzuki S, et al. Identification of a novel 2026G-->C mutation of the MRP2 gene in a Japanese patient with Dubin-Johnson syndrome. J Hum Genet 2003;48:425-9.

[287] Hirouchi M, Suzuki H, Itoda M, et al. Characterization of the cellular localization, expression level, and function of SNP variants of MRP2/ABCC2. Pharm Res 2004;21:742-8.

[288] Ito S, Ieiri I, Tanabe M, et al. Polymorphism of the ABC transporter genes, *MDR1*, *MRP1* and *MRP2/cMOAT*, in healthy Japanese subjects. Pharmacogenetics 2001;11:175-84.

[289] Mor-Cohen R, Zivelin A, Rosenberg N, *et al.* Identification and functional analysis of two novel mutations in the multidrug resistance protein 2 gene in Israeli patients with Dubin-Johnson syndrome. J Biol Chem 2001;276:36923-30.

[290] Izzedine H, Hulot JS, Villard E, *et al.* Association between *ABCC2* gene haplotypes and tenofovir-induced proximal tubulopathy. J Infect Dis 2006;194:1481-91.

[291] Lang T, Hitzl M, Burk O, *et al.* Genetic polymorphisms in the multidrug resistance-associated protein 3 (ABCC3, MRP3) gene and relationship to its mRNA and protein expression in human liver. Pharmacogenetics 2004;14:155-64.

[292] Le Saux O UZ, Tschuch C, Csiszar K, *et al.* Mutations in a gene encoding an ABC transporter cause pseudoxanthoma elasticum. Nat Genet 2000;25:223-7.

[293] Ringpfeil F LM, Christiano AM, Uitto J. Pseudoxanthoma elasticum: mutations in the MRP6 gene encoding a transmembrane ATP-binding cassette (ABC) transporter. Proc Natl Acad Sci U S A 2000;97:6001-6.

[294] Uitto J. Pseudoxanthoma elasticum-a connective tissue disease or a metabolic disorder at the genome/environment interface? J Invest Dermatol 2004;122:ix-x.

[295] Hu X, Plomp AS, van Soest S, *et al.* Pseudoxanthoma elasticum: a clinical, histopathological, and molecular update. Surv Ophthalmol 2003;48:424-38.

[296] Gheduzzi D, Guidetti R, Anzivino C, *et al.* ABCC6 mutations in Italian families affected by pseudoxanthoma elasticum (PXE). Hum Mutat 2004;24:438-9.

[297] Chassaing N, Martin L, Mazereeuw J, *et al.* Novel ABCC6 mutations in pseudoxanthoma elasticum. J Invest Dermatol 2004;122:608-13.

[298] Hu X, Peek R, Plomp A, *et al.* Analysis of the frequent R1141X mutation in the ABCC6 gene in pseudoxanthoma elasticum. Invest Ophthalmol Vis Sci 2003;44:1824-9.

[299] Hendig D, Schulz V, Eichgrun J, *et al.* New ABCC6 gene mutations in German pseudoxanthoma elasticum patients. J Mol Med 2005;83:140-7.

[300] Germain DP, Remones V, Perdu J, *et al.* Identification of two polymorphisms (c189G>C; c190T>C) in exon 2 of the human MRP6 gene (ABCC6) by screening of Pseudoxanthoma elasticum patients: possible sequence correction? Hum Mutat 2000;16:449.

[301] Gottesman MM, Fojo T, Bates SE. Multidrug resistance in cancer: role of ATP-dependent transporters. Nat Rev Cancer 2002; 2: 48-58.

[302] Teodori E, Dei S, Martelli C, *et al.* The functions and structure of ABC transporters: implications for the design of new inhibitors of Pgp and MRP1 to control multidrug resistance (MDR). Curr Drug Targets 2006; 7: 893-909.

[303] Sauna ZE, Peng XH, Nandigama K, *et al.* The molecular basis of the action of disulfiram as a modulator of the multidrug resistance-linked ATP binding cassette transporters MDR1 (ABCB1) and MRP1 (ABCC1). Mol Pharmacol 2004;65:675-84.

[304] Perego P, De Cesare M, De Isabella P, *et al.* A novel 7-modified camptothecin analog overcomes breast cancer resistance protein-associated resistance in a mitoxantrone-selected colon carcinoma cell line. Cancer Res 2001; 61: 6034-7.

[305] Vail DM, Amantea MA, Colbern GT, *et al.* Pegylated liposomal doxorubicin: proof of principle using preclinical animal models and pharmacokinetic studies. Semin Oncol 2004; 31: 16-35.

[306] Cascorbi I. Role of pharmacogenetics of ATP-binding cassette transporters in the pharmacokinetics of drugs. Pharmacol Ther 2006; 112: 457-73.

[307] Szakacs G, Paterson JK, Ludwig JA, *et al.* Targeting multidrug resistance in cancer. Nat Rev Drug Discov 2006; 5: 219-34.

CHAPTER 2

Carbapenem-Resistant *Klebsiella pneumoniae*

Renato Finkelstein*

Rambam Health Care Campus Haifa, Israel

Abstract: *Klebsiella pneumoniae* is one of the most common nosocomial pathogens. *K. pneumoniae* strains producing Extended-Spectrum β-Lactamase enzymes (ESBLs) with transferable resistance to all β-lactam (except cephamycins and carbapenems) were first detected in the mid-1980s in Western Europe. Nowadays, there is a worldwide and non-uniform spread of *K. pneumoniae* expressing ESBL phenotype with prevalence as high as 45.4 percent. For infections caused by these strains, treatment with carbapenem drugs has been associated with the best outcomes in terms of survival and bacteriologic clearance. To date, carbapenem-resistance has been unusual in isolates of *K. pneumoniae*. Nevertheless, several recent studies have well documented the emergence of carbapenem resistance in Enterobacteriacae, including *Klebsiella spp.*, which should be considered of major public concern. Resistance to carbapenems in Enterobacteriaceae is generally caused by hydrolyzing enzymes. The most important among these are carbapenemases, primarily the serine β-lactamase KPC and metallo- β-lactamase VIM. The genes coding for these enzymes are carried by plasmids that often carry other resistance factors as well, resulting in extensively drug-resistant bacteria.Outbreaks of bla (VIM-1) positive carbapenem-resistant *K. pneumoniae* (CRKP) have been reported from some European countries. In the United States, carbapenem-resistance has been observed in strains of *K. pneumoniae*-producing class A carbapenemases, namely, KPC-1, KPC-2 and KPC-3. During 2006, strains of CRKP (KPC-2 and KPC-3) spread through Israeli hospitals and became a major national outbreak. Prior exposure to carbapenem and quinolones was found to be of resistance of *K. pneumoniae* to carbapenems.Infections due to CRKP have several important implications. First, these infections are spreading worldwide rapidly and are associated with a high estimated attributable mortality. Second, to control the spread of KPC enzymes appears to be difficult. Plasmids are easily transferred and resistant genes can spread within species and even from species to species of Enterobacteriaceae. Finally, and even more worrisome is that most KPC-possessing *K. pneumoniae* isolates are resistant not only to carbapenems, but also to almost all antibiotics currently in use. The clinical usefulness of a very few drugs showing *in vitro* activity against these strains remains to be proved.

Keywords: *Klebsiella pneumoniae*, extended-spectrum β-lactamase enzymes, carbapenem, metallo- β-lactamase, plasmids, enterobacteriacae, serine β-lactamase, class A carbapenemases.

INTRODUCTION

The natural habitat of many medically important members of the family Enterobacteriaceae is the lower gastrointestinal tract of humans and other animals. Nevertheless, these organisms are quite widespread in nature and may be found, for example, in water and soil. In addition, many underlying diseases or conditions (alcoholism, diabetes mellitus and hospitalized patients) predispose for oropharyngeal colonization which is considered an important predisposing factor that allows subsequent extraintestinal infections to occur. Members of the family Enterobacteriaceae cause a wide variety of community and hospital-acquired infections which may affect normal hosts and those with preexisting illnesses. These organisms comprise the most common gram-negative isolates in microbiology laboratories, including the vast majority of urinary isolates and a large proportion of isolates from the blood, the peritoneal cavity, and the respiratory tract [1].

EPIDEMIOLOGY AND CLINICAL FEATURES OF *KLEBSIELLA* SPECIES

After *E. coli*, organisms belonging to the genus *Klebsiella* constitute the most common members of the

*Address correspondence to Renato Finkelstein: Rambam Health Care Campus Haifa, Israel; Tel: (972-4) 854-2991; Fax: (972-4) 854-3286; E-mail: rfinkelstein@rambam.health.gov.il

Enterobacteriaceae family isolated from clinical samples. Three species in the genus *Klebsiella* are associated with illness in humans: *Klebsiella pneumoniae, Klebsiella oxytoca,* and *Klebsiella granulomatis.* *K. pneumoniae*, which is the most common *Klebsiella* species, is an important cause of urinary tract infection, but also a well known pathogen causing liver abscess, and pneumoniae in otherwise healthy people. However, most infections caused by *K. pneumoniae* are acquired as a healthcare-associated infection [2]. *K. pneumoniae* is the fourth and fifth most common cause of pneumoniae and bacteremia, respectively, in intensive care patients [3]. Nosocomial infections caused by *K. pneumoniae* include also wound infections, infections of intravascular and other invasive devices, biliary tract infections, peritonitis, and meningitis. *K. pneumoniae* is second only to *E. coli* as a cause of bacteremia resulting from UTI and of gram-negative bacteremia [4-6]. Also in our institution *K. pneumoniae* is the second most common pathogen isolated from blood cultures. Of the 1549 episodes of bloodstream infections diagnosed in 2009, 165 (11%) were caused by this organism. Infections caused by *K. pneumoniae* do not have clinical features that distinguish them from those caused by other bacterial species. Nevertheless, pneumoniae caused by *K. pneumoniae* has classically been described as having particular distinguishing features, warranting the eponym Friedländer's disease. The typical clinical presentation of acute Friedländer's pneumoniae is a fulminating lobar pneumonia. This infection is described frequently in alcoholics, Hemoptysis is present in approximately 50% of cases and leukopenia is often noted. Mortality rate is high and classical radiological findings include a dense, homogeneous infiltration that may resemble a mass lesion, with bulging of the interlobar fissure, typically involving the upper lung lobes [7]. Despite these compelling descriptions, pneumoniae caused by *K. pneumoniae* cannot be distinguished on clinical grounds from that caused by other organisms, and many of the described features are likely the result of misdiagnosis, caused by culture of expectorated sputum, of anaerobic pulmonary infections [8].

RESISTANCE IN *KLEBSIELLA*

All strains of *K. pneumoniae* are intrinsically resistant to ampicillin as a result of the presence of a chromosomal gene encoding a penicillin-specific β-lactamase (9). However, *K. pneumoniae* may be susceptible to most antibiotic classes and groups. Several therapeutic options exist for treating infections caused by non-multidrug-resistant strains, including cephalosporins, penicillin/β-lactamase inhibitor combinations, trimethoprim-sulfamethoxazole, fluoroquinolones, carbapenems, aztreonam, tetracyclines, polymyxins and aminoglycosides. Unfortunately, during the past 25 years multidrug resistance has emerged and become widespread, mediated primarily *via* acquired genes that code for ESBLs, other enzymes, and additional resistance mechanisms. The emergence and spread of resistance in Enterobacteriaceae are complicating the treatment of serious infections and threatening to create species resistant to all currently available agents. There are several well-known molecular mechanisms of antimicrobial resistance in *K. pneumoniae* [10]. Enzymatic inhibition and alteration of ribosomal targets (ribosomal methylation) may confer resistance of *K. pneumoniae* to aminoglycosides. Alteration of target enzymes (DNA gyrase mutations—*gyrA*); efflux and protection of target site (plasmid-mediated *qnr* genes) may be responsible the resistance to fluoroquinolones. *K. pneumoniae* may develop resistance to β-lactam antibiotics through enzymatic inhibition, and in particular by producing extended-spectrum ß-lactamases.

EXTENDED-SPECTRUM β-LACTAMASE (ESBL) PRODUCING *KLEBSIELLA*

In Gram-negative pathogens, β-lactamase production remains the most important contributing factor to β-lactam resistance [11]. β-lactamases are bacterial enzymes that inactivate β-lactam antibiotics by hydrolysis, which results in ineffective compounds. One group of β lactamases, ESBLs, have the ability to hydrolyse and cause resistance to various types of the newer β-lactam antibiotics, including third-generation cephalosporins (*e.g.,* cefotaxime, ceftriaxone, ceftazidime), and monobactams (*e.g.,* aztreonam), but not the cephamycins (*e.g.,* cefoxitin and cefotetan) and carbapenems (*e.g.,* imipenem, meropenem, and ertapenem) [12]. Because of their broad spectrum of antimicrobial activity and their low toxicity profile, β-lactam antibiotics became one of the most prescribed drugs in the past 30 years. When first introduced, third-generation cephalosporins were stable in the presence of common β-lactamase. However, within a few years, hospital-acquired Gram-negative bacilli like *K. pneumoniae* and others began producing mutated versions of these β-lactamases that made them resistant to third-generation cephalosporins and to the monobactam aztreonam. According to the National Nosocomial Infections Surveillance (NNIS) System report, in 2003, 20.6% of all *K. pneumoniae* isolates from patients in Intensive Care Units (ICUs) in the United States were nonsusceptible to third-generation cephalosporins [13]. International studies report even higher rates of nonsusceptible *K. pneumoniae* in hospitals and particularly in ICU settings [14]. Initially found among hospitalized patients and in bacterial species more common in the intensive care setting (*e.g.*, *K. pneumoniae* and *Enterobacter cloacae*), ESBLs are now commonly found in E. coli isolates from patients in nursing homes and long term-care facilities, and even in patients with community-acquired infections. The genes that encode ESBLs are frequently found on the same plasmids as genes that encode resistance to aminoglycosides and sulfonamides, and many Enterobacteriaceae species possess changes that confer high-level resistance to quinolones. This means that ESBL-producing Enterobacteriaceae in hospitals and ICU settings are commonly multidrug resistant, which poses a particular challenge for the treatment of nosocomial infections, especially in critically ill patients [15].

CLASSIFICATION OF β-LACTAMASES

More than 350 different ß -lactamases have been identified and various definitions of extended-spectrum ß -lactamases have been in use over the past 20 years. Two major classification schemes exist for categorizing ß-lactamase enzymes: Ambler classes A through D, based on amino acid sequence homology, and Bush-Jacoby-Medeiros groups 1 through 4, based on substrate and inhibitor profile [16-17]. ESBLs arose when mutations of the genes encoding TEM-1, TEM-2, or SHV-1 gave rise to new ß -lactamases that became able to hydrolyze third-generation cephalosporins and aztreonam [12, 18]. Importantly, ESBLs are typically plasmid mediated rather than chromosomally mediated ß -lactamases. The term 'ESBL' was coined when fewer ß -lactamases were known, and served well for the TEM and SHV mutants. As the number of ß -lactamases has grown; enzymes have been called ESBLs on the basis of meeting either one of these criteria, or owing to the ability to confer resistance rather than to cause rapid hydrolysis. Recently, Livermore proposed a more comprehensive and pragmatic definition stating that ESBL is 'any ß -lactamase,' generally acquired rather than inherent to a species, that is either able to confer resistance to oxyimino-cephalosporins (but not carbapenems), or that has an increased ability to do so, as compared with classic members of its genetic family [19]. The great majority of the ESBLs encountered clinically belong to the TEM, SHV and CTX-M families. These are what are routinely sought in clinical laboratory ESBL tests, and it is their spread (particularly that of the CTX-M types) which is causing public health concern. The OXA, GES and AmpC types, those that so complicate the definition, remain extremely rare [20]. ESBLs should be distinguished from other ß -lactamase capable of hydrolyzing extended-spectrum cephalosporins. Examples include AmpC and carbapenemases. AmpC ß -lactamases hydrolyze expanded-spectrum cephalosporins, but unlike ESBLs, they are also active against cephamycins and are resistant to inhibition by clavulanate or other ß-lactamase inhibitors [21]. Carbapenemases are now recognised in classes A (*e.g.*, IMI, KPC, NMC and SME), B (*e.g.*, VIM, IMP, GIM, and SPM) and D (*e.g.*, OXA-23-like, OXA-24-like, OXA-49, OXA-51-like and OXA-58) [21-22]. Carbapenemases have broader-range activity, covering carbapenems as well as expanded-spectrum cephalosporins [20, 23].

CLINICAL SIGNIFICANCE AND TREATMENT OF ESBL PRODUCTION PATHOGENS

The question of whether ESBL production significantly increases the risk of death or any other measure of clinical failure has been addressed in a number of studies, but the issue remains unresolved [24]. Nevertheless, the multiple drug resistance associated with ESBL production has major implications for the selection of adequate therapy regimens, including an initial empirical treatment. Multiple studies in a wide range of settings, clinical syndromes, and organisms, including infections caused by ESBL-producing bacteria, have shown that failure or delay in adequate therapy results in an adverse mortality outcome [25-26]. In addition, even if an agent is selected that has activity against the bacteria *in vitro* (when tested in the laboratory), clinical efficacy in patients is not always guaranteed. This is widely believed to occur as a result of the so-called inoculum effect that occurs when the minimum inhibitory concentration of the antibiotic rises with the increasing size of the inoculum of bacteria tested [27]. This effect has been described for cephalosporins, β-lactam-β-lactamase-inhibitor combinations (*e.g.*, piperacillin-tazobactam), and to a lesser extent with the quinolones [28]. The choice of therapy for serious infection due to ESBL-producing Enterobacteriaceae is difficult by the likelihood of multidrug resistance and the fact that there are no data from large, randomized, controlled trials designed to compare one antibiotic therapy with another for infections caused by ESBL-producing organisms.

There is a marked increase in resistance to aminoglycosides when non-ESBL-producing *E. coli* and *Klebsiella* species are compared with strains that produce ESBLs, with the risk of resistance to aminoglycosides increasing by 2-3-fold [29]. Amikacin shows the greatest percentage of susceptible strains [30]. A limited amount of data suggests that efficacy is good when the aminoglycoside has a low MIC against the infecting strain. The success of aminoglycosides in general against bacteremias caused by ESBL-producing *K. pneumoniae* has been well demonstrated [31], however there are no published clinical data on amikacin that would confidently support a recommendation for its use as monotherapy for treating severe infections caused by ESBL-producing bacteria. Fluoroquinolone antibiotics have shown limited success in treating infections caused by ESBL-producing pathogens. A few publications have reported that ciprofloxacin may be successful in treating infections caused by ceftazidime-resistant Enterobacteriaceae [32, 33]. However, an increasing coresistance to fluoroquinolones has undermined the effectiveness of fluoroquinolones against ESBL-producing pathogens. In a nationwide Italian survey, among ESBL-producing strains of Enterobacteriaceae, only 58% were susceptible to ciprofloxacin [34)]. In Taiwan, concomitant ciprofloxacin resistance was observed in almost 20% of ESBL-producing *K. pneumoniae* isolates [35]. In the United States, in 1999, a cluster of 15 hospitals in Brooklyn, New York, reported that 34% of *K. pneumoniae* isolates were presumptive ESBL producers, and, of these, only 42% were susceptible to ciprofloxacin [36]. In an study to monitor worldwide antimicrobial resistance trends among aerobic and facultatively anaerobic Gram-negative bacilli isolated from intra-abdominal infections, approximately 60 % of ESBL-producing *K. pneumoniae* were resistant to ciprofloxacin [37].

Some case studies and surveillance studies suggest that piperacillin-tazobactam may have a role in treating infections caused by ESBL-producing Enterobacteriaceae. *In vitro* testing demonstrated that approximately 90% of the ESBL-producing *K. pneumoniae* isolated from patients with pneumoniae who were treated at 30 hospitals in the United States and Canada during the 1998 respiratory illness season were susceptible to piperacillin-tazobactam [38]. However, more recently only 38.6% of ESBL-producing *K. pneumoniae* isolated from intraabdominal infections were susceptible to this drug [37]. At the present time only a relatively small database of information exists on the clinical efficacy of piperacillin-tazobactam in this setting and any potential recommendation must be interpreted cautiously [24].

Cefepime is a fourth-generation cephalosporin that is more stable than third-generation cephalosporins against some ESBLs and some studies have suggested that this drug may be of clinical value for the treatment of some infections caused by bacterial strains that are resistant to third-generation cephalosporins [24]. However, a subgroup analysis from a randomized, evaluator-blind trial comparing cefepime with imipenem in patients with nosocomial pneumoniae showed that 100% of patients (10 of 10) receiving imipenem for pneumoniae caused by an ESBL producer experienced a positive clinical response compared with only 69% of patients (9 of 13) treated with cefepime [39]. Moreover, data from a number of studies strongly point to carbapenems as the drugs of choice for treating serious infections involving ESBL-producing Enterobacteriaceae. A survey of the relevant clinical literature [40], have shown that the carbapenems, especially imipenem, have a relatively high rate of clinical success among patients infected with ESBL-producing *E. coli* or *K. pneumonia*. In a prospective study of 455 consecutive episodes of *Klebsiella pneumoniae* bacteremia in 12 hospitals in 7 countries [41], 85 episodes were due to an ESBL-producing organism. Failure to use an antibiotic active against ESBL-producing *K. pneumoniae* was associated with extremely high mortality. Use of a carbapenem (primarily imipenem) was associated with significantly lower 14-day mortality than was use of other antibiotics active *in vitro*. Multivariate analysis including other predictors of mortality showed that use of a carbapenem during the 5-day period after onset of bacteremia due to an ESBL-producing organism was independently associated with lower mortality. Therefore, carbapenems have become an almost last line of defense in the treatment of infections caused by antimicrobial-resistant Enterobacteriaceae.

CARBAPENEM RESISTANCE

Carbapenems are highly stable to ß-lactamase hydrolysis, and porin penetration is facilitated by their general size and structure. As mentioned earlier, because their antimicrobial activity and successful clinical experience, carbapenems have long been the drug of choice for treating not only infections due to ESBL-producing Enterobacteriaceae, but also for treating several other infections caused by multidrug-resistant organisms. Imipenem, the first in the carbapenem class, has been used in more than 26 million patients over 20 years [42]. Therefore, it is not surprising that resistance to carbapenems developed after such a widespread use of this drug. Resistance to carbapenems may involve several combined mechanisms: modifications to outer membrane permeability and up-regulation of efflux systems associated with hyperproduction of AmpC β lactamases (cephalosporinases), or ESBLs, or production of specific carbapenem-hydrolysing β-lactamases (carbapenemases) [43]. Carbapenemases represent the most versatile family of β-lactamases, with a breadth of spectrum unrivaled by other β-lactam-hydrolyzing enzymes. Although known as "carbapenemases," many of these enzymes recognize almost all hydrolysable β-lactams, and most are resilient against inhibition by all commercially viable β-lactamase inhibitors [22, 44-45]. The most important among these carbapenemases are the serine ß-lactamase KPC, by far, the most frequent class A carbapenemases, and the metallo-ß-lactamase VIM [46]. Although the first carbapenemase-producing *Klebsiella* strain was identified in 1996 [47], until recently, carbapenem-resistant Enterobacteriaceae were rare. However, carbapenem-resistant *Klebsiella* strains have now been reported in 24 states of the United States and are endemic in parts of New York and New Jersey. In 2007 data on healthcare-associated infections reported to the Centers for Disease Control and Prevention, 8% of all *Klebsiella* isolates were reported to be carbapenem-resistant, compared to just under 1% in 2000 (48). In the United States, carbapenem resistance has been observed in strains of *K pneumoniae*-producing class A carbapenemases, namely, KPC-1, KPC-2, and KPC-3, with the last two being the predominants [47,49-55]. The genes coding for these enzymes, including *bla*KPC, are carried by plasmids which greatly facilitates its dissemination. Moreover, plasmids carrying resistance genes also may carry virulence factors, thus leading to severe infections [56]. Although KPCs are mostly identified from *K pneumoniae*, KPC enzymes have now also been reported from *E. coli*, *Salmonella cubana*, *Enterobacter cloacae*, *Proteus mirabilis* [43]. Further complicating the matter is the fact that some plasmids carrying *bla*KPC have been reported to contain genes conferring fluoroquinolone and aminoglycoside resistance as well [48]. To date, there are 6 subtypes of KPCs that have either been reported in the literature [57] or had sequences submitted to the GenBank database, although KPC subtypes 1 and 2 have recently been found to be identical [48]. Both the KPC and VIM gene families have demonstrated the potential to cause large regional and even nationwide outbreaks of carbapenem-resistant *K. pneumoniae*. Outbreaks of *bla*VIM-1positive carbapenem-resistant *K. pneumoniae* have been reported from some European countries [58-61].The first outbreak of KPC-producing *K. pneumoniae outside* the USA was from Israel [62]. A single KPC-3-producing *K. pneumoniae* clone and several KPC-2- producing *K. pneumoniae* clones are responsible for ongoing outbreaks in Israel hospitals [63-65]. The KPC-3-producing strain from Israel is genetically linked to those reported in the USA, suggesting strain exchange by travelers and patients between Israel and the USA [66]. In South America, dissemination of KPC has been reported in *K. pneumoniae* in Colombia, Brazil and Argentina [67-69]. In Europe, only a few cases have been reported. Some cases occurred among patients transferred from countries where KpC is now a well recognized pathogen (USA, Israel and Greece) [43]. Recent reports suggest that Greece, where carbapenem-resistance was until 2006 mainly the result of dissemination of the *bla*VIM-1 gene, may be another country with epidemicity of KPC-producing bacteria [70-72]. Some case-control studies have identified potential risk factors associated with carbapenem-resistance among *K. pneumoniae* isolated from both colonized and infected patients [65, 73-75]. Not surprisingly, in these studies common healthcare risk factors such as previous antibiotic treatment, including exposure to carbapenem or fluorquinolones or being treated in the intensive care unit were independently associated with acquisition of carbapenem-resistance *K. pneumoniae*. As expected, these isolates were highly resistant. Although in a study conducted at a New York hospital [73] roughly two thirds retained susceptibility to an aminoglycoside and 52% retained susceptibility to tetracycline, in Israel higher rates of resistant have been reported. In one study [65], the percentages rates of resistance of the carbapenem-resistance *K. pneumoniae* isolates ranged from 95% to 100% for piperacillin/tazobactam, third generation cephalosporins, ciprofloxacin and amikacin. The lowest rates of resistance were found for colistin, gentamicin and tigecycline (4.5%, 7%, and 15%, respectively). The minimal inhibitory concentrations of 90% of CRKP isolates (MIC90) for colistin and tigecycline were 1.5µg/ml and 4.0µg/ml, respectively. Detection of KPC-producing bacteria based only on susceptibility testing is not easy and the level of susceptibility of KPC-producing bacteria remains difficult whatever the technique used: antibiotic susceptibility testing by liquid medium or disk diffusion [43]. Clinical microbiology laboratories have often found it difficult to achieve accurate susceptibility testing results for carbapenem drugs and detection of carbapenem resistance with automatic systems may be problematic for KPC-producing *K. pneumoniae* [76]. In general, susceptibility testing using imipenem or meropenem is not sensitive enough for the detection of KPC-producing Enterobacteriaceae. Ertapenem susceptibility rates of KPC-producing *K. pneumoniae* range from 0-6%, compared with 26-29% for imipenem and 16-52% for meropenem [76-77]. Similarly in a recent study from Israel [78], KPC-producing *Enterobacter* spp were detected in all cases using ertapenem, whereas meropenem misclassifed 24% of those isolates as being susceptible. Determining resistance and susceptibility for both imipenem and meropenem with E-test is also difficult because colonies are present within the zones of inhibition and sometimes a consensus cannot be achieved on the interpretations among several different readers of the results [76]. Several confirmatory tests have been proposed. The results of double-disc synergy testing between clavulanic acid or tazobactam and any carbapenem are difficult to detect due to the low inhibition of KPC by clavulanic acid [43]. The Cloverleaf test [79, 80] (modified Hodge test) was suggested to assist in confirming the presence of carbapenemase due to its acceptable sensitivity and specificity. However, the test will not exclusively detect the KPC-type [43] and false detection of carbapenemase production has been reported [81]. Molecular diagnosis has recently been recognized as an important diagnostic tool for the rapid detection and identification of antimicrobial-resistant genes in various microorganisms. Identification of KPC-producing bacteria with these techniques should become the gold standard. However, these techniques require technical knowledge, equipment, and are costly. Thus their implementation on a routine basis should depend on the frequency of KPC-producing bacteria [82]. Alternatively, molecular confirmation tests could be restricted to reference laboratories.

TREATMENT OF INFECTIONS CAUSED BY CARBAPENEMASE-PRODUCING *K. PNEUMONIAE*

If ESBL-producing organism is a matter of multidrug-resistance, it is clear that with carbapenemase-producing *K. pneumoniae* we are heading toward a dramatic problem of extreme drug resistance. As reviewed before, and with the exception of gentamicin, tygecycline and colistin, KPC-producing *K. pneumoniae* isolates are almost always resistant to all other existing antibiotics agents. However, in-vitro susceptibility is not a guarantee of clinical success and several problems should be considered when choosing one of these agents. Infections due to KPC-producing *K. pneumoniae* occur characteristically in a healthcare setting and include serious problems such pneumonia, bacteremia, and urinary tract infection. They affect debilitated patients, usually being treated in intensive care units, and are associated with an attributable mortality of up to 33% [72]. The use of aminoglycosides (such as gentamicin) in such patients is limited by the potential of nephrotoxicy and ototoxicity, common side-effects associated with the use of these drugs. In addition, aminoglycosides alone are not considered an optimal option for treating patients with pneumonia. High failure rates were seen when aminoglycosides were used as single agents for treating pneumoniae due to *P. aeruginosa*. The failure was subsequently attributed to several factors, including low antibiotic levels achieved in the airways, inactivation of aminoglycosides in the acidic environment of the lungs, and binding of drugs to human mucus [83]. Published clinical trial data have shown tigecycline to be effective in the treatment of complicated skin, skin-structure, and intra-abdominal infections. However, the role of tigecycline in the treatment of infections due to MDR gram-negative bacilli remains undefined. Results of a small study [84] observed the evolution of resistance in one *A. baumannii* isolate, as well as persistent bacteremia with several of the organisms during therapy, raising concern about the routine use of tigecycline in the treatment of these infections until more-formal comparative data are available.Tigecycline has unusual pharmacokinetics, with low blood concentrations and comparatively higher tissue concentrations [85]. Bloodstream isolates of gram-negative bacilli may be regarded as nonsusceptible to tigecycline when the MIC exceeds the peak blood concentration found in clinical studies [85]. Furthermore, it should not be recommended for treating urinary tract infections due to its low urine concentration. This leaves polymyxins (colistin) as the sole therapeutic alternative for the previous two options. Recent studies of patients who received intravenous polymyxins for the treatment of serious *P. aeruginosa* and *A. baumannii* infections of various types, have led to the conclusion that these antibiotics have acceptable effectiveness and considerably less toxicity than was reported in old studies [86]. Nevertheless, neurotoxicity and nephrotoxicity associated with the use of these drugs still should be considered a cause of some concern. In most published experiences polymyxins were used for infections caused by Enterobacteriaceae that produce VIM or IMP carbapenemases [87, 88]. Very limited *in-vivo* data are available in the case of KPC infections [43]. However, colistin resistance [43] and panresistance (*i.e.* resistance to all antibiotic tested, including tygecycline, aminoglycosides and colistin) [89] in KPC-producing *K. pneumoniae* has been observed. Combination therapies may be an attractive option based on some *in-vitro* data, but clinical data supporting such recommendations are lacking [88].

CONCLUSIONS

Carbapenemase-producing bacteria have increasingly been isolated worldwide, mostly in the form of KPC-producing *K. pneumoniae,* which now been added to those bacteria species that became resistant to almost all classes of antibiotics by the escalating pressure of antibiotics. This phenomenon is worrying, from a public health point of view, since KPC-producing *K. pneumoniae* is prone to be the source of many hospital-acquired infections in severely ill patients, and is well-known for its ability to accumulate and transfer resistance to other microorganisms. Multidrug-resistant and even pandrug-resistant carbapenemase-producing bacteria producing bacteria may be the source of therapeutic dead-ends, since novel anti-Gram-negative molecules are not expected in the near future. New strategies for antibiotic utilization and infection control, as well as further investigations on mechanisms of antimicrobial resistance, are critical to preservation of effective therapy against gram-negative pathogens. Preventing the spread of infections due to carbapenemase-producing *K. pneumoniae* may more important than relying on last resort antibacterial drugs.

REFERENCES

[1]   Donnenberg MS. Enterobacteriaceae. In: Mandell GL, Bennett JE, Dolin R (Eds). Mandell, Douglas and Benetts's Principles and Practice of Infectious Diseases. 7th ed. 2010; pp: 2815- 2833.

[2]   Podschun R, Ullmann U. Klebsiella spp. as nosocomial pathogens: epidemiology, taxonomy, typing methods, and pathogenicity factors. Clin Microbiol Rev 1998; 11: 589-603.

[3]   Centers for Disease Control and Prevention. National Nosocomial Infections Surveillance (NNIS) System Report, data summary from January 1992 through June 2003, issued August 2003. Am J Infect Control 2003; 31: 481-98.

[4]   Bishara J, Leibovici L, Huminer D, *et al.* Five-year prospective study of bacteraemic urinary tract infection in a single institution. Eur J Clin Microbiol Infect Dis 1997; 16: 563-67.

[5]   Garcia de la Torre M, Romero-Vivas J, Martinez-Beltrán J, *et al*: *Klebsiella bacteremia*: an analysis of 100 episodes. Rev Infect Dis 1985; 7: 143-50.

[6]   Geerdes HF, Ziegler D, Lode H, *et al*: Septicemia in 980 patients at a University Hospital in Berlin: prospective studies during 4 selected years between 1979 and 1989. Clin Infect Dis 1992; 15: 991-1002.

[7]   Tzukert K, Block C, Sviri S, *et al.* A 60-Year-Old Man with Fever and a Lung Mass (Answer to the photo quiz). Clin Infect Dis 2007; 45: 937-38.

[8]   Carpenter JL: Klebsiella pulmonary infections: occurrence at one medical center and review. Rev Infect Dis 1990; 12: 672-82

[9]   Hæggman S, Löfdahl S, Burman LG: An allelic variant of the chromosomal gene for class A Beta-lactamase K2, specific for Klebsiella pneumoniae, is the ancestor of SHV-1. Antimicrob Agents Chemother 1997; 41: 2705-09.

[10]   Opal SM, Pop-Vicas A. Molecular Mechanisms of Antibiotic Resistance in Bacteria. In: Mandell GL, Bennett JE, Dolin R (Eds). Mandell, Douglas, and Benetts's Principles and Practice of Infectious Diseases. 7th ed. 2010; pp: 279-298.

[11]   Livermore DM. Bacterial resistance: origins, epidemiology, and impact. Clin Infect Dis 2003; 36 (suppl 1)**:** S11-23**.**

[12]   Bradford PA. Extended-spectrum β-lactamases in the 21st century: characterization, epidemiology, and detection of this important resistance threat. Clin Microbiol Rev 2001; 14**:** 933-51.

[13]   National Nosocomial Infections Surveillance (NNIS) System Report, data summary from January 1992 through June 2004, issued October 2004. Am J Infect Control 2004; 32: 470-85.

[14]   Paterson DL, Ko WC, Von Gottberg A, *et al.* International prospective study of *Klebsiella pneumoniae* bacteremia: implications of extended spectrum beta-lactamase production in nosocomial Infections. Ann Intern Med 2004; 140: 26-32.

[15]   Paterson DL. Resistance in Gram-Negative Bacteria: nterobacteriaceae. The American Journal of Medicine 2006; 119 (6A), S20-S28.

[16]   Ambler, RP, Coulson AF, Frere JM, *et al.* A standard numbering scheme for the class A ß-lactamases. Biochem J1991; 276: 269-270.

[17]   Bush K, Jacoby GA, Medeiros AA. A functional classification scheme for β-lactamases and its correlation with molecular structure. Antimicrob Agents Chemother 1995; 39: 1211-1233.

[18]   Rupp ME, Fey PD. Extended spectrum beta-lactamase (ESBL)-producing Enterobacteriaceae: considerations for diagnosis, prevention, and drug treatment. Drugs 2003; 63:353-365.

[19]   Livermore DM. Defining an extended-spectrum ß-lactamase. Clin Microbiol Infect 2008; 14 (Suppl. 1): 3-10.

[20]   Jacoby GA, Munoz-Price LS. The new ß -lactamases. N Engl J Med 2005; 352: 380 -91.

[21]   Livermore DM. The impact of carbapenemases on antimicrobial development and therapy. Curr Opin Invest Drugs 2002; 3: 218-24.

[22]   Nordmann P, Poirel L. Emerging carbapenemases in gram-negative aerobes. Clin Microbiol Infect 2002; 8: 321-31.

[23]   Walsh TR, Toleman MA, Poirel L, *et al.* Metallo-betalactamases: the quiet before the storm? Clin Microbiol Rev 2005; 18: 306-25.

[24]   Ramphal R, Ambrose PG. Extended-Spectrum ß-Lactamases and Clinical Outcomes: Current Data Clinical Infectious Diseases 2006; 42: S164-72.

[25]   Lautenbach E, Patel JB, Bilker WB, *et al.* Extended-spectrum β-lactamase-producing *Escherichia coli* and *Klebsiella pneumoniae*:risk factors for infection and impact of resistance on outcomes. Clin Infect Dis 2001; 32: 1162-71.

[26]   Tumbarello M, Sanguinetti M, Montuori E, *et al.* Predictors of mortality in bloodstream infections caused by extended-spectrum β-lactamaseproducing Enterobacteriaceae: importance of inadequate initial antimicrobial treatment. Antimicrob Agents Chemother 2007; 51: 1987-94.

[27]   Rice L. Evolution and clinical importance of extended-spectrum β-lactamases. Chest 2001; 119 (suppl 2): 391S-96S.

[28]   Thomson KS, Moland ES. Cefepime, piperacillin-tazobactam, and the inoculum effect in tests with extended-spectrum β-lactamaseproducing Enterobacteriaceae. Antimicrob Agents Chemother 2001; 45: 3548-54.

[29]   Jones RN, Pfaller MA. Antimicrobial activity against strains of *Escherichia coli* and *Klebsiella* spp. with resistance phenotypes consistent with an extended-spectrum ß-lactamase in Europe. Clin Microbiol Infect 2003; 9: 708-12.

[30]   Winokur PL, Canton R, Casellas JM, *et al.* Variations in the prevalence of strains expressing an extended-spectrum b-lactamase phenotype and characterization of isolates from Europe, the Americas and the Western Pacific region. Clin Infect Dis 2001; 32(Suppl 2): S94-103.

[31]   Kim YK, Pai H, Lee HJ, *et al.* Bloodstream infections by extendedspectrum ß-lactamase-producing *Escherichia coli* and *Klebsiella pneumoniae* in children: epidemiology and clinical outcome. Antimicrob Agents Chemother 2002; 46: 1481-91.

[32]   Rice LB, Willey SH, Papanicolaou GA, *et al.* Outbreak of ceftazidime resistance caused by extended-spectrum b-lactamases at a Massachusetts chronic-care facility. Antimicrob Agents Chemother 1990; 34: 2193-99.

[33]   Karas JA, Pillay DG, Muckart D, *et al.* Treatment failure due to extended spectrum beta-lactamase. J Antimicrob Chemother 1996; 37: 203-04.

[34]   Spanu T, Luzzaro F, Perilli M, *et al.* Occurrence of extended-spectrum b-lactamases in members of the family Enterobacteriaceae in Italy: implications for resistance to blactams and other antimicrobial drugs. Antimicrob Agents Chemother 2002; 46: 196-202.

[35]   Yu WL, Jones RN, Hollis RJ, *et al.* Molecular epidemiology of extendedspectrum b-lactamase-producing, fluoroquinolone-resistant isolates of *Klebsiella pneumoniae* in Taiwan. J Clin Microbiol 2002; 40: 4666-69.

[36]   Quale JM, Landman D, Bradford PA, *et al.* Molecular epidemiology of a citywide outbreak of extended-spectrum b-lactamase-producing *Klebsiella pneumoniae* infection. Clin Infect Dis 2002; 35: 834-41.

[37]   Rossi F, Baquero F, Hsueh PR, *et al. In vitro* susceptibilities of aerobic and facultatively anaerobic Gram-negative bacilli isolated from patients with intra-abdominal infections worldwide: 2004 results from SMART (Study for Monitoring Antimicrobial Resistance Trends). J Antimicrob Chemother 2006; 58: 205-10.

[38]   Mathai D, Lewis MT, Kugler KC, *et al.* Antibacterial activity of 41 antimicrobials tested against over 2773 bacterial isolates from hospitalized patients with pneumonia. I. Results from the SENTRY Antimicrobial Surveillance Program (North America, 1998). Diagn Microbiol Infect Dis 2001; 39: 105-16.

[39]   Zanetti G, Bally F, Greub G, *et al.* Cefepime *vs* imipenem-cilastatin for treatment of nosocomial pneumoniae in intensive care unit patients: a multicenter, evaluator-blind, prospective, randomized study. Antimicrob Agents Chemother 2003; 47: 3442-47.

[40]   Wong-Beringer A. Therapeutic challenges associated with extended spectrum, beta- lactamase-producing *Escherichia coli* and *Klebsiella pneumoniae*. Pharmacotherapy 2001; 21: 583-92.

[41]   Paterson DL, Ko WC, Gottberg AV, *et al.* Antibiotic Therapy for *Klebsiella pneumoniae* Bacteremia: Implications of Production of Extended-Spectrum ß-Lactamases. Clin Infec Dis 2003; 39: 31-37.

[42]   Rodloff AC, Goldstein EJC, Torres A. Two decades of imipenem therapy. J Antimicrob Chemother 2006; 58: 916-29.

[43]   Nordmann P, Cuzon G, Naas T. The real threat of *Klebsiella pneumoniae* carbapenemase-producing bacteria. Lancet Infect Dis 2009; 9: 228-36.

[44]   Livermore, DM, Woodford N. The β -lactamase threat in *Enterobacteriaceae*, *Pseudomonas* and *Acinetobacter*. Trends Microbiol 2006; 14: 413-420.

[45]   Walther-Rasmussen J, Hoiby N. OXA-type carbapenemases. J. Antimicrob. Chemother 2006; 57: 373-83.

[46]   Queenan AM, Bush K. Carbapenemases: the versatile beta-lactamases. Clin Microbiol Rev. 2007; 20(3): 440-58.

[47]   Yigit H., Queenan AM, Andersen GJ, *et al.* Novel carbapenem-hydrolyzing ß-lactamase, KPC-1, from a carbapenem-resistant strain of *Klebsiella pneumoniae*. Antimicrob Agents Chemother 2001; 45: 1151-61.

[48]   Srinivasan A, Patel JB. *Klebsiella pneumoniae* Carbapenemase- Producing Organisms: An Ounce of Prevention Really Is Worth a Pound of Cure. Infect Control Hosp Epidemiol 2008; 29: 1107-09.

[49]   Smith ME, Hanson ND, Herrera VL, *et al.* Plasmid-mediated, carbapenem-hydrolysing beta-lactamase, KPC-2, in *Klebsiella pneumoniae* isolates. J Antimicrob Chemother 2003; 51: 711-14.

[50]   Bradford PA, Bratu S, Urban C, *et al.* Emergence of carbapenem-resistant *Klebsiella* species possessing the class A carbapenem-hydrolyzing KPC-2 and inhibitor-resistant TEM-30 beta-lactamases in New York City. Clin Infect Dis 2004; 39: 55-60.

[51]   Woodford N, Tierno PM Jr., Young K, *et al.* Outbreak of *Klebsiella pneumoniae* producing a new carbapenem-hydrolyzing class A betalactamase, KPC-3, in a New York Medical Center. Antimicrob Agents Chemother 2004; 48: 4793- 99.

[52]   Bratu S, Landman D, Haag R, *et al.* Rapid spread of carbapenemresistant *Klebsiella pneumoniae* in New York City: a new threat to our antibiotic armamentarium. Arch Intern Med 2005; 165: 1430 -35

[53]   Bratu S, Mooty M, Nichani S, *et al.* Emergence of KPC-possessing *Klebsiella pneumoniae* in Brooklyn, New York: epidemiology and recommendations for detection. Antimicrob Agents Chemother 2005; 49: 3018 -20.

[54]   Bratu S, Landman D, Alam M, *et al.* Detection of KPC carbapenem-hydrolyzing enzymes in *Enterobacter* spp. from Brooklyn, New York. Antimicrob Agents Chemother 2005; 49:776-78.

[55]   Bratu S, Tolaney P, Karumudi U, *et al.* Carbapenemase-producing *Klebsiella pneumoniae* in Brooklyn, NY: molecular epidemiology and *in vitro* activity of polymyxin B and other agents. J Antimicrob Chemother 2005; 56: 128 -32.

[56]   Schwaber, MJ, Carmeli,Y. Carbapenem-Resistant Enterobacteriaceae .A Potential Threat. JAMA 2008; 300(24): 2911-13.

[57]   Queenan AM, Bush K. Carbapenemases: the versatile b-lactamases. Clin Microbiol Rev 2007; 20: 440-58.

[58]   Kassis-Chikhani N, Decré D, Gautier V, *et al.* First outbreak of multidrug-resistant *Klebsiella pneumoniae* carrying *bla*VIM-1 and *bla*SHV-5 in a French university hospital. J Antimicrob Chemother 2006; 57: 142-45.

[59]   Cagnacci S, Gualcp L, Roveta S, *et al.* Bloodstream infections caused by multidrug-resistant Klebsiella pneumoniae producing the carbapenem-hydrolysing VIM-1 metallo-beta-lactamase: first Italian outbreak. J Antimicrob Chemother 2008; 61: 296-300.

[60]   Psichogiou M, Tassios PT, Avlamis A, *et al.* Ongoing epidemic of *bla*VIM-1-positive *Klebsiella pneumoniae* in Athens, Greece: a prospective survey. J Antimicrob Chemother 2008; 61: 59-63.

[61]   Tato M, Coque TM, Garbajosa R, *et al.* Complex Clonal and Plasmid Epidemiology in the First Outbreak of Enterobacteriaceae Infection Involving VIM-1 Metallo-β-Lactamase in Spain: Toward Endemicity? Clin Infect Dis 2007; 45: 9, 1171-78.

[62]   Hussein K, Sprecher H, Mashiach T, *et al.* First outbreak of carbapenem-resistant Klebsiella pneumoniae (CRKB) in an Israeli university hospital. Rambam Health Care Campus, Haifa, Israel. The 17th European Congress of Clinical Microbiology and Infection Diseases. Munich,Germany, March 31- April 3, 2007. Presentation P-1704.

[63]   Samra Z, Ofir O, Lichtzinsky Y, *et al.* Outbreak of carbapenem-resistant *Klebsiella pneumoniae* producing KPC-3 in a tertiary medical centre in Israel. Int J Antimicrob Agents 2007; 30: 525-29.

[64]   Leavitt A, Navon-Venezia S, Chmelnitsky I, *et al.* Emergence of KPC-2 and KPC-3 in carbapenem-resistant Klebsiella pneumoniae strains in an Israeli hospital. Antimicrob Agents Chemother 2007; 51: 3026-29.

[65]   Hussein K, Sprecher H, Mashiach T, *et al.* Carbapenem-resistance among *Klebsiella pneumoniae* isolates: risk factors, molecular characteristics and susceptibility patterns. Infect Control Hosp Epidemiol 2009; 30: 666-71.

[66]   Navon-Venezia S, Leavitt A, Schwaber MJ, *et al.* First report on hyperepidemic clone of KPC-3 producing *Klebsiella pneumoniae* in Israel genetically related to a strain causing outbreaks in the United States. Antimicrob Agents Chemother 2009; 53: 818-20.

[67]   Villegas MV, Lolans K, Correa A, et al. First detection of the plasmidmediated class A carbapenemase KPC-2 in clinical isolates of Klebsiella pneumoniae from South America. Antimicrob Agents Chemother 2006; 50: 2880-82.

[68]   Peirano G, Seki LM, Val Passos VL, *et al.* Carbapenem-hydrolysing β- lactamase KPC-2 in *Klebsiella pneumoniae* isolated in Rio de Janeiro, Brazil. *J Antimicrob Chemother* 2009; 63: 265-68.

[69]   Monteiro J, Santos AF, Asensi MD, *et al.* First report of KPC-2-producing-*Klebsiella pneumoniae* in Brazil. Antimicrob Agents Chemother 2008; 53:33-34 And Pasteran FG, Otaegui L, Guerriero L, *et al. Klebsiella pneumoniae* carbapenemase-2, Buenos Aires, Argentina. *Emerg Infect Dis* 2008; 14: 1178-80.

[70]   Cuzon G, Naas T, Demachy MC, *et al.* Plasmid-mediated carbapenemhydrolyzing β-lactamase KPC in *Klebsiella pneumoniae* isolate from Greece. Antimicrob Agents Chemother 2008; 52: 796-97.

[71]   Tsakris A, Kristo I, Poulou A, *et al.* First occurrence of KPC-2-possessing *Klebsiella pneumoniae* in a Greek hospital and recommendation for detection with boronic acid disc tests. J Antimicrob Chemother 2008, 62: 1257-60.

[72]   Souli M, Galani I, Antoniadou A, *et al.* An Outbreak of Infection due to β-Lactamase *Klebsiella pneumoniae* Carbapenemase 2-Producing *K. pneumoniae* in a Greek University Hospital: Molecular Characterization, Epidemiology, and Outcomes. Clin Infect Dis 2010; 50: 364-73.

[73]   Patel G, Huprikar S, Factor SH, *et al.* Outcomes of Carbapenem-Resistant *Klebsiella pneumoniae* Infection and the Impact of Antimicrobial and Adjunctive Therapies. Infect Control Hosp Epidemiol 2008; 29: 1099-106

[74]   Falagas ME, Rafailidis PI, Kofteridis D, *et al.* Risk factors of Carbapenem-resistant *Klebsiella pneumoniae* infections: a matched case control study. J Antimicrob Chemother 2007; 60: 1124-30.

[75]   Schwaber MJ, Klarfeld-Lidji S, Navon-Venezia S, *et al.* Predictors of Carbapenem resistant Klebsiella pneumoniae acquisition among hospitalized adults, and effect of acquisition on mortality. Antimicrob Agent Chemother 2008; 52: 1028-33.

[76]   Tenover FC, Kalsi RK, Williams PP, *et al.* Carbapenem resistance in *Klebsiella pneumoniae* not detected by automated susceptibility testing. Emerg Infect Dis 2006; 12: 1209-13.

[77]   Anderson KF, Lonsway DR, Rasheed JK, *et al.* Evaluation of methods to identify the *Klebsiella pneumoniae* carbapenemase in Enterobacteriaceae. J Clin Microbiol 2007; 45: 2723-25.

[78]   Marchaim D, Navon-Venzia S, Schwaber MJ, *et al.* Isolation of imipenem-resistant *Enterobacter* species; emergence of KPC-carbapenemase, molecular characterization, epidemiology and outcomes. Antimicrob Agents Chemother 2008; 52: 1413-18.

[79]   Clinical and Laboratory Standards Institute. Performance Standards for Antimicrobial Susceptibility Testing: Nineteenth Informational Supplement M100-S19. CLSI, Wayne, PA, USA, 2009.

[80]   Orstavik I, Odegaard K. A simple test for penicillinase production in Staphylococcus aureus. Acta Pathol Microbiol Scand B Microbiol Immunol 1971; 79: 855-56.

[81]   Carvalhaes CG, Picao RC, Nicoletti AG, *et al.* Cloverleaf test (modified Hodge test) for detecting carbapenemase production in Klebsiella pneumoniae: be aware of false positive results. J Antimicrob Chemother 2010; 65: 249-51.

[82]   Cuzon G, Naas T, Demachy MC, *et al.* Plasmid-mediated carbapenemhydrolyzing β-lactamase KPC in *Klebsiella pneumoniae* isolate from Greece. Antimicrob Agents Chemother 2008; 52: 796-97.

[83]   Pier GB, Ramphal R. *Pseudomonas aeruginosa.* In: Mandell GL, Bennett JE, Dolin R (Eds). Mandell, Douglas, and Benetts's Principles and Practice of Infectious Diseases. 7th ed. 2010; pp: 2835-60.

[84]   Anthony KB, Fishman NO, Linkin DR, *et al.* Clinical and Microbiological Outcomes of Serious Infections with Multidrug-Resistant Gram-Negative Organisms Treated with Tigecycline. Clinical Infectious Diseases 2008; 46: 567-70.

[85]   Peleg AY, Potoski BA, Rea R, *et al. Acinetobacter baumannii* bloodstream infection while receiving tigecycline: a cautionary report. J Antimicrob Chemother 2006; 59: 128-31.

[86]   Falagas ME, Kasiakou SK. Colistin: the revival of polymyxins for the management of multidrug-resistant gram-negative bacterial infections. Clin Infect Dis 2005; 40: 1333-41.

[87]   Falagas ME, Grammatikos AP, Michalopoulos A. Potential of old-generation antibiotics to address current need for new antibiotics.Expert Rev Anti Infect Ther 2008; 6: 593-600.

[88]   Zavascki AP, Goldani LZ, Li J, *et al.* Polymyxin B for the treatment of multidrug-resistant pathogens: a critical review. J Antimicrob Chemother 2007; 60: 1206-15

[89]   Elemam A, Rahimian J, Mandell W. Infection with Panresistant *Klebsiella pneumoniae:* A Report of 2 Cases and a Brief Review of the Literature. Clin Infec Dis 2009; 49: 271-74

CHAPTER 3

Control of Multi-Drug Resistance

Spyros Pournaras*

Department of Microbiology, Medical School, University of Thessaly

Abstract: During the last decade, both Gram-positive and Gram-negative bacteria that are resistant to most or all available antibacterial classes are increasingly prevalent in the nosocomial environment, particularly among immunocompromised patients and those hospitalized in intensive care units. Among Gram-positive bacteria, increasing concerns are posed for health care- and community-associated methicillin-resistant *Staphylococcus aureus*, *S. aureus* with reduced susceptibility or resistance to vancomycin and vancomycin-resistant enterococci. Gram-negative bacteria have also developed multidrug resistance, which in the family of *Enterobacteriacae* is commonly due to the production of extended-spectrum β-lactamases and carbapenemases of metallo- or serine-β-lactamase type (mainly VIM-, IMP-, or KPC-types). Further, multidrug resistant non-fermenting Gram-negative bacteria such as *Pseudomonas aeruginosa* and *Acinetobacter baumannii* are common, necessitating the application of concerned efforts for their control. The control of multidrug resistant organisms requires approaches that include knowledge of their local and international epidemiological spread, accurate detection and surveillance, rational use of antibiotic treatment options and enhanced infection control measures. In the following sections of this chapter, such approaches will be presented for each category of the aforementioned major multidrug resistant bacteria.

Keywords: Gram-positive, *Acinetobacter baumannii*, VIM-, IMP-, KPC, methicillin-resistant *Staphylococcus aureus*, *serine-β-lactamase*, *Pseudomonas aeruginosa*, epidemiological spread.

INTRODUCTION

Since the introduction of each new class of antibiotics, the emergence of resistance to that or also to other classes has been followed over time, rendering hospitalized patients vulnerable to infections that are treated not effectively by the available agents. Even the newest classes of antimicrobial agents, with more potent and broader activity against Multidrug Resistant (MDR) organisms, have been associated with varying degrees of resistance. Multidrug resistance is usually considered as resistance to three or more antimicrobial classes. During the last decade, both Gram-positive and Gram-negative bacteria that are resistant to most or even all available antibacterial classes have become increasingly prevalent nosocomial pathogens, particularly among immunocompromised patients and those hospitalized in intensive care units. Among Gram-positive bacteria, the most significant concerns are posed for health care- and community-associated Methicillin-Resistant *Staphylococcus Aureus* (MRSA), *S. aureus* with reduced susceptibility or resistance to vancomycin and Vancomycin-Resistant Enterococci (VRE). MDR Gram-negative bacteria have also become prevalent. In the *Enterobacteriacae* family, multidrug resistance mostly involves isolates producing Extended-Spectrum β-Lactamases (ESBLs) and carbapenemases of metallo- or serine-β-lactamase type (mainly VIM-, IMP-, or KPC-types). Currently also, non-fermenting Gram-negative bacteria such as *Pseudomonas aeruginosa* and *Acinetobacter baumannii* are commonly resistant to all available antibiotics, including the newer agents. The increasing emergence of these MDR bacteria necessitates efforts for their early recognition and containment [1].

The clinical importance of resistant organisms in health care settings consists of the associated increases in morbidity and mortality, length of hospitalization, cost of health care and the limited therapeutic options; therefore, the control of their dissemination is an important patient safety activity. The infection-related morbidity and mortality have decreased significantly during the last decades due to earlier and better

***Address correspondence to Spyros Pounaras:** Department of Microbiology, Medical School, University of Thessaly; Tel: + 30 241350 2929; Fax: + 30 241350 1570; Email: sppournaras@yahoo.gr

diagnosis, as well as improved management, however, a recent increase in cases of antibacterial failure has been observed [2]. Until recently, the medical community worldwide has seemed incapable of reacting to the issue of antibiotic resistance. Although we still need a better understanding of the factors involved in the emergence and spread of antibiotic resistance, action has to be implemented promptly. The essentials of better control of antibiotic resistance are already well known and in essence include the knowledge of the local and international epidemiology, the accurate detection, the active surveillance, the rational use of newer antibacterial agents and the enhanced infection control measures. Some general infection control measures include use of alcohol-based hand rubs by patients and health care workers, processes to identify colonized or infected patients, adherence of routine hand-hygiene practices for all patients, contact precautions such as gowns and gloves when providing care to colonized or infected patients with active somatic secretions, housekeeping and equipment cleaning, disinfecting and sterilizing and consultation with public health officials or infection control personnel [3]. In this chapter, such aspects and more specific control measures will be presented for each category of MDR bacteria.

MULTIDRUG RESISTANT GRAM-POSITIVE BACTERIA

MRSA

S. aureus is a natural inhabitant of the nose, skin, intestine and genital tract. The nose harbours methicillin-susceptible *Staphylococcus aureus* (MSSA) in approximately 30% of individuals and MRSA in approximately 2-5%. MRSA isolates first arose in the 1960s and for the following 20 years were rather limited; however, after the 1980s, there was an increase in the isolation of MRSA [4]. The frequency of MRSA infections continues to rise in hospitals, increasing patients' morbidity and mortality. The majority of MRSA infections have been mainly Hospital-Associated (HA-MRSA) up to the 1990s, with the isolates being commonly resistant not only to β-lactam antibiotics but also to most non-β-lactam antibiotics, except vancomycin [2]. However, starting from the beginning of the 2000's, multi-drug-susceptible MRSA have also appeared intra-hospitally [5]. More recently, MRSA has emerged as a significant cause of Community-Associated (CA) *S. aureus* infections in the United States and globally. These strains were initially phenotypically and genetically distinct from those established in healthcare settings, suggesting that they arose de novo in the community. The majority of CA-MRSA infections are purulent skin and soft tissue infections, but they also include bloodstream infections, pneumonia, and musculoskeletal infections. CA-MRSA strains typically belong to a few genetic lineages, suggesting that they possess factors conferring unusual fitness, such as the Panton-Valentine leukocidin and other putative toxins, of which the relative contribution to the virulence of the strains is still unclear [6]. A constant characteristic of CA-MRSA strains has been their susceptibility to multiple non-β-lactam antibacterial agents and lower level of resistance or phenotypic susceptibility to oxacillin [7].

MRSA are considered the *S. aureus* isolates that either have oxacillin Minimum Inhibitory Concentration (MIC) > 2 mg/L or harbour the *mecA* gene [8]. As the presence of the *mecA* gene is not always accompanied by elevated oxacillin MICs [7], MRSA isolates are preferably defined as those harbouring this gene or expressing its protein product, the altered penicillin-binding protein PBP2a. The *mecA* gene is found on the Staphylococcal Cassette Chromosome (SCC). Different strains of MRSA have *SCC*mec numbered I to VI. *SCC*mec types I to III are typically found in HA-MRSA [9], while CA-MRSA characteristically carries the two smallest *SCC*mec types IV [10] and V [11]. Methicillin resistance in *mecA*-positive isolates is due to the production of PBP2a, which shows low affinity for β-lactams [12]; these isolates are resistant to all β-lactam antibiotics and β-lactam/β-lactamase inhibitors.

Identification

A prerequisite for the control of MRSA is the accurate identification of an isolate as *S. aureus* and its distinction from Coagulase-Negative Staphylococci (CoNS). Various tests can be used to identify *S. aureus*, such as production of protein A, cell-bound clumping factor, extracellular coagulase and heat-stable nuclease, while molecular methods have been developed more recently. In addition, the results of susceptibility testing to oxacillin may be equivocal and again in this instance further molecular testing is appropriate. This holds particularly true in cases of "MRSA" strains that appear oxacillin-susceptible (OS-

MRSA) [2]. In such cases, the amplification of the gene *mecA* by PCR is the "gold standard" for the detection of MRSA. The PCR tests for detection of *mecA* can be combined with simultaneous PCR detection of an *S. aureus*-specific target to allow rapid identification of MRSA isolates [13, 14].

Screening for MRSA

The control of MRSA usually necessitates the screening for MRSA carriers. Several screening methods have been proposed for the detection of MRSA, including solid agar media, without or with prior broth enrichment to enhance detection by overnight incubation before plating on solid agar. However, comparative studies of currently available media assessed with clinical specimens are very limited. Most media contain an indicator to distinguish *S. aureus*, inhibitory substances to aid the selection of *S. aureus* from other organisms and oxacillin or, more recently, cefoxitin to select for methicillin-resistant strains. Inhibitory substances have included NaCl, polymyxin B, aztreonam, tellurite and desferrioxamine [15]. Recently developed chromogenic agars for identifying *S. aureus* have been also utilized and had variable sensitivity and specificity in screening for MRSA [16, 17], but the performance was good with cefoxitin as a selective agent [17].

Molecular methods have been also applied for the screening of samples for MRSA. The majority of these have relied on multiplexed PCR primers to detect genes identifying strains as *S. aureus* (*nuc* and *fem* are frequently used) and *mecA* [13]. However, the methods are generally only applicable to identification of purified cultures of staphylococci and they should not be used directly on samples, as they could detect also possibly co-existing CoNS carrying the *mecA* gene or MSSA.

Treatment Options

Most *S. aureus* strains produce a β-lactamase, which inactivates all β-lactams, with the exception of oxacillin and, further, as soon as oxacillin was used clinically, oxacillin resistance of *S. aureus* strains was emerged. Unfortunately, the use of different types of antibiotics over the years has led to the emergence of multiantibiotic-resistant MRSA strains, as the result of mutations in genes coding for target proteins and through acquisition of resistance genes against multiple unrelated antibiotics [18].

Vancomycin remains the standard treatment for serious MRSA infections and is thus the second most commonly used antibiotic in US hospitals. It retains excellent use against MRSA and in 50 years of use, only 6 clinical vancomycin resistant MRSA strains have been found. However, several concerns have been raised, including vancomycin heteroresistance, "MIC creep" and prolonged MRSA bacteremia in many patients despite adequate vancomycin treatment [19]. In cases of vancomycin failures, the use of linezolid or daptomycin is likely to be required. Linezolid is the only available oral agent for these infections and is preferred for pneumonia and also for complicated skin and soft-tissue infections [20], rifampicin and fusidic acid oral combination therapy may be also used. Daptomycin has been associated with elevated levels of creatine kinase, its optimal dosing is still not clear and it is inactivated by lung surfactant. Daptomycin seems to perform slightly better than vancomycin for MRSA infections. Finally, co-trimoxazole use may be problematic because of a potential for severe reactions and clindamycin is associated with *Clostridium difficile* colitis [21].

Control

Control measures that have been used for the containment of MRSA include the education of healthcare workers, with emphasis on hand-washing practices; the Active Surveillance Cultures (ASCs), the contact isolation of MRSA-positive patients and antibiotic stewardship. However, despite these interventions, MRSA is still endemic in many hospitals worldwide and there is increasing evidence that a multidisciplinary approach is required towards that direction. Some of these approaches follow. In general, the measures required to control MRSA in hospitals where the infection is very common may be different from those required in institutions with lower prevalence. On the basis of existing evidence, only Intensive Care Units (ICU) should preferably apply extensive screening. Screening for MRSA carriage and isolation of the positive patients seems to have a significant role in the prevention of cross-transmission. MRSA colonization can be determined by culturing nasal and either pharyngeal, inguinal or rectal samples [22]. It has been suggested previously that the risk of infection after MRSA colonization was four times higher compared with MSSA colonization [23], while colonization with CA-MRSA strains increases the risk of infection as well [24]. Many studies indicate that intensive concerted interventions including screening and isolation can substantially reduce MRSA infections [25], but the optimal approach to prevent transmission of MRSA is not yet defined [26].

A significant variable of the MRSA control attempts is the active surveillance of patients, followed by contact precautions and decolonization. It has been widely shown previously that the rates of hospital MRSA infections were considerably reduced after the application of MRSA screening at admission and thereafter in a regular weekly basis [27]. Nevertheless, there are also a few studies that showed a minimal impact of active surveillance cultures to the reduction of MRSA infections [28].

Another aspect of the MRSA control that still remains questionable is the screening of healthcare workers [29]. There is little evidence to suggest that exclusion of MRSA-positive personnel would reduce the MRSA infections. The routine screening of staff for MRSA is time-consuming and costly and would also have practical and ethical considerations. However, screening of staff might have a role during outbreaks [30].

Due to the increased cost required for screening all patients, a targeted active surveillance of medical or surgical patients at risk might be more reasonable. Risk factors for MRSA colonization at patient admission commonly include previous use of antibiotics (quinolones, cephalosporins and carbapenems), previous exposure to health care environment, advanced age, dialysis, chronic illnesses, skin lesions, intravenous drug use, homelessness, prison stay, promiscuity [31]. Most of these situations also predispose for MRSA infections, both in the community and in the hospital setting. Before starting active surveillance cultures, laboratories should be prepared for the heavy workload and the need for rapid results and hospital authorities should monitor the effectiveness of the interventions and make decisions about their rationale. Some countries have maintained low endemic levels of MRSA by implementing nationwide control measures targeting MRSA, such as the search and destroy strategy. This approach, further to the measures shown above, includes contact isolation for MRSA positive patients, pre-emptive isolation and screening for high-risk patients, screening of all patients and healthcare workers and keeping carriers away from work until decontamination, and closing wards when more than one patient carries MRSA. It has been suggested that a combined approach of screening and isolation is effective, and that MRSA prevalence might be reduced to <1% in high-endemicity settings by a search and destroy strategy and stepwise interventions [30, 32].

Finally, as far the control of CA-MRSA in the community, there is a general feeling among infection control policy makers and clinicians that aggressive control would be almost impossible to achieve. However, in Europe, Denmark still implements a 'search-and-destroy' strategy even in the community [33] and in Switzerland a voluntary CA-MRSA surveillance system has been implemented to ensure adequate case investigation and secondary prevention [34]. Also, although current US guidelines do not recommend contact tracing or systematic decontamination with topical medications [35], it is believed that they could be effective in controlling the spread of CA-MRSA, at least in settings with non-endemic CA-MRSA and good public health infrastructures [36]. Overall, the potential to control CA-MRSA in the community is still limited and may be targeted at high-risk groups only. Preventive strategies may rely on active surveillance, contact tracing, eradicating the carriage status and hygiene counseling in low-hygiene populations [37].

STAPHYLOCCOCUS AUREUS WITH REDUCED SUSCEPTIBILITY OR RESISTANCE TO VANCOMYCIN

Clinical *S. aureus* isolates that demonstrate reduced susceptibility to vancomycin were firstly reported in 1997 and followed by multiple reports from many regions worldwide. The Clinical Laboratory Standards Institute has developed guidelines to define susceptibility to vancomycin for *S. aureus* isolates. According to these guidelines, isolates with MIC ≤ 4 mg/L are considered susceptible, isolates with MIC 8-16 mg/L intermediate (VISA), and isolates with MIC ≥32 mg/L resistant (VRSA) [8]. In addition to *S. aureus* isolates that are identified as VISA or VRSA, there are strains of *S. aureus* that are referred to as "heteroresistant." These strains are phenotypically susceptible to vancomycin (MIC ≤ 4 mg/L) but they contain subpopulations for which the vancomycin MIC is in the intermediate range. The clinical significance of heteroresistance is controversial and is under active investigation [38].

Vancomycin was first released in 1958 and subsequently has been the treatment of choice for serious MRSA infections, which are becoming increasingly common globally. For many years there was no indication that vancomycin resistance in *S. aureus* was likely to be a problem. Therefore, initial reports of reduced vancomycin susceptibility in clinical isolates of *S. aureus* from Japan in 1997 generated significant concern in the medical community [39, 40]. Since that time, there has been uncertainty regarding optimal laboratory detection and the clinical relevance of reduced vancomycin susceptibility in *S. aureus*. Also, there have been changes in the CLSI breakpoints for vancomycin against *S. aureus* and increasing concern regarding the efficacy of vancomycin for the treatment of *S. aureus* infections. The proposed mechanisms of resistance described for VISA and VRSA strains are distinctly different from each other. There is evidence that VISA strains have a thickened cell wall, which results in the elevation of vancomycin MICs to 8-16 mg/L [41]. In contrast, the clinical isolates of VRSA do not produce a thickened cell wall but contain the *vanA* gene and exhibit true vancomycin resistance (MIC ≥ 32 μg/ml). Since 2002, nine clinical isolates of VRSA—all carrying the *vanA* gene complex—were reported in the United States [42, 43]. Moreover, VRSA also have been reported from India, where two strains were found [44]. The DNA sequence of the *vanA* gene isolated from the VRSA isolates is usually identical to that from enterococci, suggesting that transfer of this genetic element has occurred as a portentous evolutionary development [2]. In particular, these strains harboured a plasmid-borne Tn1546 element following conjugation from a glycopeptide-resistant *Enterococcus* strain. In the second step, Tn1546 transposed to a resident plasmid in five strains; the acquired plasmid behaved as a suicide gene delivery vector, and the incoming DNA had been rescued by illegitimate recombination. Competition growth experiments in the absence of inducer between the MRSA recipient and isogenic VRSA transconjugant revealed a disadvantage for the transconjugant, accounting, in part, for the low level of dissemination of the VRSA clinical isolates [43].

Risk factors for hVISA and VISA

Not surprisingly, the main risk factors for infection with VISA and hVISA appear to be prior MRSA infection or colonization and exposure to vancomycin [39, 45]. Additionally, most VISA and hVISA infections occur in patients with serious underlying disease such as malignancy, diabetes, renal failure, or recent major surgery [46]. A high bacterial load, which occurs with infections such as abscesses or infection of prosthetic joints, may also confer to the development of hVISA infection during glycopeptide therapy, as large numbers of organisms are present and the levels of antibiotics into the infected areas may be limited [46]. In such circumstances, a proportion of bacteria may survive and the vancomycin treatment may fail. Some data also suggests that low serum levels of vancomycin early in the treatment course of MRSA infections may also be associated with the emergence of VISA and hVISA [46]. As independent predictors associated with higher vancomycin MICs and reduced *in vitro* bactericidal activity of vancomycin against *S. aureus* (rather than hVISA or VISA per se), were shown to be a prior vancomycin exposure and residence in ICU [47, 48]. Finally, the true VRSA strains are very limited and involve mainly patients harbouring simultaneously Vancomycin-Resistant Enteococci (VRE).

Identification

Possible methods for defining the vancomycin MIC include CLSI-approved methods (agar dilution and broth MIC) [8], Etest MIC using a 0.5 Mc- Farland standard and commercial automated tests. The 2-McFarland-standard macromethod Etest is a screening tool for hVISA and VISA but is not a true vancomycin or teicoplanin MIC and its results should not be reported as a true MIC. Subtle but potentially important variability in vancomycin MIC results is obtained with different methods [49, 50].

There is currently no standardized method for the accurate detection of hVISA [51], which makes laboratory testing and interpretation of the clinical significance of hVISA difficult. Given the low inoculum used for CLSI broth and agar dilution methods, the hVISA phenotype may not be detected. Methods to detect hVISA therefore tend to rely on the testing higher inocula (such as 10^8 CFU for population analysis) and methods to promote the growth of the resistant subpopulation, such as prolonged incubation (usually 48 h). From a laboratory point of view, population analysis is currently considered to be the gold standard for hVISA confirmation [52].

Treatment Options

A number of antimicrobials with activity against *S. aureus* retain activity *in vitro* against hVISA and VISA. In a few cases, therapy with oral rifampin and fusidic acid was an important component of therapy for the successful treatment of hVISA and VISA infections in patients who had failed vancomycin therapy [52]. Strains of *S. aureus* and coagulase-negative staphylococci with reduced vancomycin susceptibility commonly retain susceptibility to linezolid. Although linezolid resistance has been reported for *S. aureus* [53], rates of resistance remain very low [54]. Also, although linezolid is essentially bacteriostatic against *S. aureus in vitro*, a number of serious cases of MRSA, hVISA, and VISA infections, including endocarditis, have been treated successfully with linezolid. As far as daptomycin, there has been an association between hVISA and VISA and reduced susceptibility. It appears that vancomycin exposure per se can induce low-level daptomycin resistance or heteroresistance [55] even though these changes appear to be strain specific and may be unstable [56]. Quinupristin-Dalfopristin (QD) is also active against MRSA and has also demonstrated *in vitro* activity against a range of hVISA and VISA strains (MIC90 for hVISA and VISA of 1 μg per ml) [57]. Finally, tigecycline has very good *in vitro* activity against MSSA and MRSA strains (MIC90 of 0.12 to 1 μg per ml), including a small number of VISA strains but it has not been extensively tested against hVISA and VISA strains [58].

Control of hVISA, VISA, VRSA

Although humans are the main reservoir of *S. aureus* non-susceptible to glycopeptides, these organisms are capable to colonise the environment and persist, despite repeated and concerted eradication efforts. In a large-scale VISA outbreak that occurred in a French ICU [59], conventional preventive isolation measures had been implemented when the index patient developed an MRSA ventilator-associated pneumonia. Hospital workers used gowns and gloves and washed their hands after each patient contact; however, new cases continued to emerge, necessitating the implementation of extraordinary measures to control the outbreak. These included restricting patient admissions, twice-daily environmental disinfection and use of a hydroalcoholic solution to decontaminate the hands of hospital workers. This report underlined the real dangers of MRSA with reduced glycopeptides susceptibility, as 5 of the 21 VISA-positive patients died in the ICU either directly or partly as a result of VISA infection (22). VISA/VRSA infections require additional efforts compared with MRSA, including wearing a gown on entry into the patient's room, use of an alcohol rub when washing hands on exiting the room, one-to-one nursing and routine contact investigation while the patient is in hospital. During outpatient follow-up, the patient should be seen as the last patient of the day, all healthcare workers should come to a single location, and cleaning and disinfection of the room should be conducted when the patient departs. Whereas MRSA patients should be placed in contact isolation indefinitely whenever there is a need to utilise healthcare resources, VISA and VRSA patients should be placed in special isolation for the term of their life. Long-term residential care presents a particular problem with respect to preventing the dissemination of VISA and VRSA. It is believed that chronic leg or decubitus ulcers in the elderly are the primary source of VRSA and potentially of VISA. Concern therefore arises over the practical issue of adhering to hospital control measures in these institutions and what to do when patients are transferred from long-term facilities to community or tertiary care facilities. Also, the rational and restricted use of vancomycin, teicoplanin and any other glycopeptides is essential to prevent or limit the continued emergence of hVISA, VISA and VRSA. In this context, the increasing occurrence of serious infections caused by community-acquired MRSA, which are susceptible to most non-β-lactams, requires therapy with drugs other than glycopeptides, to decrease the selective pressure for glycopeptide resistance [60].

Overall, several commercially available antibiotics that have demonstrated activity against VISA and VRSA have been referred above. Whilst their use will have an important future role in limiting the impact of infection, the prevention of dissemination must be a constant focus, not only of hospital workers but also of those working in residential care and other healthcare environments. In this context, the rapid identification of patients harbouring VRSA, VISA or hVISA, the prompt isolation and the adherence to infection control protocols are are very important in controlling the dissemination of these pathogens [60].

VRE

Enterococci are important hospital-acquired pathogens. Isolates of *Enterococcus faecalis* and *Enterococcus faecium* are the third- to fourth-most prevalent nosocomial pathogen worldwide [61]. Vancomycin-Resistant Enterococci (VRE) were first identified as hospital-associated pathogens in Europe during the mid-1980s and have rapidly disseminated worldwide [62]. In 2006, the European Antimicrobial Resistance Surveillance System (EARSS) reported vancomycin-resistance rates among enterococci ranging from none in Iceland, Norway, Romania, Bulgaria, Denmark and Hungary, to 42% of *Enterococcus faecium* strains in Greece [63]. A surveillance study conducted in US hospitals from 1995 through 2002 showed that 9% of nosocomial bloodstream infections were caused by enterococci and that 2% of *E. faecalis* isolates and 60% of *E. faecium* isolates were vancomycin-resistant [64] .The majority of reported hospital outbreaks have occurred in the USA. Conversely, asymptomatic carriage among healthy people is relatively common in Europe compared to the USA [62, 65, 66].

As far as European hospitals, since the mid 1990s, Norway, Denmark and Iceland have only experienced sporadic cases and minor outbreaks of VRE infection or colonisation, often among patients transferred from hospitals in higher-prevalence countries. In the United Kingdom (UK), bacteraemia caused by VRE is monitored by four complementary surveillance proGrammes. Based on data from all surveillance proGrammes, estimates for the proportion of enterococcal bacteraemia attributable to VRE for the UK as a whole in 2007 are 8.5-12.5% for all enterococci, 20 - 25% for *E. faecium* and 1.6-2.5% for *E. faecalis* [67-69]. In France, only sporadic cases or outbreaks with a limited number of cases due to VRE were reported before 2005, with the incidence of glycopeptide resistance in *E. faecium* from bacteraemia to remain below 5% [67]. Despite this low proportion, large outbreaks affecting several hundreds of patients occurred in 2005 in a few hospitals and these prompted the French authorities to recommend in 2005 and 2006 notification of all cases of infections/ colonisations due to VRE. The highest rates of VRE associated with nosocomial infections in Europe were reported in some countries of southern Europe; levels up to 45% were reported recently from Greece and Portugal [67]. As also observed in most geographical regions, *vanA E. faecium* isolates were the species mainly responsible for the high rates of infections caused by VRE in Greece, Portugal and Italy [67, 70-73].

Infections and Resistance Profile

Initially thought of as commensal microorganisms, enterococci have emerged as significant human pathogens, currently being the third most common nosocomial bloodstream pathogen in the USA [74]. They have relatively low virulence, but may cause urinary tract and intraabdominal infections, bacteraemias and endocarditis. The bacteria can disseminate by direct or indirect contact within a particular institution. Enterococci can also be spread between hospitals by healthcare professionals who work at more than one institution or by patients who were previously infected at another institution [75]. Enterococcal infections occur predominantly in patients with immunodeficiencies, either due to their underlying illness or to immunosuppressive therapy and in patients with vascular catheters or urinary catheters. It has been reported that 60% of enterococcal infections are nosocomial, with half of them occurring in ICUs, most probably because of the selection of these organisms by the use of broad-spectrum antibiotics, such as cephalosporins, which lack enterococcal activity [76].

The first patients infected with plasmid-mediated Vancomycin-Resistant Enterococci (VRE) were reported from France and England in 1986 [76]. Remarkably, vancomycin resistance is more common in *E. faecium* than in *E. faecalis* [77, 78]. Since the initial descriptions, VRE (predominantly of the VanA phenotype) have emerged as important nosocomial pathogens worldwide [74, 79-82]. The first VRE outbreaks in US hospitals often resulted from dissemination of a single strain, especially in ICUs and nephrology wards [82, 83].

Resistance mechanisms: There are six recognized phenotypes of vancomycin resistance, VanA, VanB, VanC, VanD, VanE and VanG [84]. Two of these (VanA and VanB) are mediated by newly acquired gene clusters not previously found in enterococci. VanA and VanB resistance phenotypes were described primarily in *E. faecalis* and *E. faecium*. VanA-resistant strains possess inducible, high-level resistance to vancomycin (MICs ≥64 mg/ml) and teicoplanin (MICs ≥16 mg/ml). Resistance can be induced by glycopeptides (vancomycin, teicoplanin, avoparcin, and ristocetin) and by nonglycopeptide agents such as bacitracin, polymyxin B, and robenidine, a drug used to treat infections in poultry. Vancomycin resistance has been best described to occur *via* the *vanA* gene cluster found on the transposon Tn*1546* that is transferable to other susceptible enterococci by conjugation [85].

VanB isolates were initially believed to be inducibly resistant to more modest levels of vancomycin (MICs, 32 to 64 mg/ml) but are susceptible to teicoplanin. However, resistance to teicoplanin develops rapidly during antibiotic exposure. It is now known that levels of vancomycin resistance among VanB isolates may range from 4 to > 1,000 mg/L whereas susceptibility to teicoplanin is retained. VanB resistance determinants are chromosomally mediated but may also reside on large mobile elements [86]. The VanC resistance phenotype was described in *E. casseliflavus* and *E. gallinarum*, which demonstrate intrinsic, low-level resistance to vancomycin (MICs, 4-32 mg/L) and are susceptible to teicoplanin [85].

Screening Methods

Clinical cultures with VRE only represent a small proportion of the isolates carried by the hospitalized patients. It has been estimated that, for every patient with VRE isolated from clinical cultures, at least 10 other patients will be colonised [87]. Asymptomatic carriers may remain unnoticed for long periods of time, facilitating the widespread dissemination of VRE within hospitalized patients. Several microbiological screening methods have been developed for VRE using stool specimens and rectal or perirectal swabs. Isolation of VRE from heavily contaminated specimens, such as faeces, can be hampered due to inhibition of VRE growth by the indigenous intestinal flora [88]. Many laboratories have applied direct inoculation of swabs on vancomycin-containing agar plates for selective isolation of VRE. The use of solid media instead of broth offers the advantage of a rapid assessment of colony morphology, but low VRE numbers may not be detected [87]. Detection can be optimised by inoculating faecal samples or swabs in broth enrichment, such as Enterococcosel broth with vancomycin and aztreonam, followed by subculture on agar plates containing vancomycin. This method is more time-consuming, but has been recommended for surveillance cultures from patients [88] and environmental surfaces [89].

Treatment Options

Following identification of VRE infections, the first step in treatment is surgical (such as abscess drainage) or other intervention, depending on the site of infection. For instance, bacteraemia has been treated successfully without the use of antimicrobial agents and with only removal of an indwelling intravenous catheter [75]. Failure to clear the bacterium with removal of catheters alone will mandate initiation of antimicrobial therapy. There are several therapeutic options for VRE urinary tract infections that are not useful for other infections or bacteraemias. Lower urinary tract infections can be treated with fosfomycin or nitrofurantoin, agents that achieve adequate levels in the urine, but not in the blood. There are fewer therapeutic options for serious deep-seated visceral infections and bacteraemias. Anecdotal reports have noted the effectiveness of doxycycline, which was also used successfully in the ICU of the University Hospital of Larissa for VRE infections (E. Zakynthinos, personal communication). Chloramphenicol has been used for the treatment of VRE bacteraemia and other serious infections [90]. Teicoplanin is effective against VRE that express the VanB phenotype, rather than the VanA phenotype, but resistance frequently emerges during therapy. The introduction of quinupristin/dalfopristin and linezolid has greatly increased the therapeutic options for the treatment of serious VRE infections. Quinupristin/dalfopristin, a combination of a streptoGramin A (dalfopristin) and a streptoGramin B (quinupristin), has proved effective for therapy of VRE infections due to *Enterococcus faecium*, but *Enterococcus faecalis* are intrinsically resistant [75]. Linezolid is bacteriostatic against enterococci but has become the drug of choice for many types of VRE infection. Linezolid is approved in some countries for serious VRE infections, including bacteraemias, urinary tract infections, and skin and soft tissue infections [91, 92]. Linezolid has also been reported to cure VRE endocarditis and other serious intravascular infections [93]. A major advantage of linezolid is the availability of both parenteral and oral formulations. The most serious side effect noted with linezolid therapy is bone marrow suppression, with thrombocytopenia to be especially common [94, 95]. Linezolid-resistant VRE isolates have been increasingly isolated, correlated with heavy linezolid consumption [96]. Several other new agents have been available during the last few years for the treatment of VRE infections, such as daptomycin, a lipopeptide antimicrobial agent that is bactericidal for VRE and tigecycline that also has good, even bacteriostatic, activity against VRE [97, 98]. Widespread hospital use of antibiotics, particularly ticarcillin/clavulanate, third-generation cephalosporins, and vancomycin have been shown to select for VRE, while piperacillin/tazobactam possibly has had a protective effect against VRE [2]. Despite the therapeutic restrictions caused by the MDR of VRE, the significance of vancomycin resistance for clinical outcome is still under debate, while in patients with neutropenia VRE bacteremia is associated with increased mortality [99].

Control

Given the sparse armamentarium available for treating serious VRE infections and the reports of resistance to newer agents, new approaches to the prevention of infection are needed. Decolonization of the gastrointestinal (GI) tract, the primary reservoir for VRE, could decrease environmental contamination and thus help reducing the nosocomial spread of VRE. The ideal agent for VRE decolonization should not be used against VRE infections, have low potential for resistance development, be unlikely to cause cross resistance with other agents used against VRE, have narrow spectrum of activity, have bactericidal activity, be given orally and not systemically absorbed and be well tolerated. For that purpose, several studies have been reported using bacitracin. Two early, uncontrolled trials showed that the combination of bacitracin with doxycycline appeared to be effective in decolonization of VRE from the GI tract, but three subsequent studies showed bacitracin to be ineffective [98]. In the only randomized, placebo-controlled, blinded study that compared treatment with 50,000 U zinc bacitracin capsules with placebo, given to six patients in each group four times daily for 10 days, VRE was eradicated from stool in only two patients in each group after 3 weeks [100]. Novobiocin has also been tried for VRE decolonization in a small number of oncology patients, some of whom were also bacteraemic. Tetracycline, doxycycline or rifampicin was added to the non-absorbable agent; in only one of eight patients VRE was cleared from stool, and novobiocin was poorly tolerated. It should be mentioned that persistence of VRE in the GI tract for long periods appears to be the rule [101].

Until the decolonization of GI tract proves to be effective, isolation precautions recommended by the US Hospital Infection Control Practices Advisory Committee (HICPAC) should be used for VRE-colonized patients. Several studies have shown that isolation precautions lead to decreased transmission of VRE [102]. Precautions include the use of a private room for colonized patients and dedicated equipment to be kept in the room for that patient's care. Clean, non-sterile gloves and disposable gowns should be worn by those entering the room. The requirement for gowns remains controversial, as they are costly, take additional time and can be uncomfortably warm [103]. However, gowns have been shown to be helpful in an outbreak situation and probably increase healthcare workers' recognition of their personal role in the transmission of VRE. Careful attention to hand cleansing, even though gloves are worn, cannot be overemphasized. The recommendations for such strict precautions have been generated, in part, by the important role played by the environment in the transmission of VRE [104, 105] and the recognition that patients remain persistently colonized for extremely long periods [101]. Environmental contamination by VRE is common; the highest concentrations of organisms occur on bed rails, over-the-bed tables, bed linen, urinals and bedpans [75].

The US Hospital Infection Control Practices Advisory Committee (HICPAC) guidelines for the prevention and control of the spread of VRE also focus on the early detection of VRE carriage by the microbiology laboratory and the prudent use of antibiotics [76]. An active infection control proGramme, including surveillance cultures and the isolation of infected patients, reduced the overall prevalence of VRE in healthcare facilities in three US states in 3 years from 2.2% to 0.5% [106]. Enhanced infection control measures, such as weekly surveillance cultures, observation of hand-washing practices and cohorting of patients and nurses, also decreased the incidence of VRE bacteraemia, antibiotic use and healthcare costs [107]. Further, reducing the antibiotic pressure seems to be a logical approach for the control of VRE, as multiple studies have identified antibiotics as a risk factor for acquisition. Changes in specific prescribing practice in ICUs were associated with decreased vancomycin use and VRE prevalence, when compared with ICUs in which no unit-specific changes had been implemented [108]. In contrast, VRE prevalence increased steadily over a 10-year period, despite significant reductions in cephalosporin use, without undertaking aggressive infection control interventions [109]. A proGramme combining the restricted use of vancomycin, cephalosporins and clindamycin and the use of gowns for VRE-colonised patients was associated with a considerable decrease in VRE prevalence [76]. Overall, despite the formulation of guidelines and reports of successful interventions, the incidence of VRE infections was increasing in the USA [74]. A simple explanation is that, despite all the guidelines, endemicity persists because of poor hand hygiene compliance. It may also be argued that control measures have been implemented too late; the existing reservoir of VRE within hospitals is now too large for successful infection control [76].

MULTIDRUG RESISTANT GRAM-NEGATIVE BACTERIA

MDR Enterobacteriacae

In Gram-negative pathogens, β-lactamase production is the main mechanism involved in acquired β-lactam resistance. Four molecular classes of β-lactamases have been described: A, B, C, and D. Classes A, C, and D are enzymes with a serine moiety in the active centre that catalyzes hydrolysis of the β-lactam ring through an acyl-intermediate of serine, whereas the class B enzymes require a metal cofactor (*e.g.* zinc in the natural form) to function, and for this reason, they are also referred to as Metallo-β-Lactamases (MBLs) [110]. *Enterobacteriaceae* are important causes of serious hospital infections and are becoming more resistant to available antibiotics. A significant and increasing concern is caused by the resistance of *Enterobacteriacae* to most or all commercial β-lactam antibiotics, caused by ESBLs and carbapenemases of the MBL- or *Klebsiella pneumoniae* carbapenemase (KPC)-type [2]. The organisms that harbour those β-lactamases are also frequently resistant to many other antibacterial classes. Due to these reasons, in this chapter we will focus on the aspects of resistance and control of Gram-negative organisms that produce these types of potent β-lactamases.

Epidemiology

The ESBLs are Ambler molecular class A β-lactamases that are capable of hydrolyzing expanded-spectrum cephalosporins and aztreonam and are inhibited by β-lactamase-inhibitors such as clavulanate, sulbactam and tazobactam [111]. The first description of ESBLs was in 1983 and since then enterobacterial species possessing ESBLs have become common worldwide [111]. ESBLs have been reported in many different genera of *Enterobacteriaceae* however, they are most common in *Klebsiella pneumoniae* and *Escherichia coli*. In the '80s and '90s, the most common β-lactamases were belonging to the TEM and SHV variants, but in the last decade CTX-M enzymes are the most prevalent ESBLs in clinical isolates [112]. The real prevalence of ESBL producers may be unappreciated since they commonly have MIC values for expanded-spectrum cephalosporins and aztreonam lying within the standard breakpoints for susceptibility (*e.g.*, 2-8 mg/L) [2]. The distribution of ESBL producers varies in different regions. As far as Europe, yearly national surveillance and published studies in northern European countries (Denmark, Norway and Sweden) show increasing trends of ESBLs [113]. In southern Europe, the prevalence of ESBL producers in Spain and Portugal has increased over time, with a predominance of CTX-M-producing *E. coli* causing community acquired UTIs [114, 115]. Also in Spain, a shift in the proportion of ESBL-producing *Klebsiella* isolates recovered from outpatients (7% to 31%) was observed between the periods 1989 to 2000 and 2001 to 2004 [116]. In Italy, the prevalence of ESBL producers among clinical isolates has also increased over the last decade, with TEM and SHV-12 enzymes to predominate and non-TEM, non-SHV enzymes to emerge. More recently, however, it is reported that enzymes of the CTX-M-type are more commonly detected [117-119]. In France, the prevalence of ESBL production in *Enterobacteriaceae* reported in different multicentre studies is under 1%, with a progressive increase in the occurrence of CTX-M enzymes linked to *E. coli* expansion [120]. In United Kingdom, a recent dramatic increase in ESBL-producing organisms is being observed both in hospitals and in the community, mainly caused by the CTX-M-15 enzyme [121]. The sudden worldwide increase of CTX-M-producing *E. coli* is mainly due to CTX-M-15-enzymes and molecular epidemiology studies suggested that such isolates mostly belong to a single CTX-M-15-producing *E. coli* clone, named ST131. As far as the USA, ESBLs are commonly detected and, interestingly, the predominant enzymes belong to the SHV family [122]. CTX-M β-lactamases were thought to be uncommon in North America [122], but recent studies indicate that their prevalence is also increasing [123]. Finally, the prevalence of ESBLs is particularly high in other regions, such as Asia, where ESBL producers are commonly detected not only from hospitalised [124] but also from healthy people [125].

Carbapenems are considered as the treatment of choice for severe infections due to ESBL producers. The increasing occurrence of ESBL infections has ultimately led to the overuse of carbapenems and subsequently to the selection of pathogens that survive by producing carbapenem-hydrolyzing enzymes. The production of carbapenemases, although relatively common among Gram-negative non-fermenting bacteria, still remains uncommon in *Enterobacteriaceae* in a global basis [126]. However, outbreaks of carbapenemase-producing *Enterobacteriaceae* (CRE) are increasing in several regions [127, 128]. Among carbapenemases, those of KPC-type are plasmid-borne class A ESBLs that hydrolyze carbapenems, penicillins, cephalosporins, and aztreonam. Although detected originally in the United States, they are now reported in Latin America, China, Europe and, endemically, in Israel and Greece [127]. Organisms bearing these resistance factors currently present the most significant challenge in the Gram-negative resistance to date. The other most common carbapenemase produced by *Enterobacteriacae* is the Verona-imipenemase (VIM)-type MBL. It should be noted that sporadic isolates and small outbreaks of VIM-producing *Enterobacteriacae* have been reported in some European and Mediterranean countries [129, 130]. However, Greece seems to be the only country to date, where such clinical strains are isolated in high numbers [131].

Infections-Treatment Options

Since 2000, *Escherichia coli* producing ESBLs of the CTX-M-type (especially CTX-M-15) have emerged worldwide as important causes of community-onset Urinary Tract Infections (UTIs) and bloodstream infections. ESBL producers are commonly resistant to different antibiotic families including not only β-lactams, but also fluoroquinolones, aminoglycosides and trimethoprim-sulfamethoxazole, which contribute to the selection and persistence of multidrug-resistant ESBL strains and plasmids in both clinical and community settings [132, 133]. Due to the multidrug resistance, infections due to ESBL-producing *Enterobacteriaceae* are associated with a delay in initiation of appropriate antibacterial therapy, which consequently prolongs hospital stays, increases hospital costs and appears to be associated with higher patient mortality [113].

The carbapenems are widely considered the drugs of choice for the treatment of severe infections due to ESBL-producing *Enterobacteriaceae*, although comparative clinical trials are lacking. Other agents in use for the treatment of ESBL-associated UTIs include fosfomycin, nitrofurantoin, quinolones and temocillin and their use should be encouraged to reduce the use of carbapenems for serious community-acquired UTIs [134]. Infections due to *Enterobacteriaceae* producing carbapenemases of KPC- and VIM-types are usually systemic and not site-specific. Risk factors for acquiring infections with these bacteria include prolonged hospitalization, ICU stay, invasive devices, immunosuppression and previous exposure of antibiotics, including, but not limited to, carbapenems [135, 136]. Both in Israel and in the USA, a high mortality rate, ranging from 38% to 57%, has been attributed to KPC-producing *K. pneumoniae* infections [136, 137], but a lower attributable mortality of approximately 25% was reported from Greece [138-140].

Resistance Phenotypes and Detection

The ESBL-producing isolates are commonly resistant to other antimicrobial classes. Their resistance to fluoroquinolones has increased over time, initially in *K. pneumoniae* and later also in *E. coli* [132]. This increase has correlated with the increase of the plasmid-mediated *qnr* genes (*qnrA*, *qnrB* or *qnrS*), of acetylases affecting the action of certain fluroquinolones [*aac(6')-Ib-cr*] or of systems pumping fluoroquinolones out of the bacteria (*qepA*) [141, 142]. Very recent studies indicate that the *aac(6')-Ib-cr* gene seems to be confined to *E. coli* ST131 that is mainly linked to CTX-M-15 isolates, whereas *qnr* genes are mostly associated with enzymes from the CTX-M-9 or CTX-M-1 groups [141-143]. Several ESBL producers also carry genes encoding resistance to aminoglycosides, trimethoprim or sulfonamides and are located on integrons or transposons associated with different ESBL plasmids [142-145]. Of particular concern is the recovery of plasmids coding for ESBLs that express a low level of resistance to β-lactams [146] or contain silenced antibiotic resistance genes [147], as they may serve as reservoirs of antibiotic resistance determinants not detected by phenotype [113]. The detection of ESBL production is thus complicated, affecting the control efforts, by the apparent susceptibility of several ESBL producers to third- and fourth-generation cephalosporins and monobactams. In addition, the sensitivity and specificity of tests to detect ESBLs can vary with the cephalosporin tested, while the detection of ESBLs in *Enterobacteriaceae* that commonly possess AmpC β-lactamase, such as *Enterobacter*, *Citrobacter freundii*, *Serratia*, *Morganella morganii* and *Providencia,* can be particularly problematic. Due to these reasons, specific detection schemes have been implemented for the accurate detection of ESBLs [148]. These tests rely on the synergy of clavulanate with cefotaxime, ceftazidime or cefepime for cases where the co-production of an AmpC enzyme is suspected. The accurate detection of β-lactamases is especially important, since there is evidence that the therapeutic response of β-lactam antibiotics for phenotypically susceptible ESBL producers is uncertain [2]. The spread of KPC and MBL producers may be also underestimated because these enzymes do not always confer obvious carbapenem resistance [2]. The accurate detection of MBLs is based on tests using EDTA, which inhibits their activity, in combination with carbapenems [149]. KPC enzymes were initially detected by nonspecific tests like the modified Hodge test, but more recently the specific boronic acid disk tests have been implemented for the accurate detection of KPC producers [150]. Finally, the combination of EDTA and boronic acid has been proposed to detect the co-production of MBL and KPC enzymes [151, 152] that was also recently emerged [152, 153].

Control

Overall, the prevalence of ESBL-producing *Enterobacteriaceae* is increased worldwide, both in nosocomial and community settings. Of concern is the wide representation of CTX-M enzymes, particularly among community-acquired *E. coli* isolates, the wide spread of successful clones and multiresistant plasmids and the spread of ESBL producers that also express MBLs or AmpCs and resistance to fluoroquinolones or aminoglycosides. These evolutions constitute a public health problem that requires the implementation of specific interventions at different levels. Towards that direction, the use of broad spectrum cephalosporins and fluoroquinolones should be particularly limited, in order to restrict the selection and persistence of predominant ESBL clones or plasmids. Furthermore, the detection methods should be improved and introduced to all microbiology laboratories, to identify not only the high-level resistant bacteria, but also ESBL producers with apparent susceptibility to extended spectrum β-lactams. A surveillance of a possible faecal carriage in community-patients is important to detect a circulation of epidemic clones and to monitor ESBL trends. The control of ESBL producers ideally should be intensive prior to the establishment of endemicity in the community setting, when their restriction would be impossible [113].

As far as the CRE, the accurate detection of carbapenemase production in *Enterobacteriaceae,* particularly *Klebsiella* spp. and *Escherichia coli* is of utmost importance for the application of infection control measures. All acute care facilities should review microbiology records for the preceding 6-12 months to ensure that previously unrecognized CRE cases have not occurred. When a case of hospital-associated CRE is identified, the hospitals should conduct point prevalence surveys by active surveillance cultures in units with patients at high risk (*e.g.* ICUs, units where previous cases have been identified and units where patients are exposed to broad-spectrum antimicrobials) to identify possible additional patients colonized with CRE. The recommended surveillance culture methodology is mainly focused at detecting carbapenem resistance or carbapenemase production in *Klebsiella* spp. and *E. coli*, because these organisms represent the majority of CRE encountered in most regions worldwide [110].

The infection control measures in settings with absence or occasional occurrence of CRE include screening of all patients in contact with an index case, epidemiological investigation in cases of nosocomial cross-transmission with more than two secondary cases, education of staff and stringent infection control. In settings with ongoing outbreaks or endemic occurrence of CRE, the suggested control measures should include actions at the hospital level, such as cohorting of carriers or continuous active surveillance, but also interventions to the national level. The surveillance of carbapenemase producers at the national level requires the co-ordinated action of i) health-care specialists, which should introduce surveillance and control guidelines and intervention tools and ii) reference laboratories, which should confirm suspected cases, investigate the molecular epidemiology and implement adequate detection and quality assurance methods [138].

MDR *Pseudomonas aeruginosa*

P. aeruginosa is an environmental Gram-negative rod that accounts for about 12% of all bacterial nosocomial infections [154]. *P. aeruginosa* is recognised as a major pathogen associated with invasive devices, mechanical ventilation, operations or burn wounds in immunocompromised or immunocompetent hosts [155]. *P. aeruginosa* has particularly troublesome properties, such as innate resistance to multiple unrelated antibiiotic families, the ability to develop resistance through mutations and high virulence [156, 157]. MDR strains of *P. aeruginosa* may express unrelated resistance mechanisms and typically exhibit several mechanisms simultaneously. Carbapenems have been widely used to treat pseudomonal infections, but resistance to these agents due to the production of carbapenemases is increasing worldwide [2]. Carbapenem resistance is commonly accompanied by simultaneous resistance to almost all available antibiotics. Due to that reason, we will focus in this chapter more on the resistance of *P. aeruginosa* to carbapenems.

Infections

P. aeruginosa is ubiquitous in the environment due to its ability to grow in nutrient-poor conditions (including distilled water) and extreme temperatures. Moisture plays a critical role in the epidemiology of this pathogen. *P. aeruginosa* is frequently isolated from hydrotherapy pools, Jacuzzis and spas, swimming pools or contact lens solutions. The water supply in hospitals may also be an important source for colonization and infections, *via* faucets contaminated during hand washing [158]. Although patterns may vary among institutions, *P. aeruginosa* has been identified as the second most common cause of hospital-acquired, healthcare-associated and ventilator-associated pneumonia [159]. Numerous studies have identified *P. aeruginosa* as an important pathogen also in bum patients [160]. *P. aeruginosa* is responsible for approximately 6% of all surgical site infections and 9.5% of surgical site infections in ICUs reported to the US National Nosocomial Infections Surveillance System from 1986 to 2003 were due to *P. aeruginosa* [161]. Further, *P. aeruginosa* is a common cause of nosocomial Urinary Tract Infections (UTIs), accounting for up to 16.3% of UTIs in ICU patients [159]. Nosocomial bloodstream infections have been reported to be due to *P. aeruginosa* in 4-6% of cases [162], but higher rates occur in burn ICUs [154]. *P. aeruginosa* is an important pathogen in immunodeficient patients. For instance, *P. aeruginosa* is the most commonly identified cause of septicaemia in patients with primary immunodeficiencies [163], while transplant patients have higher rates of *P. aeruginosa* bacteraemia compared with the general hospital population. Lastly, *P. aeruginosa* is particularly important in cystic fibrosis patients, which commonly have chronic and recurrent pulmonary infections by *P. aeruginosa* [154].

Resistance Mechanisms and Phenotypes

Resistance to β-lactams and carbapenems due to Carbapenemase Production (CP, mainly MBLs) and also resistance to all other antibiotics, is now common in many parts of the world. Carbapenem resistance due to a MBL (IMP-1) was initially detected in a *P. aeruginosa* isolate from Japan in 1990 and since that time IMP enzymes have been observed throughout the world. During the last decade, VIM-type MBLs are also increasingly detected among *P. aeruginosa* isolates. A large outbreak due to VIM-producing multiresistant *P. aeruginosa* was initially reported from Greece in 2000 and since then pseudomonads expressing VIM-2 enzymes have been identified as causing hospital outbreaks worldwide [2]. MBLs of SPM- and GIM-types have also been found in *P. aeruginosa* from Brazil and Germany, respectively. Carbapenem resistance in *P. aeruginosa* can also occur through a range of other mechanisms, including the loss of specific porins and overexpression of efflux pumps [164]. *P. aeruginosa* isolates usually also harbour mechanisms of resistance to aminoglycosides and quinolones. This multidrug resistance often leaves colistin as the only agent available [138].

P. aeruginosa is intrinsically resistant to many structurally unrelated antimicrobial agents [165] because of the low permeability of its outer membrane (1/100 of the permeability of the *E. coli* outer membrane) [166], the constitutive expression of various efflux pumps with wide substrate specificity [164] and the naturally occurring chromosomal AmpC β-lactamase [167, 168]. The natural resistance of the species relates to the following β-lactams: penicillin G; aminopenicillins, including combinations with β-lactamase inhibitors and first and second generation cephalosporins. *P. aeruginosa* easily acquires additional resistance mechanisms, which leads to serious therapeutic problems. The susceptible *P. aeruginosa* phenotype (called wild-type) includes susceptibility to carboxypenicillins, ureidopenicillins, third generation- and fourth generation-cephalosporins, aztreonam, imipenem and meropenem [169]. There are several basic resistance phenotypes: (i) The intrinsic, resistant to carbenicillin, phenotype is characterized by a 4- to 8-fold increase of the wild-type MIC for most of the β-lactams, including meropenem but not imipenem. No production of chromosomal AmpC β-lactamase above the basic level is found. This phenotype includes resistance to non-β-lactams like quinolones, trimethoprim, tetracycline and chloramphenicol. The cause for the rise in MIC is the low outer membrane permeability combined with activation or derepression of efflux systems [169]. (ii) The second phenotype affects all β-lactams except cephems (cefepime and cefpirome) and carbapenems. The change is due to derepression of the AmpC β-lactamase [170]. (iii) In the third phenotype, penicillins (in particular ticarcillin, azlocillin and piperacillin) are affected more than cephalosporins, resulting from production of OXA-type β-lactamases [169]. These narrow-spectrum oxacillinases confer resistance to carboxypenicillins and ureidopenicillins, but not to expanded-spectrum cephalosporins and aztreonam [171]. (iv) The fourth phenotype is characterized by increased MICs to carbapenems; resistance to other β-lactams is not affected because strains exhibiting this phenotype have a decreased level of the carbapenem-specific porin OprD [164]. Other resistance phenotypes are determined mainly by the production of plasmid- or integron-encoded Extended-Spectrum β-Lactamases (ESBLs) from different molecular classes. In *P. aeruginosa*, all possible mechanisms determining resistance to β-lactams, such as enzymatic inactivation, active efflux, changes in outer membrane permeability and synthesis of PBPs with lower affinity to β-lactams, may exist simultaneously or in combinations [172].

Detection

The detection of carbapenem resistance of *P. aeruginosa*, more importantly due to CP, is a matter of major importance for the clinical laboratory, to allow the selection of appropriate therapeutic schemes and the implementation of infection control measures. A number of simple phenotypic tests have been described and evaluated as methodologies for the specific detection of carbapenemase-producing organisms. The clover leaf method (or modified Hodge test) has been extensively used as a general phenotypic method for detecting carbapenemase activity [148]. It is based on the inactivation of a carbapenem by whole cells or cell extracts of the carbapenemase-producing organisms, which enables a carbapenem-susceptible indicator strain to extend growth towards a carbapenem disk, along the streak of inoculum of the test strain or extract. The assay is sensitive for the detection of a CP-mediated mechanism of carbapenem resistance but does not provide information regarding the type of carbapenemase involved. For that reason, several inhibitor-based tests have been developed for the specific detection of MBL producers. These are based on the synergy between MBL inhibitors – such as EDTA [173], mercaptopropionic or mercaptoacetic acid [174] and dipicolinic acid [175] and a carbapenem (imipenem and/or meropenem) and/or an oxyimino-cephalosporin (ceftazidime) as indicator β-lactam compounds. These tests take advantage of the metalloenzyme dependence on zinc ions, and use the chelating agents to inhibit β-lactam hydrolysis. For that purpose, the Double-Disk Synergy Test (DDST) and the Combined Disk Test (CDT), using different amounts of EDTA and, in the case of DDST, different distances between the disks, exhibit high sensitivity even with isolates with low carbapenem resistance levels. Zinc supplementation of the culture medium may increase the sensitivity of the method [176]. The Etest MBL strip is also based on synergy between EDTA and imipenem and was found to have good sensitivity and specificity for detecting MBL-producing *P. aeruginosa* [177], although its specificity might be impaired by the intrinsic antibacterial activity of EDTA

[178-180]. The risk of obtaining false or ambiguous results with the use of mechanism-based β-lactamase inhibitors is certainly higher than in the case of ESBL detection. Therefore, the results should be interpreted cautiously and it is strongly recommended to have them confirmed with reference methodologies such as spectrophotometric or molecular assays. Hydrolysis of carbapenems in the presence or absence of inhibitors (*i.e.* EDTA for MBLs, tazobactam or clavulanic acid for KPCs, NaCl for most CHDLs), performed with crude cell extracts or partially purified enzymes, could provide additional information concerning the enzyme type. The molecular methods such as conventional and real-time PCR and sequencing have been commonly used for the identification of carbapenemase genes in research laboratories and reference centres. Nowadays, some of these methods, mostly PCR, are routinely performed in some clinical laboratories in order to circumvent the problems of the phenotypic detection of carbapenemase-producing organisms. This methodology allows detection of the carbapenemase-encoding genes directly from clinical samples. Commercial kits of this type seem to be promising, and their thorough evaluation in multicentre studies must be considered [181].

Treatment Options

P. aeruginosa remains one of the most important and difficult to treat nosocomial pathogens. MDR strains are increasingly being reported and, in these cases, the choice of therapy is often very limited, especially when looking for antimicrobial combinations against severe infections. An additional matter of concern is represented by the fact that no new antimicrobial agents, active against MDR strains of *P. aeruginosa*, are in advanced stages of development. While the medical community awaits the development of new drugs, MDR *P. aeruginosa* strains represent an increasing threat, and every effort should be made to preserve as long as possible, or to restore, the efficacy of currently available agents [182].

In-vitro susceptibility data are essential for the selection of antimicrobial chemotherapy for *P. aeruginosa* infections, because of the frequency and variability of acquired resistance shown by clinical isolates. Susceptibility testing is well standardised for most anti-pseudomonal agents, but there are no recommended breakpoints for susceptibility testing of polymyxin B or colistin. MIC determination is preferable in the case of these drugs because the correlation with disk diffusion testing is relatively poor [183]. As *P. aeruginosa* can be a lethal pathogen, empirical regimens adequate for *P. aeruginosa* coverage should always be initiated prior to receipt of the results of cultures and susceptibility testing when infection by this species is suspected. For the selection of empirical regimens, several aspects should be considered, including: (i) the nature and source of the infection (hospital- or community-acquired), (ii) information concerning the resistance phenotypes prevailing in the individual setting, (iii) pharmacokinetic parameters, (iv) underlying risk factors (*e.g.* diseases, length of hospitalisation, ICU admissions, previous antimicrobial chemotherapy) and (v) hospital prescription policies.

Antibiotics are usually used as monotherapy in UTIs caused by *P. aeruginosa*, with the exception of upper urinary infections or UTIs accompanied by bacteraemia. Antibiotic combinations with at least two different anti-pseudomonal drugs are normally recommended for severe *P. aeruginosa* infections, such as endocarditis, nosocomial pneumonia and bacteraemia [184]. The rationale for combination chemotherapy is essentially to reduce the chances of selecting resistant mutants during therapy, as well as to exploit the potential synergistic activity of some agents [165]. The experiences from different countries have shown that hospital transmission and cross-infections by carbapenemase-producing *P. aeruginosa* can be responsible for increased adverse outcomes [138].

Control

The most troublesome property of *P. aeruginosa* is its ability to acquire resistance during treatment of an infection. Unfortunately, the appearance of novel antibiotics with antipseudomonal activity is not anticipated in the near future. Therefore, further to the general infection control measures that apply also for MDR pseudomonads and are refered in the previous sections of this chapter, the only feasible option in the next few years is to retard the emergence of resistance through optimizing therapy with the available drugs. Towards this direction, the prevention of the resistance emergence requires the consideration of potential resistant subpopulations. Resistant subpopulations could be derived through mutations and usually require the contribution of multiple resistance mechanisms [185]. Therefore, the antibiotic selection based upon the susceptibility of the original clinical isolate does not always prevents the resistance emerging during therapy and some investigators have proposed the replacement of the MIC by the mutant prevention concentration. However, this approach has not been adopted by clinical laboratories. A more widely used approach is the combination of antibacterial agents to treat serious *P. aeruginosa* infections. The primary focus of combination therapy against *P. aeruginosa*, as also noted above, is to prevent the emergence of resistance, with an antipseudomonal β-lactam plus an aminoglycoside to be the treatment of choice [186]. Also, the combination of levofloxacin plus imipenem or other carbapenems has been suggested to prevent the emergence of resistance of *P. aeruginosa* [187]. Therefore, search for more effective combinations and clinical trials are absolutely needed.

To control the multidrug resistance of *P. aeruginosa*, it is also critical that we look for novel strategies. A possible challenge would be to elucidate the regulation of bacterial resistance mechanisms. Hoewever, although an amount of knowledge has been accumulated towards understanding the mechanisms by which *P. aeruginosa* regulates AmpC, OprD and efflux pumps, the means by which *P. aeruginosa* coregulates different resistance mechanisms are still obscure [188].

MDR *Acinetobacter baumannii*

The genus *Acinetobacter* comprises Gram-negative, aerobic, catalase-positive, oxidase-negative, nonfermenting and nonmotile opportunistic pathogens with a GC content of 39-47%. *A. baumannii* is the species most commonly causing disease; they may cause severe MDR infections and have become increasingly prevalent among hospitalized patients during the last 15 years. The resistance of *A. baumannii* to antibiotics is due to combined mechanisms, including cell membrane impermeability, increased expression of efflux pumps and production of β-lactamases of several types. Carbapenems, such as imipenem and meropenem, have been preferred for use in serious *A. baumannii* infections; however, the incidence of infections with carbapenem-resistant strains of *A. baumannii* is increasing and they often cause high morbidity and mortality rates [189]. Outbreaks caused by such strains have been identified in several ICUs worldwide and in many instances have been associated with strains that are resistant to all available antibacterial agents including carbapenems, except colistin [190, 191]. In this chapter, similarly with *P. aeruginosa*, we will focus more on carbapenem-resistant *A. baumannii* isolates.

Epidemiology

A. baumannii infections have been a substantial clinical issue in many parts of Europe. Several hospital outbreaks of *A. baumannii* infections have occurred and been investigated in several European countries using molecular epidemiological typing methods [192] and clonal multidrug-resistant *A. baumannii* have been shown to spread on a national or international scale. For instance, the so-called Southeast clone and the OXA-23 clones 1 and 2 have been spread in Southeast England [193] and a multiresistant *A. baumannii* clone has been disseminated in multiple centers in France [194]. Furthermore, three international *A. baumannii* clones (the so-called European clones I, II, and III) have been reported from hospitals in Northern Europe as well as southern European countries [195] and also in Eastern Europe [196].

Carbapenem resistance in *A. baumannii* is now a significant issue in many European countries. The prevalence of carbapenem resistance in various European countries appears to be highest in Turkey, Greece, Italy, Spain, and England, while it is still rather low in Germany and Netherlands and increasing in Eastern Europe [197]. The evolution of carbapenem resistance among *A. baumannii* in Greece is of interest, as it was rare up to 1998 [198]. However, acinetobacters were one of the most frequent pathogens in Greek hospitals and the majority of them were multiresistant to other antibiotics, leading to an extensive use of carbapenems [198]. In this respect, starting from early 2000, isolates with low-level carbapenem resistance have gradually emerged [199], while during the following years carbapenem resistant *A. baumannii* have become very common in most Greek hospitals [200]. In the United States, *A. baumannii* infections are an increasing cause of concern, especially in the ICUs, where 7% of pneumonias were due to *Acinetobacter* in 2003, compared to 4% in 1986 ($P < 0.001$) [201]. Numerous US hospitals have reported clonal outbreaks of MDR- or pandrug-resistant *A. baumannii* [202] and also, US surveillance studies have demonstrated significant trends in the emergence of multidrug-resistant *Acinetobacter* strains [201]. Furthermore, a significant concern has been caused by the *A. baumannii* infections of US military personnel who have fought in Iraq or Afghanistan [203]. An increase in infections with *A. baumannii* was first observed in U.S. military personnel in March 2003, soon after the start of operations in Iraq. These isolates were MDR, with carbapenem resistance, varying from 10 to 37%, to be due mainly to the production of OXA-23 or OXA-58 carbapenemase. The *A. baumannii* strains from injured military personnel from the United States were clonally related with strains from the United Kingdom [204].

Infections

The majority of *A. baumannii* isolates are recovered from the respiratory tracts of hospitalized patients and it is, thus, very difficult to distinguish colonization from true infection. However, it is evident that one of the most common hospital infections due to *A. baumannii* is the Ventilator-Associated Pneumonia (VAP). Furthermore, *A. baumannii* was responsible for 1.3% of nosocomial bloodstream infections in a large report from the United States [201]. *A. baumannii* may also occasionally cause skin and soft tissue infections, being responsible for as much as 2.1% of ICU-acquired skin/soft tissue infections [201] and commonly affects patients in burn units. *A. baumannii* is also an occasional cause of nosocomial UTIs [201] mainly involving patients with catheters, while is an increasing pathogen of meningitis following neurosurgical operations [205].

Mechanisms of Antimicrobial Resistance

A. baumannii usually expresses a MDR phenotype that currently includes most or all available antibiotics [206]. The exposure of *A. baumannii* to the selective pressure of potent antimicrobials in the ICUs, has gradually led to a global prevalence of *A. baumannii* strains that are resistant to all β-lactams, including carbapenems. Genetic elements that contribute to the overexpression of β-lactamases in *A. baumannii*, such as cephalosporinases (AmpCs) or oxacillinases (OXA-51-like or OXA-58) include the IS elements, known as IS*Aba1* or IS*Aba3* [207]. ESBLs have also been described in *A. baumannii*, but their actual prevalence is difficult to be assessed due to the difficulties in their laboratory detection, caused by the inherent production of AmpC enzymes. The major concern is caused by the production of carbapenemases, which include the serine oxacillinases (Ambler class A) and the MBLs [167].

The first reported OXA-type enzyme with potent carbapenemase activity was a plasmid-encoded enzyme described in 1985 that was initially named ARI-1 and later named bla_{OXA-23} [208]. This enzyme type now contributes to the carbapenem resistance of *A. baumannii* worldwide [209, 210]. Among OXA-type carbapenemases, OXA-27 and OXA-49 belong to the bla_{OXA-23} gene cluster of *A. baumannii* [211]. Two other clusters of acquired OXA-type carbapenemases include the $bla_{OXA-24-like}$ (OXA-24, -25, -26, and -40) and the $bla_{OXA-58-like}$ enzymes [212]. The bla_{OXA-58} was identified more recently, is often plasmid mediated [213], has been reported to cause hospital outbreaks in many ICUs worldwide [200] and has been identified more frequently among carbapenem- resistant compared with -susceptible *A. baumannii* isolates [214]. Finally, the cluster of OXA-51-like enzymes (OXA-51, -64, -65, -66, -68, -69, -70, -71, -78, -79, -80, and -82), differs from the other OXA-type carbapenemases in that it is chromosomally located and inherent in *A. baumannii* [215]. As far as MBLs, they are less commonly identified in *A. baumannii* than the OXA-type carbapenemases, but their carbapenem-hydrolyzing activities are 100- to 1,000-fold more potent. These enzymes are hydrolyzing all β-lactams (including carbapenems) except aztreonam. Three types of MBL enzymes have been identified in *A. baumannii*, including IMP [216], VIM [217] and SIM [218] types.

Nevertheless, carbapenem resistance has been commonly attributed also to non-enzymatic mechanisms, including changes in Outer Membrane Proteins (OMPs) [219], multidrug efflux pumps [220], and alterations in the PBPs [219]. Relative to other Gram-negative pathogens, very little is known about the porins of the *A. baumannii* outer membrane. Recently, the loss of a 29-kDa protein, also known as CarO, was shown to be associated with carbapenem resistance. Another OMP, the Omp25, was identified in association with CarO, but it lacked pore-forming capabilities [221]. The efflux systems of *A. baumannii* (the mostly studied is the RND-type pump AdeABC) extrude a broad range of substrates, including aminoglycosides, erythromycin, chloramphenicol, tetracyclines, fluoroquinolones and trimethoprim, but affect carbapenems in a lesser extent [220].

An intriguing characteristic of *A. baumannii* that may contribute to the emergence of carbapenem resistance is the recently reported heteroresistance to carbapenems, which probably hampers its efficient killing and may lead to the selection of resistant populations [222].

Treatment of Infections

A. baumannii is one of the most difficult to treat pathogens [223]. Prior to the 1970s, it was possible to treat *Acinetobacter* infections with several antibiotics, including aminoglycosides, β-lactams, and tetracyclines. However, resistance to all known antibiotics has now emerged in *A. baumannii* [224]. Antibiotic selection for empirical therapy is thus challenging and must rely on the susceptibility data of each hospital. Carbapenems have been the agents of choice for serious *A. baumannii* infections, but their clinical utility is now frequently affected by the emergence of resistance. Among the remaining treatment alternatives, sulbactam has clinically relevant antimicrobial activity against *Acinetobacters* [225] mediated by its binding to PBP 2. The emergence of *A. baumannii* strains resistant to all routinely tested antimicrobials has led to the use of colistin that demonstrates concentration-dependent bactericidal activity against *A. baumannii*, even though heterogeneous resistance has also emerged [226].

Of the recently licensed antimicrobials, tigecycline has been promising, but clinical data are still limited. Other agents with activity against Gram-negative organisms including *A. baumannii* include doripenem, a new parenteral carbapenem, and the next generation of cephalosporins with activity against MRSA, ceftobiprole and ceftaroline. The use of combination therapy to treat multidrug- or pandrug- resistant Gram-negative organisms has also been investigated, as it is anticipated not only to improve the efficacy of therapy but also to prevent the emergence of resistance [227].

Control

A. baumannii is particularly capable of surviving for a long time in the hospital environment and this is due to its resistance to major antimicrobial drugs and resistance to desiccation and to disinfectants. Resistance to antibiotics may provide certain *A. baumannii* strains with a selective advantage in the ICU environment with an extensive exposure to potent antimicrobials. The resistance rates of epidemic *A. baumannii* strains have been reported to be significantly higher compared with sporadic *A. baumannii* strains [228]. The recently observed increase in carbapenem-resistant *A. baumannii* strains was associated almost exclusively with hospital outbreaks [229]. To control the spread of *A. baumannii* in the hospital, it is necessary to identify potential reservoirs of the organism and the modes of transmission. To distinguish the outbreak strain from epidemiologically unrelated acinetobacters, molecular typing of isolates is required. For that purpose, a wide array of typing systems have been developed, including plasmid profiling, ribotyping [230], PFGE [231], RAPD analysis [232], REP-PCR [233], AFLP analysis; integrase gene PCR, infrequent-restriction-site PCR and most recently, MLST and multilocus PCR-ESI-MS [234].

The ability of multidrug-resistant *A. baumannii* to cause outbreaks has been clearly demonstrated. Only one or two strain types were identified in multiple reported outbreaks, using PFGE or PCR-based typing methods [235]. For instance, In New York City, two strain types accounted for >80% of carbapenem-resistant isolates [236]. This clearly demonstrates the importance of infection control approaches in response to outbreaks of multidrug-resistant *A. baumannii* infections. The following infection control interventions are appropriate with regard to *A. baumannii* outbreaks:

i)   Molecular epidemiologic investigations, to determine if a clonal outbreak strain is present.

ii) Environmental cultures, to determine if a common environmental source is present, which should be removed. Numerous potential sources have been identified in prior studies, including ventilator tubing, suction catheters, humidifiers, containers of distilled water, urine collection jugs, multidose vials of medication, intravenous nutrition, moist bedding articles, inadequately sterilized reusable arterial pressure transducers, and computer keyboards [236].

iii) Enhanced environmental cleaning, to eliminate the organism from the patient's environment.

iv)	Contact isolation (use of gloves and gowns) and improved hand hygiene. Cohorts of patients or staff have been also used, but patients should be preferably nursed in single rooms with dedicated personnel.

v)	Antibiotic management processes should be used to restrict the use of last-resort antibiotics. Numerous studies have assessed antibiotic risk factors for infection with multidrug-resistant *A. baumannii*, although only a few have examined risk factors for emergence of pandrug resistance. Although exposure to any antibiotic active against Gram-negative bacteria has been associated with the emergence of multidrug-resistant *A. baumannii*, broad-spectrum cephalosporins, carbapenems and fluoroquinolones have been implicated most frequently [197].

REFERENCES

[1]	Rice LB. The clinical consequences of antimicrobial resistance. Curr Opin Microbiol 2009; 12: 476-81.

[2]	Pournaras S, Iosifidis E, Roilides E. Advances in antibacterial therapy against emerging bacterial pathogens. Semin Hematol 2009; 46: 198-11.

[3]	Matlow AG, Morris SK. Control of antibiotic-resistant bacteria in the office and clinic. CMAJ 2009; 180: 1021-24.

[4]	Duckworth GJ, Lothian JL, Williams JD. Methicillin-resistant *Staphylococcus aureus*: report of an outbreak in a London teaching hospital. J Hosp Infect 1988; 11: 1-15.

[5]	Pournaras S, Slavakis A, Polyzou A, *et al.* Nosocomial spread of an unusual methicillin-resistant *Staphylococcus aureus* clone that is sensitive to all non-β-lactam antibiotics, including tobramycin. J Clin Microbiol 2001; 39: 779-81.

[6]	Nygaard TK, DeLeo FR, Voyich JM. Community-associated methicillin-resistant *Staphylococcus aureus* skin infections: advances toward identifying the key virulence factors. Curr Opin Infect Dis 2008; 21: 147-52.

[7]	Ikonomidis A, Michail G, Vasdeki A, *et al. In vitro* and *in vivo* evaluations of oxacillin efficiency against mecA-positive oxacillin-susceptible *Staphylococcus aureus*. Antimicrob Agents Chemother 2008; 52: 3905-08.

[8]	Clinical and Laboratory Standards Institute. Methods for dilution antimicrobial susceptibility tests for bacteria that grow aerobically. 9th ed. CLSI approved standard M7-A7: CLSI; 2009.

[9]	de Lencastre H, Oliveira D, Tomasz A. Antibiotic resistant Staphylococcus aureus: a paradigm of adaptive power. Curr Opin Microbiol 2007; 10: 428-35.

[10]	Daum RS, Ito T, Hiramatsu K, *et al.* A novel methicillin-resistance cassette in community-acquired methicillin-resistant Staphylococcus aureus isolates of diverse genetic backgrounds. J Infect Dis 2002; 186: 1344-47.

[11]	Ito T, Ma XX, Takeuchi F, *et al.* Novel type V staphylococcal cassette chromosome mec driven by a novel cassette chromosome recombinase, *ccrC*. Antimicrob Agents Chemother 2004; 48: 2637-51.

[12]	Chambers HF, Sachdeva M. Binding of β-lactam antibiotics to penicillin-binding proteins in methicillinresistant *Staphylococcus aureus*. J Infect Dis 1990; 161: 1170-76.

[13]	Brown DF, Edwards DI, Hawkey PM. Guidelines for the laboratory diagnosis and susceptibility testing of methicillin-resistant *Staphylococcus aureus* (MRSA). J Antimicrob Chemother 2005; 56: 1000-18.

[14]	Grisold AJ, Leitner E, Mühlbauer G, *et al.* Detection of methicillin-resistant *Staphylococcus aureus* and simultaneous confirmation by automated nucleic acid extraction and real-time PCR. J Clin Microbiol 2002; 40: 2392-7.

[15]	Safdar N, Narans L, Gordon B, *et al.* Comparison of culture screening methods for detection of nasal carriage of methicillin-resistant *Staphylococcus aureus*: a prospective study comparing 32 methods. J Clin Microbiol 2003; 41: 3163-66.

[16]	Davies S, Zadik PM, Mason CM, *et al.* Methicillin-resistant *Staphylococcus aureus*: evaluation of five selective media. Br J Biomed Sci 2000; 57: 269-72.

[17]	Perry JD, Davies A, Butterworth LA, *et al.* Development and evaluation of a chromogenic agar medium for methicillin-resistant *Staphylococcus aureus*. J Clin Microbiol 2004; 42: 4519-23.

[18]	Starleton PD, Taylor P. Methicillin resistance in *Staphylococcus aureus*: mechanisms and modulation. Sci Prog 2002; 85: 57-72.

[19]   Tenover FC, Moellering RCJr. The rationale for revising the Clinical and Laboratory Standards Institute vancomycin minimal inhibitory concentration interpretive criteria for *Staphylococcus aureus*. Clin Infect Dis 2007; 44: 1208-15.

[20]   Wunderink RG, Rello J, Cammarata SK, *et al.* Linezolid *vs* vancomycin: analysis of two double-blind studies of patients with methicillin-resistant *Staphylococcus aureus* nosocomial pneumonia. Chest 2003; 124: 1789-97.

[21]   Bartlett JG. Methicillin-resistant *Staphylococcus aureus* infections, Top HIV Med 2008; 16: 151-55.

[22]   Batra R, Eziefula AC, Wyncoll D, *et al.* Throat and rectal swabs may have an important role in MRSA screening of critically ill patients. Intensive Care Med 2008; 34: 1703-06.

[23]   Safdar N, Bradley EA. The risk of infection after nasal colonization with *Staphylococcus aureus*. Am J Med 2008; 12: 310-15.

[24]   Ellis MW, Griffith ME, Dooley DP, *et al.* Targeted intranasal mupirocin to prevent colonization and infection by community-associated methicillin- resistant *Staphylococcus aureus* strains in soldiers: a cluster randomized controlled trial. Antimicrob Agents Chemother 2007; 51: 3591-98.

[25]   Cooper BS, Stone SP, Kibbler CC, *et al.* Isolation measures in the hospital management of methicillin resistant *Staphylococcus aureus* (MRSA): systematic review of the literature. BMJ 2004; 329: 533-38.

[26]   McGinigle KL, Gourlay ML, Buchanan IB. The use of active surveillance cultures in adult intensive care units to reduce methicillin-resistant *Staphylococcus aureus*-related morbidity, mortality, and costs: a systematic review. Clin Infect Dis 2008; 46: 1717-25.

[27]   Clancy M, Graepler A, Wilson M, *et al.* Active screening in high-risk units is an effective and cost-avoidant method to reduce the rate of methicillin-resistant *Staphylococcus aureus* infection in the hospital. Infect Control Hosp Epidemiol 2006; 27: 1009-17.

[28]   Nijssen S, Bonten MJ, Weinstein RA. Are active microbiological surveillance and subsequent isolation needed to prevent the spread of methicillin-resistant *Staphylococcus aureus*? Clin Infect Dis 2005; 40: 405-09.

[29]   Simpson AH, Dave J, Cookson B. The value of routine screening of staff for MRSA. J Bone Joint Surg Br 2007; 89: 565-66.

[30]   Tacconelli E. Methicillin-resistant *Staphylococcus aureus:* source control and surveillance organization. Clin Microbiol Infect 2009; 15: 31-38.

[31]   Haley CC, Mittal D, Laviolette A, *et al.* Methicillin-resistant *Staphylococcus aureus* infection or colonization present at hospital admission: multivariable risk factor screening to increase efficiency of surveillance culturing. J Clin Microbiol 2007; 45: 3031-38.

[32]   Bootsma MC, Diekmann O, Bonten MJ. Controlling methicillin-resistant *Staphylococcus aureus*: quantifying the effects of interventions and rapid diagnostic testing. Proc Natl Acad Sci 2006; 103: 5620-25.

[33]   Larsen A, Stegger M, Goering R, *et al.* Emergence and dissemination of the methicillin resistant *Staphylococcus aureus* USA300 clone in Denmark (2000-2005). Euro Surveill 2007; 12: 22-24.

[34]   Aramburu C, Harbarth S, Liassine N, *et al.* Community-acquired methicillin-resistant *Staphylococcus aureus* in Switzerland: first surveillance report. Euro Surveill 2006; 11: 42-43.

[35]   Gorwitz RJ. A review of community-associated methicillin-resistant *Staphylococcus aureus* skin and soft tissue infections. Pediatr Infect Dis J 2008; 27: 1-7.

[36]   Wiese-Posselt M, Heuck D, Draeger A, *et al.* Successful termination of a furunculosis outbreak due to lukS-lukF-positive, methicillin-susceptible *Staphylococcus aureus* in a German village by stringent decolonisation, 2002-2005. Clin Infect Dis 2007; 44: 88-95.

[37]   Navarro MB, Huttner B, Harbarth S. Methicillin-resistant *Staphylococcus aureus* control in the 21st century: beyond the acute care hospital. Curr Opin Infect Dis 2008; 21: 372-79.

[38]   Cosgrove SE, Carroll KC, Perl TM. *Staphylococcus aureus* with reduced susceptibility to vancomycin. Clin Infect Dis 2004; 39: 539-45.

[39]   Hiramatsu, K, Aritaka N, Hanaki H, *et al.* Dissemination in Japanese hospitals of strains of *Staphylococcus aureus* heterogeneously resistant to vancomycin. Lancet 1997; 350: 1670-73.

[40]   Hiramatsu, K, Hanaki H, Ino T, *et al.* Methicillin-resistant *Staphylococcus aureus* clinical strain with reduced vancomycin susceptibility. J Antimicrob Chemother 1997; 40: 135-36.

[41]   Appelbaum PC. The emergence of vancomycin-intermediate and vancomycin-resistant *Staphylococcus aureus*. Clin Microbiol Infect 2006; 12: 16-23.

[42]   Sung JM, Lindsay JA. *Staphylococcus aureus* strains that are hypersusceptible to resistance gene transfer from enterococci. Antimicrob Agents Chemother 2007; 51: 2189-91.

[43] Perichon B, Courvalin P. VanA-type vancomycin-resistant *Staphylococcus aureus*. Antimicrob Agents Chemother 2009; 53: 4580-87.

[44] Tiwari HK, Sen MR. Emergence of vancomycin resistant *Staphylococcus aureus* (VRSA) from a tertiary care hospital from northern part of India. BMC Infect Dis 2006; 6: 156.

[45] Fridkin SK, Hageman J, McDougal LK, *et al.* Epidemiological and microbiological characterization of infections caused by *Staphylococcus aureus* with reduced susceptibility to vancomycin, United States, 1997-2001. Clin Infect Dis 2003; 36: 429-39.

[46] Charles PG, Ward PB, Johnson PD, *et al.* Clinical features associated with bacteremia due to heterogeneous vancomycin-intermediate *Staphylococcus aureus*. Clin Infect Dis 2004; 38: 448-51.

[47] Lodise TP, Miller CD, Graves J, *et al.* Predictors of high vancomycin MIC values among patients with methicillin-resistant *Staphylococcus aureus* bacteraemia. J Antimicrob Chemother 2008; 62: 1138-41.

[48] Moise PA, Smyth DS, El-Fawal N, *et al.* Microbiological effects of prior vancomycin use in patients with methicillin-resistant *Staphylococcus aureus* bacteraemia. J Antimicrob Chemother 2008; 61: 85-90.

[49] Leonard SN, Rossi KL, Newton KL, *et al.* Evaluation of the Etest GRD for the detection of *Staphylococcus aureus* with reduced susceptibility to glycopeptides. J Antimicrob Chemother 2009; 63: 489-92.

[50] Swenson JM, Anderson KF, Lonsway DR, *et al.* Accuracy of commercial and reference susceptibility testing methods for detecting vancomycin-intermediate *Staphylococcus aureus*. J Clin Microbiol 2009; 47: 2013-17.

[51] Liu C, Chambers HF. *Staphylococcus aureus* with heterogeneous resistance to vancomycin: epidemiology, clinical significance, and critical assessment of diagnostic methods. Antimicrob Agents Chemother 2003; 47: 3040-45.

[52] Howden BP, Davies JK, Johnson PD, *et al.* Reduced vancomycin susceptibility in *Staphylococcus aureus*, including vancomycin intermediate and heterogeneous vancomycin-intermediate strains: resistance mechanisms, laboratory detection, and clinical implications. Clin Microbiol Rev 2010; 23: 99-139.

[53] Kola A, Kirschner P, Gohrbandt B, *et al.* An infection with linezolid-resistant *S. aureus* in a patient with left ventricular assist system. Scand J Infect Dis 2007; 39: 463-65.

[54] Tillotson GS, Draghi DC, Sahm DF, *et al.* Susceptibility of *Staphylococcus aureus* isolated from skin and wound infections in the United States 2005-07: laboratory-based surveillance study. J Antimicrob Chemother 2008; 62: 109-15.

[55] Tenover FC, Sinner SW, Segal RE, *et al.* Characterisation of a *Staphylococcus aureus* strain with progressive loss of susceptibility to vancomycin and daptomycin during therapy. Int J Antimicrob Agents 2009; 33: 564-68.

[56] Rose WE, Leonard SN, Sakoulas G, *et al.* Daptomycin activity against *Staphylococcus aureus* following vancomycin exposure in an *in vitro* pharmacodynamic model with simulated endocardial vegetations. Antimicrob Agents Chemother 2008; 52: 831-36.

[57] Leuthner KD, Cheung CM, Rybak MJ. Comparative activity of the new lipoglycopeptide telavancin in the presence and absence of serum against 50 glycopeptide non-susceptible staphylococci and three vancomycin-resistant *Staphylococcus aureus*. J Antimicrob Chemother 2006; 58: 338-43.

[58] Huang YT, Liao CH, Teng LJ, *et al.* Comparative bactericidal activities of daptomycin, glycopeptides, linezolid and tigecycline against blood isolates of Gram-positive bacteria in Taiwan. Clin Microbiol Infect 2008; 14: 124-29.

[59] de Lassence A, Hidri N, Timsit JF, *et al.* Control and outcome of a large outbreak of colonization and infection with glycopeptides intermediate *Staphylococcus aureus* in an intensive care unit. Clin Infect Dis 2006; 42: 170-78.

[60] Appelbaum PC. Reduced glycopeptide susceptibility in methicillin-resistant *Staphylococcus aureus* (MRSA). Int J Antimicrob Agents 2007; 30: 398-408.

[61] Werner G, Coque TM, Hammerum AM, *et al.* Emergence and spread of vancomycin resistance among enterococci in Europe. Euro Surveill 2008; 13: 19046.

[62] Tacconelli E, Cataldo MA. Vancomycin-resistant enterococci (VRE): transmission and control. Int J Antimicrob Agents 2008; 31: 99-106.

[63] European Antimicrobial Resistance Surveillance System. Susceptibility results for *Enterococcus faecium* isolates in 2006. Available at: http://www.rivm.nl/earss/database/

[64] Wisplinghoff H, Bischoff T, Tallent SM, *et al.* Nosocomial bloodstream infections in US hospitals: analysis of 179 cases from a prospective nationwide surveillance study. Clin Infect Dis 2004; 39: 309-17.

[65] van den Braak N, Ott A, van Belkum A, *et al.* Prevalence and determinants of fecal colonization with vancomycin-resistant *Enterococcus* in hospitalized patients in The Netherlands. Infect Control Hosp Epidemiol 2000; 21: 520-24.

[66]   Gambarotto K, Ploy MC, Turlure P, *et al.* Prevalence of vancomycin-resistant enterococci in fecal samples from hospitalized patients and non hospitalized controls in a cattle-rearing area of France. J Clin Microbiol 2000; 38: 620-24.

[67]   The European Antimicrobial Resistance Surveillance System. EARSS results. Available from: http://www.rivm.nl/earss/result/.

[68]   Brown DFJ, Hope R, Livermore DM, *et al.* Nonsusceptibility trends among enterococci and non-pnemococcal streptococci from bacteraemias in the UK and Ireland, 2001 to 2006. J Antimicrob Chemother 2008; 62: 75-85.

[69]   British Society for Antimicrobial Chemotherapy (BSAC). Resistance Surveillance Project. Available from: Http://www.bsac.org.uk/resistance_surveillance.cfm.

[70]   Maniatis AN, Pournaras S, Kanellopoulou M, *et al.* Dissemination of clonally unrelated erythromycin- and glycopeptides- resistant *Enterococcus faecium* isolates in a tertiary Greek hospital. J Clin Microbiol 2001; 39: 4571-74.

[71]   Novais C, Sousa JC, Coque TM, *et al.* Molecular characterization of glycopeptide-resistant *Enterococcus faecium* isolates from Portuguese hospitals. Antimicrob Agents Chemother 2005; 49: 3073-79.

[72]   Routsi C, Platsouka E, Willems RJ, *et al.* Detection of enterococcal surface protein gene (*esp*) and amplified fragment length polymorphism typing of glycopeptide-resistant *Enterococcus faecium* during its emergence in a Greek intensive care unit. J Clin Microbiol 2003; 41: 5742-46.

[73]   Stampone L, Del GM, Boccia D, *et al.* Clonal spread of a vancomycin-resistant *Enterococcus faecium* strain among bloodstream-infecting isolates in Italy. J Clin Microbiol 2005; 43: 1575-80.

[74]   Centers for Disease Control and Prevention. National nosocomial infections surveillance (NNIS) system report, data summary from January 1990 to May 1999. Am J Infect Control 1999; 27: 520-32.

[75]   Kauffman CA, Therapeutic and preventative options for the management of vancomycin-resistant enterococcal infections. J Antimicrob Chemother 2003; 51: 23-30.

[76]   Mascini EM, Bonten MJ. Vancomycin-resistant enterococci: consequences for therapy and infection control. Clin Microbiol Infect 2005; 4: 43-56.

[77]   Bhavnani SM, Drake JA, Forrest A, *et al.* A nationwide, multicenter, case-control study comparing risk factors, treatment, and outcome for vancomycin-resistant and - susceptible enterococcal bacteremia. Diagn Microbiol Infect Dis 2000; 36: 145-58.

[78]   Krcmery V, Bilikova E, Svetlansky I, *et al.* Is vancomycin resistance in enterococci predictive of inferior outcome of enterococcal bacteremia? Clin Infect Dis 2001; 32: 1110-12.

[79]. Murray BE. Vancomycin-resistant enterococcal infections. N Engl J Med 2000; 342: 710-21.

[80]   Descheemaker P, Ieven M, Chapelle S, *et al.* Prevalence and molecular epidemiology of glycopeptide-resistant enterococci in Belgian renal dialysis units. J Infect Dis 2000; 181: 235-41.

[81]   Von Gottberg A, Van Nierop W, Duse A, *et al.* Epidemiology of glycopeptide-resistant enterococci colonizing high-risk patients in hospitals in Johannesburg, Republic of South Africa. J Clin Microbiol 2000; 38: 905-09.

[82]   Manson JM, Keis S, Smith JMB, *et al.* Clonal lineage of vanA-type *Enterococcus faecalis* predominates in vancomycin-resistant enterococci isolated in New Zealand. Antimicrob Agents Chemother 2003; 47: 204-10.

[83]   Lai KK, Fontecchio SA, Kelley AL, *et al.* The changing epidemiology of vancomycin-resistant enterococci. Infect Control Hosp Epidemiol 2003; 24: 264-68.

[84]   Fines M, Perichon B, Reynolds P, *et al.* VanE, a new type of acquired glycopeptide resistance in *Enterococcus faecalis* BM4405. Antimicrob Agents Chemother 1999; 43: 2161-64.

[85]   Cetinkaya Y, Falk PS, Mayhall CG. Effect of gastrointestinal bleeding and oral medications on acquisition of vancomycin-resistant *Enterococcus faecium* in hospitalized patients. Clin Infect Dis 2002; 35: 935-42.

[86]   Quintiliani R Jr, Courvalin P. Conjugal transfer of the vancomycin resistance determinant *vanB* between enterococci involves the movement of large genetic elements from chromosome to chromosome. FEMS Microbiol Lett 1994; 119: 359-63.

[87]   D'Agatha EMC, Gautam S, Green WK, *et al.* High rate of false-negative results of the rectal swab culture method in detection of gastrointestinal colonization with vancomycin-resistant enterococci. Clin Infect Dis 2002; 34: 167-72.

[88]   Donskey CJ, Hume ME, Callaway TR, *et al.* Inhibition of vancomycin-resistant enterococci by an *in vitro* continuous-flow competitive exclusion culture containing human stool flora. J Infect Dis 2001; 184: 1624-27.

[89]   Reisner BS, Shaw S, Huber ME, *et al.* Comparison of three methods to recover vancomycin-resistant enterococci (VRE) from perianal and environmental samples collected during a hospital outbreak of VRE. Infect Control Hosp Epidemiol 2000; 21: 775-79.

[90]   Ricaurte JC, Boucher HW, Turett GS, *et al.* Chloramphenicol treatment for vancomycin-resistant *Enterococcus faecium* bacteremia. Clin Microbiol Infect 2001; 7: 17-21.

[91]   Chien JW, Kucia ML, Salata RA. Use of linezolid, an oxazolidinone, in the treatment of multi-drug resistant Gram-positive bacterial infections. Clin Infect Dis 2000; 30: 146-51.

[92]   Diekema DJ, Jones RN. Oxazolidinone antibiotics. Lancet 2001; 358:1975-82.

[93]   Babcock HM, Ritchie DJ, Christiansen E, Starlin R, Little R, Stanley S. Successful treatment of vancomycin-resistant *Enterococcus* endocarditis with oral linezolid. Clin Infect Dis 2001; 32: 1373-75.

[94]   Green SL, Maddox JC, Huttenbach ED. Linezolid and reversible myelosuppression. JAMA 2001; 285: 1291.

[95]   Attassi K, Hershberger E, Alam R, *et al.* Thrombocytopenia associated with linezolid therapy. Clin Infect Dis 2002; 34: 695-98.

[96]   Scheetz MH, Knechtel SA, Malczynski M, *et al.* Increasing incidence of linezolid-intermediate or -resistant, vancomycin-resistant *Enterococcus faecium* strains parallels increasing linezolid consumption. Antimicrob Agents Chemother 2008; 52: 2256-59.

[97]   Gales AC, Jones RN. Antimicrobial activity and spectrum of the new glycylcycline, GAR-936 tested against 1,203 recent clinical bacterial isolates. Diagn Microbiol Infect Dis 2000; 36: 19-36.

[98]   Hachem R, Raad I. Failure of oral antimicrobial agents in eradicating gastrointestinal colonization with vancomycin-resistant enterococci. Infect Control Hosp Epidemiol 2002; 23: 43-44.

[99]   Diaz-Granados CA, Jernigan JA. Impact of vancomycin resistance on mortality among patients with neutropenia and enterococcal bloodstream infection. J Infect Dis 2005; 191: 588-95.

[100] Mondy KE, Shannon W, Mundy LM. Evaluation of zinc bacitracin capsules *vs* placebo for enteric eradication of vancomycin-resistant *Enterococcus faecium*. Clin Infect Dis 2001; 33: 473-76.

[101] Baden LR, Thiemke W, Skolnik A, *et al.* Prolonged colonization with vancomycin-resistant *Enterococcus faecium* in long-term care patients and the significance of "clearance". Clin Infect Dis 2001; 33: 1654-60.

[102] Montecalvo MA, Jarvis WR, Uman J, *et al.* Infection-control measures reduce transmission of vancomycin-resistant enterococci in an endemic setting. Ann Intern Med 1999; 131: 269-72.

[103] Lai KK, Kelley AL, Melvin ZS, *et al.* Failure to eradicate vancomycin-resistant enterococci in a university hospital and the cost of barrier precautions. Infect Control Hosp Epidemiol 1998; 19: 647-52.

[104] Weber DJ, Rutala WA. Role of environmental contamination in the transmission of vancomycin-resistant enterococci. Infect Control Hosp Epidemiol 1997; 18: 306-09.

[105] Bonten MJ, Hayden MK, Nathan C, *et al.* Epidemiology of colonisation of patients and environment with vancomycin-resistant enterococci. Lancet 1996; 348: 1615-19.

[106] Ostrowsky BE, Trick WE, Sohn AH, *et al.* Control of vancomycin-resistant enterococcus in health care facilities in a region. N Engl J Med 2001; 344: 1427-33.

[107] Montecalvo MA, Jarvis WR, Uman J, *et al.* Costs and savings associated with infection control measures that reduced transmission of vancomycin-resistant enterococci in an endemic setting. Infect Control Hosp Epidemiol 2001; 22: 437-42.

[108] Fridkin SK, Lawton R, Edwards JR, *et al.* Monitoring antimicrobial use and resistance: comparison with a national benchmark on reducing vancomycin use and vancomycin-resistant enterococci. Emerg Infect Dis 2002; 8: 702-07.

[109] Lautenbach E, LaRosa LA, Marr AM, *et al.* Changes in the prevalence of vancomycin- resistant enterococci in response to antimicrobial formulary interventions: impact of progressive restrictions on use of vancomycin and third-generation cephalosporins. Clin Infect Dis 2003; 36: 440-46.

[110] Centers for Disease Control and Prevention (CDC). Guidance for control of infections with carbapenem-resistant or carbapenemase-producing *Enterobacteriaceae* in acute care facilities. MMWR Morb Mortal Wkly Rep 2009; 58: 256-60.

[111] Paterson DL, Bonomo RA. Extended-spectrum β-lactamases: a clinical update. Clin Microbiol Rev 2005; 18: 657-86.

[112] Canton R, Coque TM. The CTX-M β-lactamase pandemic. Curr Opin Microbiol 2006; 9: 466-75.

[113] Coque TM, Baquero F, Canton R. Increasing prevalence of ESBL-producing *Enterobacteriaceae* in Europe. Euro Surveill 2008; 13: 19044.

[114] Oteo J, Navarro C, Cercenado E, *et al.* Spread of *Escherichia coli* strains with high-level cefotaxime and ceftazidime resistance between the community, long-term care facilities, and hospital institutions. J Clin Microbiol 2006; 44: 2359-66.

[115] Mendonca N, Leitao J, Manageiro V, *et al.* Spread of extended-spectrum β-lactamase CTX-M-producing *Escherichia coli* clinical isolates in community and nosocomial environments in Portugal. Antimicrob Agents Chemother 2007; 51: 1946-55.

[116] Valverde A, Grill F, Coque TM, *et al.* High rate of intestinal colonization with extended-spectrum-β-lactamase-producing organisms in household contacts of infected community patients. J Clin Microbiol 2008; 46: 2796-99.

[117] Mugnaioli C, Luzzaro F, De Luca F, *et al.* CTX-M-type extended-spectrum β-lactamases in Italy: molecular epidemiology of an emerging countrywide problem. Antimicrob Agents Chemother 2006; 50: 2700-06.

[118] Carattoli A, Garcia-Fernandez A, Varesi P, *et al.* Molecular epidemiology of *Escherichia coli* producing extended-spectrum β-lactamases isolated in Rome, Italy. J Clin Microbiol 2008; 46: 103-08.

[119] Caccamo M, Perilli M, Celenza G, *et al.* Occurrence of extended spectrum β-lactamases among isolates of *Enterobacteriaceae* from urinary tract infections in southern Italy. Microb Drug Resist 2006; 12: 257-64.

[120] Galas M, Decousser JW, Breton N, *et al.* Nationwide study of the prevalence, characteristics, and molecular epidemiology of extended-spectrum-β-lactamase producing *Enterobacteriaceae* in France. Antimicrob Agents Chemother 2008; 52: 786-89.

[121] Livermore DM, Canton R, Gniadkowski M, *et al.* CTX-M: changing the face of ESBLs in Europe. J Antimicrob Chemother 2007; 59: 165-67.

[122] Bush K. Extended-spectrum β-lactamases in North America, 1987-2006. Clin Microbiol Infect 2008; 14: 134-43.

[123] McGettigan SE, Hu B, Andreacchio K, *et al.* Prevalence of CTX-M β-lactamases in Philadelphia, Pennsylvania. J Clin Microbiol 2009; 47: 2970-74.

[124] Ko WC, Hsueh PR. Increasing extended-spectrum β-lactamase production and quinolone resistance among Gram-negative bacilli causing intra-abdominal infections in the Asia/Pacific region: data from the Smart Study 2002-2006. J Infect 2009; 59: 95-103.

[125] Lo WU, Ho PL, Chow KH, *et al.* Faecal carriage of CTX-M- type extended-spectrum β-lactamase-producing organisms by children and their household contacts. J Infect 2010; 60: 286-92.

[126] Deshpande LM, Jones RN, Fritsche TR, *et al.* Occurrence and characterization of carbapenemase-producing *Enterobacteriaceae*: report from the SENTRY antimicrobial surveillance proGram (2000-2004). Microb Drug Resist 2006; 12: 223-30.

[127] Nordmann P, Cuzon G, Naas T. The real threat of *Klebsiella pneumoniae* carbapenemase-producing bacteria. Lancet Infect Dis 2009; 9: 228-36.

[128] Vatopoulos A. High rates of metallo-β-lactamase-producing *Klebsiella pneumoniae* in Greece- a review of the current evidence. Euro Surveill 2008; 13: 8023.

[129] Poirel L, Naas T, Nicolas D, *et al.* Characterization of VIM-2, a carbapenem-hydrolyzing metallo-β-lactamase and its plasmid- and integron-borne gene from a *Pseudomonas aeruginosa* clinical isolate in France. Antimicrob. Antimicrob Agents Chemother 2000; 44: 891-97.

[130] Pournaras S, Maniati M, Petinaki E, *et al.* Hospital outbreak of multiple clones of *Pseudomonas aeruginosa* carrying the unrelated metallo-β-lactamase gene variants bla_{VIM-2} and bla_{VIM-4}. J Antimicrob Chemother 2003; 51: 1409-14.

[131] Ikonomidis A, Tokatlidou D, Kristo I, *et al.* Outbreaks in distinct regions due to a single *Klebsiella pneumoniae* clone carrying bla_{VIM-1} metallo-β-lactamase gene. J Clin Microbiol 2005; 43: 5344-47.

[132] Canton R, Novais A, Valverde A, *et al.* Prevalence and spread of extended-spectrum β-lactamase-producing Enterobacteriaceae in Europe. Clin Microbiol Infect 2008; 14: 144-53.

[133] Morosini MI, Garcva-Castillo M, Coque TM, *et al.* Antibiotic co-resistance in extended-spectrum-β-lactamase-producing *Enterobacteriaceae* and *in vitro* activity of tigecycline. Antimicrob Agents Chemother 2006; 50: 2695-99.

[134] Pitout JD. Infections with extended-spectrum β-lactamase-producing *Enterobacteriaceae*: changing epidemiology and drug treatment choices. Drugs 2010; 70: 313-33.

[135] Schwaber MJ, Klarfeld-Lidji S, Navon-Venezia S, *et al.* Predictors of carbapenem-resistant *Klebsiella pneumoniae* acquisition among hospitalized adults and effect of acquisition on mortality. Antimicrob Agents Chemother 2008; 52: 1028-33.

[136] Patel G, Huprikar S, Factor SH, *et al.* Outcomes of carbapenem-resistant *Klebsiella pneumoniae* infection and the impact of antimicrobial and adjunctive therapies. Infect Control Hosp Epidemiol 2008; 29: 1099-106.

[137] Woodford N, Tierno PM Jr, Young K, *et al.* Outbreak of *Klebsiella pneumoniae* producing a new carbapenem-hydrolyzing class A β-lactamase, KPC-3, in a New York medical center. Antimicrob Agents Chemother 2004; 48: 4793-99.

[138] Carmeli Y, Akova M, Cornaglia G, *et al.* Controlling the spread of carbapenemase-producing Gram-negatives: therapeutic approach and infection control. Clin Microbiol Infect 2010; 16: 102-11.

[139] Souli M, Galani I, Antoniadou A, *et al.* An outbreak of KPC-2-producing *Klebsiella pneumoniae* in a Greek university hospital: molecular characterization, epidemiology and outcomes. Clin Infect Dis. 2010; 50: 364-73.

[140] Maltezou HC, Giakkoupi P, Maragos A, *et al.* Outbreak of infections due to KPC-2-producing *Klebsiella pneumoniae* in a hospital in Crete (Greece). J Infect 2009; 58: 213-19.

[141] Nordmann P, Poirel L. Emergence of plasmid-mediated resistance to quinolones in *Enterobacteriaceae.* J Antimicrob Chemother 2005; 56: 463-69.

[142] Cattoir V, Poirel L, Nordmann P. Plasmid-mediated quinolone resistance pump QepA2 in an *Escherichia coli* isolate from France. Antimicrob Agents Chemother 2008; 52: 3801-04.

[143] Jones GL, Warren RE, Skidmore SJ, *et al.* Prevalence and distribution of plasmid-mediated quinolone resistance genes in clinical isolates of *Escherichia coli* lacking extended-spectrum β-lactamases. J Antimicrob Chemother 2008; 62: 1245-51.

[144] Novais A, Canton R, Valverde A, *et al.* Dissemination and persistence of $bla_{CTX-M-9}$ are linked to class 1 integrons containing CR1 associated with defective transposon derivatives from Tn402 located in early antibiotic resistance plasmids of IncHI2, IncP1-alpha, and IncFI groups. Antimicrob Agents Chemother 2006; 50: 2741-50.

[145] Machado E, Ferreira J, Novais A, *et al.* Preservation of integron types among *Enterobacteriaceae* producing extended-spectrum β-lactamases in a Spanish hospital over a 15-year period (1988 to 2003). Antimicrob Agents Chemother 2007; 51: 2201-04.

[146] Sunde M, Tharaldsen H, Slettemeas JS, *et al. Escherichia coli* of animal origin in Norway contains a bla_{TEM-20}-carrying plasmid closely related to bla_{TEM-20} and bla_{TEM-52} plasmids from other European countries. J Antimicrob Chemother 2009; 63: 215-16.

[147] Enne VI, Delsol AA, Roe JM, *et al.* Evidence of antibiotic resistance gene silencing in *Escherichia coli.* Antimicrob Agents Chemother 2006; 50: 3003-10.

[148] Clinical and Laboratory Standards Institute. Performance standards for antimicrobial susceptibility testing, 19th informational supplement. M100-S19. 2009. Clinical and Laboratory Standards Institute, Wayne, PA.

[149] Franklin C, Liolios L, Peleg AY. Phenotypic detection of carbapenems susceptible metallo-β-lactamase-producing Gram-negative bacilli in the clinical laboratory. J Clin Microbiol 2006; 44: 3139-44.

[150] Tsakris A, Kristo I, Poulou A, *et al.* Evaluation of boronic acid disk tests for differentiating KPC-possessing *Klebsiella pneumoniae* isolates in the clinical laboratory. J Clin Microbiol 2009; 47: 362-67.

[151] Pournaras S, Poulou A, Tsakris A. Inhibitor-based methods for the detection of KPC carbapenemase-producing *Enterobacteriaceae* in clinical practice by using boronic acid compounds. J Antimicrob Chemother 2010; 65: 1319-21.

[152] Pournaras S, Poulou A, Voulgari E, *et al.* Detection of the new metallo-β-lactamase VIM-19 along with KPC-2, CMY-2 and CTX-M-15 in *Klebsiella pneumoniae.* J Antimicrob Chemother 2010 Jun 3 [Epub ahead of print]

[153] Giakkoupi P, Pappa O, Polemis M, *et al.* Emerging *Klebsiella pneumoniae* isolates co-producing KPC-2 and VIM-1 carbapenemases. Antimicrob Agents Chemother 2009; 53: 4048-50.

[154] Driscoll JA, Brody SL, Kollef MH. The epidemiology, pathogenesis and treatment of *Pseudomonas aeruginosa* infections. Drugs 2007; 67: 351-68.

[155] Giamarellou H, Kanellakopoulou K. Current therapies for *Pseudomonas aeruginosa.* Crit Care Clin 2008; 24: 261-78.

[156] Livermore DM. Multiple mechanisms of antimicrobial resistance in *Pseudomonas aeruginosa*: our worst nightmare? Clin Infect Dis 2002; 34: 634-40.

[157] Souli M, Galani I, Giamarellou H. Emergence of extensively drug - resistant and pandrug - resistant Gram - negative bacilli in Europe. Euro Surveill 2008; 20: 13: 19045.

[158] Navon-Venezia S, Ben-Ami R, Carmeli Y. Update on *Pseudomonas aeruginosa* and *Acinetobacter baumannii* infections in the healthcare setting. Curr Opin Infect Dis 2005; 18: 306-13.

[159] Gaynes R, Edwards JR, National Nosocomial Infections Surveillance System. Overview of nosocomial infections caused by Gram-negative bacilli. Clin Infect Dis 2005; 41: 848-54.

[160] Erol S, Altoparlak U, Akcay MN, *et al.* Changes of microbial flora and wound colonization in burned patients. Bums 2004; 30: 357-61.

[161] Weiss CA 3rd, Statz CL, Dahms RA, *et al.* Six years of surgical wound infection surveillance at a tertiary care center: review of the microbiologic and epidemiological aspects of 20,007 wounds. Arch Surg 1999; 134: 1041-48.

[162] Harbarth S, Ferriere K, Hugonnet S, *et al.* Epidemiology and prognostic determinants of bloodstream infections in surgical intensive care. Arch Surg 2002; 137: 1353-59.

[163] Lee WI, Jaing TH, Hsieh MY, *et al.* Distribution, infections, treatments and molecular analysis in a large cohort of patients with primary immunodeficiency diseases (PIDs) in Taiwan. J Clin Immunol 2006; 26: 274-83.

[164] Livermore DM. Of pseudomonas, porins, pumps and carbapenems. J Antimicrob Chemother 2001; 47: 247-50.

[165] Mesaros N, Nordmann P, Plesiat P. *Pseudomonas aeruginosa*: resistance and therapeutic options at the turn of the new millenium. Clin Microbiol Infect 2007; 13: 560-78.

[166] Livermore DM. Penicillin-binding proteins, porins and outer-membrane permeability of carbenicillin-resistant and -susceptible strains of *Pseudomonas aeruginosa*. J Med Microbiol 1984; 18: 261-70.

[167] Queenan AM, Bush K. Carbapenemases: the versatile β-lactamases. Clin Microbiol Rev 2007; 20: 440-58.

[168] Nordmann P, Guibert M. Extended-spectrum β-lactamases in *Pseudomonas aeruginosa*. J Antimicrob Chemother 1998; 42: 128-31.

[169] Pechere JC, Kohler T. Patterns and modes of β-lactam resistance in *Pseudomonas aeruginosa*. Clin Microbiol Infect 1999; 5: 15-18.

[170] Livermore, DM. b-lactamases in laboratory and clinical resistance. Clin Microbiol Rev 1995; 8: 557-84.

[171] Bert F, Branger C, Lambert-Zechovsky N. Identification of PSE and OXA β-lactamase genes in *Pseudomonas aeruginosa* using PCR-restriction fragment length polymorphism. J Antimicrob Chemother 2002; 50: 11-18.

[172] Strateva T, Yordanov D. *Pseudomonas aeruginosa* - a phenomenon of bacterial resistance. J Med Microbiol 2009; 58: 1133-48.

[173] Yong D, Lee K, Yum JH, *et al.* Imipenem-EDTA disk method for differentiation of metallo-β-lactamase-producing clinical isolates of *Pseudomonas spp.* and *Acinetobacter spp.* J Clin Microbiol 2002; 40: 3798-801.

[174] Lee K, Lim YS, Yong D, *et al.* Evaluation of the Hodge test and the imipenem-EDTA double-disk synergy test for differentiating metallo-β-lactamase-producing isolates of *Pseudomonas spp.* and *Acinetobacter spp.* J Clin Microbiol 2003; 41: 4623-29.

[175] Kimura S, Ishii Y, Yamaguchi K. Evaluation of dipicolinic acid for detection of IMP- or VIM-type metallo-β-lactamase-producing *Pseudomonas aeruginosa* clinical isolates. Diagn Microbiol Infect 2005; 53: 241-44.

[176] Giakkoupi P, Vourli S, Polemis M, *et al.* Supplementation of growth media with Zn^{2+} facilitates detection of VIM-2-producing *Pseudomonas aeruginosa*. J Clin Microbiol 2008; 46: 1568-69.

[177] Walsh TR, Bolmstrom A, Qwarnstrom A, *et al.* Evaluation of a new Etest for detecting metallo-β-lactamases in routine clinical testing. J Clin Microbiol 2002; 40: 2755-59.

[178] Chu YW, Cheung TK, Ngan JY, *et al.* EDTA susceptibility leading to false detection of metallo-β-lactamase in *Pseudomonas aeruginosa* by Etest and an imipenem-EDTA disk method. Int J Antimicrob Agents 2005; 26: 340-41.

[179] Ratkai C, Quinteira S, Grosso F, *et al.* Controlling for false positives: interpreting MBL Etest and MBL combined disc test for the detection of metallo-β-lactamases. J Antimicrob Chemother 2009; 64: 657-58.

[180] Samuelsen O, Buaro L, Giske CG, *et al.* Evaluation of phenotypic tests for the detection of metallo-β-lactamase-producing *Pseudomonas aeruginosa* in a low prevalence country. J Antimicrob Chemother 2008; 61: 827-30.

[181] Miriagou V, Cornaglia G, Edelstein M, *et al.* Acquired carbapenemases in Gram-negative bacterial pathogens: detection and surveillance issues. Clin Microbiol Infect 2010; 16: 112-22.

[182] Rossolini GM, Mantengoli E. Treatment and control of severe infections caused by multiresistant *Pseudomonas aeruginosa*. Clin Microbiol Infect 2005; 4:17-32.

[183] Gales AC, Reis AO, Jones RN. Contemporary assessment of antimicrobial susceptibility testing methods for polymyxin B and colistin: review of available interpretative criteria and quality control guidelines. J Clin Microbiol 2001; 39: 183-90.

[184] Lutz F, Xiong G, Jungblut R, *et al.* Pore-forming cytotoxin of *Pseudomonas aeruginosa*: the molecular effects and aspects of pathogenicity. Antibiot Chemother 1991; 44: 54-58.

[185] Ikonomidis A, Tsakris A, Kantzanou M, *et al.* Efflux systems overexpression and decreased OprD contribute to the carbapenem heterogeneous growth in *Pseudomonas aeruginosa*. FEMS Microbiol Lett 2008; 279: 36-39.

[186] Juan C, Macia MD, Gutierrez O, *et al.* Molecular mechanisms of β-lactam resistance mediated by AmpC hyperproduction in *Pseudomonas aeruginosa* clinical strains. Antimicrob Agents Chemother 2005; 49: 4733-38.

[187] Lister PD, Wolter DJ, Wickman PA, *et al.* Levofloxacin/imipenem prevents the emergence of high-level resistance among *Pseudomonas aeruginosa* strains already lacking susceptibility to one or both drugs. J Antimicrob Chemother 2006; 57: 999-1003.

[188] Lister PD, Wolter DJ, Hanson ND. Antibacterial-Resistant *Pseudomonas aeruginosa*: Clinical impact and complex regulation of chromosomally encoded resistance mechanisms. Clin Microbiol Rev 2009; 22: 582-610.

[189] Lee NY, Lee HC, Ko NY, *et al.* Clinical and economic impact of multidrug resistance in nosocomial *Acinetobacter baumannii* bacteremia. Infect Control Hosp Epidemiol 2007; 28: 713-19.

[190] Chan PC, Huang LM, Lin HC, *et al.* Control of an outbreak of pandrug-resistant *Acinetobacter baumannii* colonization and infection in a neonatal intensive care unit. Infect Control Hosp Epidemiol 2007; 28: 423-29.

[191] Van Looveren M, Goossens H. Antimicrobial resistance of *Acinetobacter* spp. in Europe. Clin Microbiol Infect 2004; 10: 684-704.

[192] Fournier PE, Richet H. The epidemiology and control of *Acinetobacter baumannii* in health care facilities. Clin Infect Dis 2006; 42: 692-99.

[193] Coelho JM, Turton JF, Kaufmann ME, *et al.* Occurrence of carbapenem-resistant *Acinetobacter baumannii* clones at multiple hospitals in London and Southeast England. J Clin Microbiol 2006; 44: 3623-27.

[194] Naas T, Coignard B, Carbonne A, *et al.* VEB-1 extended-spectrum β-lactamase-producing *Acinetobacter baumannii*, France. Emerg Infect Dis 2006; 12: 1214-22.

[195] Nemec A, Dijkshoorn L, Van der Reijden TJ. Long-term predominance of two pan-European clones among multi-resistant *Acinetobacter baumannii* strains in the Czech Republic. J Med Microbiol 2004; 53: 147- 53.

[196] Wroblewska MM, Towner KJ, Marchel H, *et al.* Emergence and spread of carbapenem-resistant strains of *Acinetobacter baumannii* in a tertiary-care hospital in Poland. Clin Microbiol Infect 2007; 13: 490-96.

[197] Peleg AY, Seifert H, Paterson DL. *Acinetobacter baumannii*: emergence of a successful pathogen. Clin Microbiol Rev 2008; 21: 538-82.

[198] Maniatis AN, Pournaras S, Orkopoulou S, *et al.* Multi-resistant *Acinetobacter baumannii* isolates in intensive care units in Greece. Clin Microbiol Infect 2003; 9: 547-53.

[199] Tsakris A, Tsioni C, Pournaras S, *et al.* Spread of low-level carbapenem-resistant *Acinetobacter baumannii* clones in a tertiary care Greek hospital. J Antimicrob Chemother 2003; 52: 1046-47.

[200] Pournaras S, Markogiannakis A, Ikonomidis A, *et al.* Outbreak of multiple clones of imipenem-resistant *Acinetobacter baumannii* isolates expressing OXA-58 carbapenemase in an intensive care unit. J Antimicrob Chemother 2006; 57: 557-61.

[201] Gaynes R, Edwards JR. Overview of nosocomial infections caused by Gram-negative bacilli. Clin Infect Dis 2005; 41: 848-54.

[202] Landman, D, Bratu S, Kochar S, *et al.* Evolution of antimicrobial resistance among *Pseudomonas aeruginosa*, *Acinetobacter baumannii* and *Klebsiella pneumoniae* in Brooklyn, N.Y. J Antimicrob Chemother 2007; 60: 78-82.

[203] Scott P, Deye G, Srinivasan A, *et al.* An outbreak of multidrug-resistant *Acinetobacter baumannii-calcoaceticus* complex infection in the US military health care system associated with military operations in Iraq. Clin Infect Dis 2007; 44: 1577-84.

[204] Turton JF, Kaufmann ME, Gill MJ, *et al.* Comparison of *Acinetobacter baumannii* isolates from the United Kingdom and the United States that were associated with repatriated casualties of the Iraq conflict. J Clin Microbiol 2006; 44: 2630-44.

[205] Palabiyikoglu I, Tekeli E, Cokca F, *et al.* Nosocomial meningitis in a university hospital between 1993 and 2002. J Hosp Infect 2006; 62: 94-97.

[206] Perez F, Hujer AM, Hujer KM, *et al.* Global challenge of multidrug-resistant *Acinetobacter baumannii*. Antimicrob Agents Chemother 2006; 51: 3471-84.

[207] Ruiz M, Marti S, Fernandez-Cuenca F, *et al.* Prevalence of IS (*Aba1*) in epidemiologically unrelated *Acinetobacter baumannii* clinical isolates. FEMS Microbiol Lett 2007; 274: 63-66.

[208] Garcia-Penuela, E, Aznar E, Alarcon T, *et al.* Susceptibility pattern of *Acinetobacter baumannii* clinical isolates in Madrid *vs* Hong Kong. Rev Esp Quimioter 2006; 19: 45-50.

[209] Corvec S, Poirel L, Naas T, *et al.* Genetics and expression of the carbapenem-hydrolyzing oxacillinase gene bla_{OXA-23} in *Acinetobacter baumannii*. Antimicrob Agents Chemother 2007; 51: 1530-33.

[210] Valenzuela JK, Thomas L, Partridge SR, *et al*. Horizontal gene transfer in a polyclonal outbreak of carbapenem-resistant *Acinetobacter baumannii*. J Clin Microbiol 2007; 45: 453-60.

[211] Brown S, Amyes S. OXA (β)-lactamases in *Acinetobacter*: the story so far. J Antimicrob Chemother 2006; 57: 1-3.

[212] Giordano, A, Varesi P, Bertini A, *et al*. Outbreak of *Acinetobacter baumannii* producing the carbapenem-hydrolyzing oxacillinase OXA-58 in Rome, Italy. Microb Drug Resist 2007; 13: 37-43.

[213] Poirel L, Marque S, Heritier C, *et al*. OXA-58, a novel class D β-lactamase involved in resistance to carbapenems in *Acinetobacter baumannii*. Antimicrob Agents Chemother 2005; 49: 202-08.

[214] Tsakris A, Ikonomidis A, Pournaras S, *et al*. Carriage of OXA-58 but not of OXA-51 correlates with carbapenem resistance in *Acinetobacter baumannii*. J Antimicrob Chemother 2006; 58: 1097-99.

[215] Coelho J, Woodford N, Afzal-Shah M, *et al*. Occurrence of OXA-58-like carbapenemases in *Acinetobacter* spp. collected over 10 years in three continents. Antimicrob Agents Chemother 2006; 50: 756-58.

[216] Sader HS, Castanheira M, Mendes RE, *et al*. Dissemination and diversity of metallo-β-lactamases in Latin America: report from the SENTRY Antimicrobial Surveillance ProGram. Int J Antimicrob Agents 2005; 25: 57-61.

[217] Tsakris A, Ikonomidis A, Pournaras S, *et al*. VIM-1 Metallo-β-lactamase in *Acinetobacter baumannii*. Emerg Infect Dis 2006; 12: 981-83.

[218] Lee K, Yum JH, Yong D, *et al*. Novel acquired metallo-β-lactamase gene, $bla_{(SIM-1)}$, in a class 1 integron from *Acinetobacter baumannii* clinical isolates from Korea. Antimicrob Agents Chemother 2005; 49: 4485-91.

[219] Siroy A, Cosette P, Seyer D, *et al*. Global comparison of the membrane subproteomes between a multidrug-resistant *Acinetobacter baumannii* strain and a reference strain. J Proteome Res 2006; 5: 3385-98.

[220] Heritier C, Poirel L, Lambert T, *et al*. Contribution of acquired carbapenem-hydrolyzing oxacillinases to carbapenem resistance in *Acinetobacter baumannii*. Antimicrob Agents Chemother 2005; 49: 3198-202.

[221] Siroy A, Molle V, Lemaitre-Guillier C, *et al*. Channel formation by CarO, the carbapenem resistance-associated outer membrane protein of *Acinetobacter baumannii*. Antimicrob Agents Chemother 2005; 49: 4876-83.

[222] Ikonomidis A, Neou E, Gogou V, *et al*. Heteroresistance to meropenem in carbapenem-susceptible *Acinetobacter baumannii*. J Clin Microbiol 2009; 47: 4055-59.

[223] Talbot GH, Bradley J, Edwards JE, *et al*. Bad bugs need drugs: an update on the development pipeline from the Antimicrobial Availability Task Force of the Infectious Diseases Society of America. Clin Infect Dis 2006; 42: 657-58.

[224] Falagas ME, Bliziotis IA. Pandrug-resistant Gram-negative bacteria: the dawn of the post-antibiotic era? Int. J. Antimicrob. Agents 2007; 29: 630-36.

[225] Levin AS. Multiresistant *Acinetobacter* infections: a role for sulbactam combinations in overcoming an emerging worldwide problem. Clin Microbiol Infect 2002; 8: 144-53.

[226] Owen RJ, Li J, Nation RL, *et al*. *In vitro* pharmacodynamics of colistin against *Acinetobacter baumannii* clinical isolates. J Antimicrob Chemother 2007; 59: 473-77.

[227] Chait R, Craney A, Kishony R. Antibiotic interactions that select against resistance. Nature 2007; 446: 668-71.

[228] Koeleman JG, van der Bijl MW, Stoof J, *et al*. Antibiotic resistance is a major risk factor for epidemic behavior of *Acinetobacter baumannii*. Infect Control Hosp Epidemiol 2001; 22: 284-8.

[229] Coelho JM, Turton JF, Kaufmann ME, *et al*. Occurrence of carbapenem-resistant *Acinetobacter baumannii* clones at multiple hospitals in London and Southeast England. J Clin Microbiol 2006; 44: 3623-27.

[230] Brisse S, Milatovic D, Fluit AC, *et al*. Molecular surveillance of European quinolone-resistant clinical isolates of *Pseudomonas aeruginosa* and *Acinetobacter* spp. using automated ribotyping. J Clin Microbiol 2000; 38: 3636-45.

[231] Bou G, Cervero G, Dominguez MA, *et al*. PCR-based DNA fingerprinting (REP-PCR, AP-PCR) and pulsed-field gel electrophoresis characterization of a nosocomial outbreak caused by imipenem- and meropenem-resistant *Acinetobacter baumannii*. Clin Microbiol Infect 2000; 6: 635-43.

[232] Koeleman JG, Stoof J, Biesmans DJ, *et al*. Comparison of amplified ribosomal DNA restriction analysis, random amplified polymorphic DNA analysis, and amplified fragment length polymorphism fingerprinting for identification of *Acinetobacter* genomic species and typing of *Acinetobacter baumannii*. J Clin Microbiol 1998; 36: 2522-29.

[233] Huys G, Cnockaert M, Nemec A, *et al*. Repetitive-DNA-element PCR fingerprinting and antibiotic resistance of pan-European multi-resistant *Acinetobacter baumannii* clone III strains. J Med Microbiol 2005; 54: 851-56.

[234] Ecker JA, Massire C, Hall TA, *et al*. Identification of *Acinetobacter* species and genotyping of *Acinetobacter baumannii* by multilocus PCR and mass spectrometry. J Clin Microbiol 2006; 44: 2921-32.

[235] Villegas MV, Hartstein AI. *Acinetobacter* outbreaks, 1977- 2000. Infect Control Hosp Epidemiol 2003; 24: 284-95.

[236] Quale J, Bratu S, Landman D, *et al*. Molecular epidemiology and mechanisms of carbapenem resistance in *Acinetobacter baumannii* endemic in New York City. Clin Infect Dis 2003; 37: 214-20.

CHAPTER 4

Multi-Drug Resistance Among Gram-Negative Bacteria in Thailand

Pattarachai Kiratisin*

Department of Microbiology, Faculty of Medicine Siriraj Hospital, Mahidol University

Abstract: Trends of resistance among gram-negative bacteria are progressively on the rise and it appears that control measures may not yet be successfully achieved. Multi-drug resistant bacteria often complicate treatment options and result in unfavorable morbidity. Thailand experiences the emergence of various resistant phenotypes in the last decade. For example, extended-spectrum β-lactamase (ESBL)-producing bacteria have reached ca. 40% among *Escherichia coli* and *Klebsiella pneumoniae* isolates. The rapidly spread of ESBL family, CTX-M, is highly endemic in this area. It is noteworthy that ESBL producers are now recognized as a cause of community-onset infection, and thus indicating a more difficult situation to control. In addition, probably due to a heavy use of carbapenem agents against ESBL producers, carbapenem-resistant *Enterobacteriaceae* have recently emerged. *Pseudomonas aeruginosa* and *Acinetobacter baumannii* are predominantly nosocomial pathogens. They are notorious for their extreme resistance to available antimicrobial agents, in which ca. 30% and 70%, respectively, of our clinical isolates are classified as "extensive drug resistance". This leads to an unwilling use of colistin, a high toxicity drug with a little experience for use in human. Although it is effective against these organisms, it is unfortunate that colistin-resistant isolates have lately been identified, likely reflecting an increased use of colistin. An inefficiency of antimicrobial stewardship program and a lack of policy for controlling antibiotic purchase over the counter are believe to, at least in part, contribute to this abrupt expansion of resistant bacteria. In this chapter, various resistant phenotypes among gram-negative bacteria posing a health care problem in Thailand, as well as their resistant genotypic characteristics and molecular epidemiology, will be discussed.

Keywords: *Escherichia coli*, *Klebsiella pneumoniae*, *Acinetobacter baumannii*, ESBL producers, carbapenem-resistant, ESBL family, CTX-M, multidrug resistant bacteria, Extensive drug resistance.

INTRODUCTION

Antimicrobial resistance among pathogenic bacteria has always been a therapeutic problem. Although infection control practices and several antimicrobial resistance monitoring programs have been implemented, expansion of resistance spectrum and rapid spread of resistant bacteria remain to be seriously concerned due to the increase of highly resistant strains. In Thailand, prevalence of carbapenem-resistant *Acinetobacter baumannii* in a national survey has exceeded 60 percent, dramatically rising from two percent a decade ago [1]. Isolates of *A. baumannii* that are resistant to at least three classes of antimicrobial agents, known as Multidrug Resistant (MDR) bacteria and are resistant to all except only one or two agents, known as extensive drug resistant (XDR) bacteria [2], are widespread in several tertiary care hospitals and often cause infection among patients admitted to intensive care unit resulting in a high mortality rate. Approximately 40 percent of *Escherichia coli* and *Klebsiella pneumoniae* clinical isolates are currently reported to produce Extended Spectrum β-Lactamase (ESBL). A number of reports have addressed the emergence of ESBL producers among community-onset infections, thus raising awareness of the extent of these resistant bacteria. *Pseudomonas aeruginosa* with MDR phenotype has long been an eminent threat for nosocomial infections, especially for patients with hospital-acquired pneumonia and ventilator-associated pneumonia. Rate of resistance to anti-pseudomonal penicillins and carbapenems among *P. aeruginosa* has reached approximately 30 percent. Infections due to these highly resistant gram-negative bacteria have not only limited treatment options but are also inevitably associated with higher complicated morbidities and mortality rates. Inadequate infection control measures, lack of effective surveillance and appropriate

*Address correspondence to Pattarachai Kiratisin: Department of Microbiology, Faculty of Medicine Siriraj, Hospital Mahidol University; Tel: +66-2-419-7058; Fax: +66-2-411-3106; Email: sipkr@mahidol.ac.th

Asad U. Khan and Raffaele Zarrilli (Eds)

antimicrobial stewardship programs, and unrestricted antimicrobial sales over the counter at the least contribute to the emergence and dissemination of high-level resistant bacterial strains in this country. Data on molecular epidemiology of resistant bacteria are limited in Thailand, and thus endemic resistant strains could be underreported. In this chapter, information regarding major MDR bacteria in Thailand, including *Enterobacteriaceae, P. aeruginosa* and *A. baumannii*, will be discussed in terms of prevalence, susceptibility patterns, clinical relevance, molecular characterization of resistance genes and epidemiology.

ENTEROBACTERIACEAE

The family *Enterobacteriaceae*, possibly the most common gram-negative bacteria causing infection in humans, can be resistant to several classes of antimicrobial agents through a number of mechanisms. Resistance to β-lactam antibiotics in *Enterobacteriaceae* is mostly mediated by various β-lactamase enzymes. Although several β-lactamases have been identified from these bacteria, the most concern are enzymes with potent activity against broad spectrum cephalosporins such as Extended Spectrum β-Lactamases (ESBLs) and AmpC β-lactamases and against carbapenems such as *Klebsiella Pneumoniae Carbapenemases* (KPCs) and metallo-β-lactamases. Many studies have reported that an increased use of broad spectrum cephalosporins, including in Thailand, is likely a significant predisposing factor for acquiring infection due to ESBL-producing bacteria and probably other resistant phenotypes. ESBL producers are highly prevalent in Thailand while information regarding the production of other β-lactamases remains limited. Variants of β-lactamases with extended hydrolytic activity against oxyimino-cephalosporins and aztreonam are known as ESBLs. A majority of these enzymes belong to β-lactamases in the molecular class A or functional class 2be and a few belong to molecular class D or functional group 2d (*e.g.* OXA types) with characteristics of being inhibited by β-lactamase inhibitors but lacking hydrolytic activity against cephamycins and carbapenems [3, 4].

During the last decade, a number of ESBL variants have been increasingly recognized (see http://www.lahey.org/Studies for updated list) and their rapid spread among gram-negative bacteria has become a serious health threat in many regions including Thailand. Prevalence of ESBL producers appears to significantly rise in Thailand, particularly among tertiary-care health services and critically ill patients [5]. Surveys at several provincial government-based hospitals throughout the country by the Thai Ministry of Health during a 10-year period (1998-2007) suggesting that overall prevalence of ESBL-producing *K. pneumoniae* has risen from 26% to 41%, whereas prevalence ESBL-producing *E. coli* more strikingly increases from 6% to 35% as shown in Fig. **1** (modified from reference [1]). Additional surveys at other medical centers or university hospitals in Thailand revealed the prevalence of ESBL-producing *E. coli and K. pneumoniae* ranging between 5.1-40.1% and 12.7-44.4%, respectively [5-8].

Although a major portion of ESBL-producing isolates were derived from respiratory tract and urinary tract clinical samples, they were also recovered commonly from blood and other sterile body parts indicating their versatility in causing human infection. A recent Asia-Pacific survey among intra-abdominal infections due to gram-negative bacteria showed that approximately 50.8% and 45.5% of *E. coli* and *K. pneumoniae* isolates, respectively, from Thailand were ESBL positive while overall prevalence in this region was approximately 42.2% and 35.8%, respectively [9]. The data also indicated that prevalence of ESBL producers causing intra-abdominal infection in Thailand was in the third rank in the Asia Pacific region after India and China. Detection of ESBL production in fact remains problematic. Based on the guideline by the Clinical and Laboratory Standards Institute (CLSI), ESBL production is screened by the reduction of susceptibility to broad spectrum cephalosporins or aztreonam and is confirmed by the synergistic effect of clavulanate on ceftazidime or ceftriaxone [10]. However, some ESBL-producing isolates may demonstrate low-level resistance to testing cephalosporins and may not meet the screening or confirmatory criteria, thus resulting in a false-negative report [11]. It was also demonstrated that 8.9% and 20.3% of *E. coli* (n = 4, 515) and *K. pneumoniae* (n = 2, 303) isolates collected for an ESBL surveillance program in the Asia Pacific region passed the screening test but failed the confirmatory test [12].

A majority of ESBL confirmatory-negative isolates (62% for *E. coli* and 75% for *K. pneumoniae*) carried a plasmid-mediated AmpC β-lactamase gene which likely falsifies the result of clavulanate synergy test because AmpC β-lactamase is not inhibited by clavulanate [13]. This also suggested that production of multiple types of β-lactamases is not uncommon in this region and detection of resistant phenotype among isolates in the Asia Pacific region should be carefully interpreted. Recently, CLSI has revised its guideline by reducing Minimal Inhibitory Concentration (MIC) breakpoints for *Enterobacteriaceae* against some cephalosporins and suggesting that routine testing and report of ESBL detection may not be necessary with these new lower breakpoints [10]. In concordance with the guideline by the European Committee on Antimicrobial Susceptibility Testing (EUCAST) organized by the European Society for Clinical Microbiology and Infectious Diseases, this revision was based on the pharmacokinetic-pharmacodynamic data presumably that most isolates producing ESBL and other β-lactamases such as AmpC would demonstrate cephalosporin MIC above the new cut-off breakpoints. However, MIC evaluation of various species of *Enterobacteriaceae* clinical isolates from Thai patients (n = 505) including *E. coli* and *K. pneumoniae* that carried ESBL genes revealed that approximately 1.7%, 2.6% and 23.4% of isolates had MIC lower than new CLSI breakpoints of cefotaxime (1 μg/mL), ceftriaxone (1 μg/mL) and ceftazidime (4 μg/mL), respectively [13a]. Therefore, these new lower breakpoints may not be able to reliably cover all ESBL-producing *Enterobacteriaceae* and use of cephalosporin against these ESBL producers is controversial. Most laboratories in Thailand have not yet adopted these new breakpoints for interpretation of susceptibility and remain to perform and report ESBL detection as previously recommended. More clinical data regarding the correlation of *in vitro* MIC and treatment outcome are warranted to further refine the guideline for ESBL detection. However, detection of ESBL production is still recommended for the purpose of antimicrobial resistance monitoring and infection control [10].

In consistence with the rising trend of ESBL producers, a Thai national survey also reported that both ESBL-producing *E. coli* and *K. pneumoniae* have continuingly increased their resistance to fluoroquinolones and aminoglycosides during 1998-2007 as shown in Table **1**. Resistance to ciprofloxacin and gentamicin among *E. coli* isolates increased 0.51 and 1.96 folds, respectively, while *K. pneumoniae* isolates increased 2.22 and 1.73 folds, respectively. It is additionally of concerns that up to 44.5% and 77.3% of ESBL-producing *E. coli* and *K. pneumoniae*, respectively, express MDR phenotype [5] which causes more difficulty and limitation to select an appropriate choice of antimicrobial agent for treatment. A study of ESBL producers isolated from Thai patients demonstrated that ESBL producers had significant higher resistant rates, when compared to non-ESBL-producing isolates, to various antimicrobial agents including fluoroquinolones, aminoglycosides, tetracycline, trimethoprim/sulfamethoxazole and chloramphenicol [5]. This phenomenon is truly evident from a recent survey during the last five years (2006-2010) at the largest university hospital in Bangkok, Siriraj Hospital, that ESBL-producing *E. coli* and *K. pneumoniae* are significantly more resistant to ciprofloxacin and gentamicin than non-ESBL producing strains as shown in Fig. **2**.

Characterization of ESBL molecular type at major university hospitals in Thailand identified CTX-M as the most predominant family in Thailand. A survey at two major university hospitals showed that up to 99.6% and 99.2% of ESBL-producing *E. coli* and *K. pneumoniae*, respectively, carried a gene in this family [8]. CTX-M has recently become an emerging ESBL family which is globally spread within a short period [14]. Several types of *bla*CTX-M genes were identified in which, similar to reports from other countries, *bla*CTX-M-14 and *bla*CTX-M-15 were most widespread [8]. Interestingly, a new variant of CTX-M, which, in general, exclusively affects cefotaxime but not ceftazidime, with an increased hydrolytic activity against ceftazidime, namely CTX-M-55, was firstly identified in Thailand from both patients with community-onset infection and hospital acquired infection [15]. Insertion sequence IS*Ecp1* is commonly identified in the upstream region of *bla*CTX-M gene and is believed to serve as a promoter or facilitate expression of this gene [16, 17]. Although the distribution of ESBL genes in the TEM and SHV families has been shown in many countries, they are much less common than the CTX-M family in Thailand. Detection of *bla*VEB gene, specifically *bla*VEB-1, among *Enterobacteriaceae* has been more exclusively reported from Thailand and its neighboring countries such as Vietnam [8, 18-21]. A survey of enterobacterial isolates from clinical specimens in Thailand revealed that a gene encoding for VEB-1, *bla*VEB-1, was mostly embedded as a part of class 1 integron on self-conjugative plasmids, posing a threat of rapid transfer even among non-clonally related isolates [21, 22]. Such plasmids also carried both other β-lactam and non-β-lactam resistance determinants, which should be worrisome for the spread of MDR phenotype. Class 1 integrons with MDR determinants were also commonly found from fecal isolates of farm animals in Thailand indicating a possible reservoir of isolates with resistance genes in animals that are capable of horizontal transfer to humans [23].

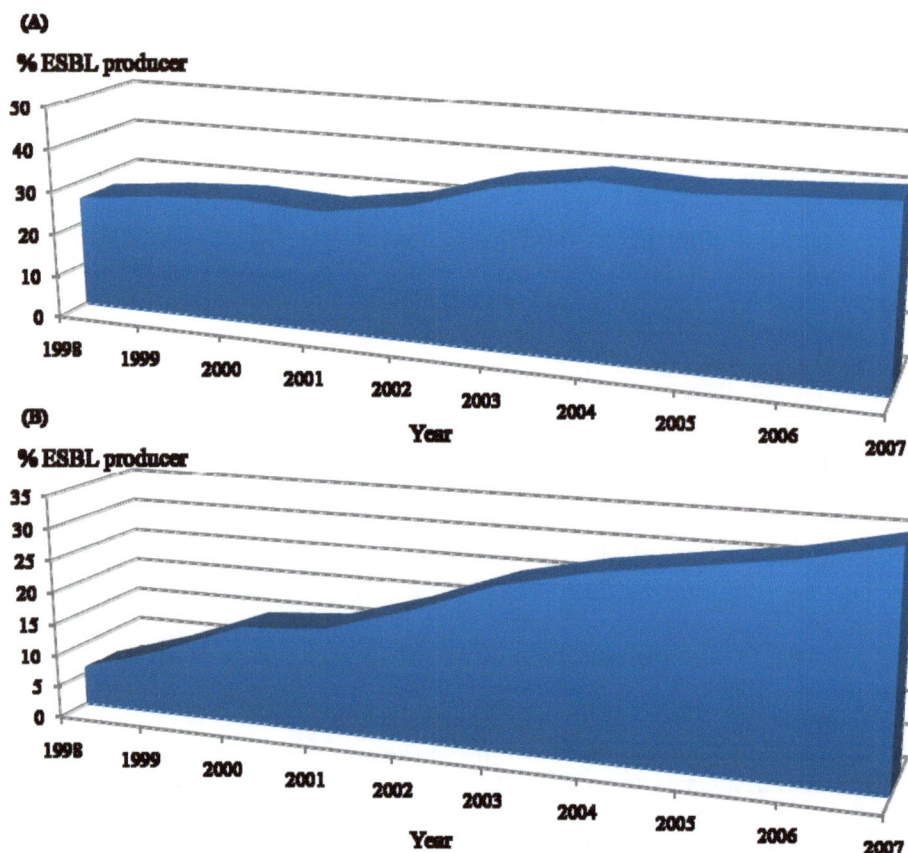

Figure 1: Estimated prevalence of ESBL-producing *K. pneumoniae* (**A**) and *E. coli* (**B**) in Thailand from a national survey of provincial government-based hospitals (modified from reference [1]).

Table 1: Trends of Percent Resistance to Ciprofloxacin and Gentamicin among ESBL-producing *E. coli* and *K. pneumoniae* in Thailand During 1998-2007.[a]

Year	Percent Resistance			
	E. coli		*K. pneumoniae*	
	Ciprofloxacin	Gentamicin	Ciprofloxacin	Gentamicin
1998	35	23	18	26
1999	35	23	20	28
2000	40	25	28	27
2001	40	28	27	26
2002	37	30	28	27
2003	41	33	30	31
2004	40	35	33	35
2005	44	38	38	38
2006	46	42	38	42
2007	48	45	40	45

[a]Modified from reference [1].

In addition to *E. coli* and *K. pneumoniae*, other members of the family *Enterobacteriaceae* are also recognized for their ESBL production. CLSI provides the ESBL detection guideline for only *E. coli*, *K. pneumoniae*, *Klebsiella oxytoca* and *Proteus mirabilis* [10]. This is probably due to unreliability of ESBL detection in other genera that various β-lactamases, including AmpC types, may be co-produced and disturb the synergistic effect of clavulanate to interpret ESBL production. A study of 143 *Enterobacteriaceae* isolates other than *Escherichia* spp. and *Klebsiella* spp. recovered from Thai patients that were not susceptible to at least a broad spectrum cephalosporin revealed that up to 99.3% of these isolates harbored one or multiple types of ESBL genes [24]. *bla*$_{\text{CTX-M}}$ gene was also the most predominant ESBL family among these bacteria at the prevalence of 87.3% in which 61.3% carried *bla*$_{\text{CTX-M-15}}$. Unlike *E. coli* and *K. pneumoniae* that TEM-type ESBL gene was rarely present in Thai isolates, *bla*$_{\text{TEM-116}}$ gene was widespread among *Citrobacter* spp., *Enterobacter* spp., *Morganella* spp., *Proteus* spp., *Providencia* spp., *Salmonella* spp. and *Serratia* spp., and was the only TEM-type ESBL gene identified in these genera. It was notably that 69% of these ESBL gene carrying isolates were also detected for up to three types of plasmid-mediated AmpC β-lactamase genes except for *Serratia* spp. and *Providencia* spp. The CIT and ACC groups, based on grouping category by multiplex PCR method [25], were more commonly found than other groups of plasmid-mediated AmpC β-lactamase genes. When testing for ESBL phenotype according to the method recommended by the CLSI, both isolates carrying ESBL with and without plasmid-mediated AmpC β-lactamase genes may yield either positive or negative results. However, ESBL gene carrying isolates that possessed one or more plasmid-mediated AmpC β-lactamase genes significantly resulted in negative ESBL confirmatory test as compared to isolates that had no plasmid-mediated AmpC β-lactamase gene [13a]. This phenomenon is also evident among *E. coli* and *K. pneumoniae* isolates. Detection of AmpC β-lactamase production based on its properties of non-susceptibility to cefoxitin and beta-lactamase inhibitors may not be adequate because other resistance mechanisms may interfere with the interpretation of these phenotypes. Use of aminophenylboronic acid testing (*i.e.* this substance inhibits the activity of AmpC β-lactamase) may help detect the production of AmpC β-lactamase with a better accuracy and specificity but remains to be validated [27].

Among healthcare-associated infection due to ESBL-producing bacteria, prior exposure to broad spectrum cephalosporins and transfer from other health care facility were identified to be related risk factors [28]. A survey among health care-associated infection due to ESBL-producing *E. coli* and *K. pneumoniae* revealed that several isolates harbored multiple ESBL genes, often in different families, up to three genes [8]. The only risk factor for acquiring infection due to isolates harboring multiple ESBL genes were patients who had been exposed to three or more classes of antibiotics and these patients were likely received inadequate empirical antimicrobial therapy [29]. Infection control measures with effective antimicrobial stewardships therefore play a key role to limit the emergence and spread of these ESBL-producing bacteria among health care-associated infection. Community-onset infection due to ESBL-producing bacteria has recently become an emerging problem. The mortality rate related to ESBL-producing *E. coli*, shown in a Thai study [30], was up to 30% in which bloodstream infection appeared to be the sole predictor of mortality according to a multivariable analysis. In addition, several factors were determined to be associated risks for acquiring community-onset infection due to ESBL-producing *E. coli* including diabetes, prior colonization of ESBL-producing *E. coli*, recent antibiotic administration and previous treatment with broad spectrum cephalosporins or fluoroquinolones [31]. Both *bla*$_{\text{CTX-M-15}}$ and *bla*$_{\text{CTX-M-55}}$ genes were identified among ESBL-producing *E. coli* isolates from patients with community-onset infection [8, 31].

It is also very interesting that ESBL genes, particularly *bla*$_{\text{CTX-M}}$, were detected among isolates, mostly *E. coli*, from fecal samples of healthy Thai population in a remote community who have been minimally exposed to antimicrobial treatment at a high prevalence (up to 60 percent) [32]. It is unclear how resistance genes that are predominant among hospital-acquired clinical isolates are widely distributed in a low selective pressure community. One assumption that could be made is the heavy use of antimicrobial agents in animal feeds. Such agents may be carried over to humans *via* animal products. It was also demonstrated in a study that commensal bacteria carrying class 1 integrons with MDR phenotype were present among healthy animal farmers [23]. Therefore, it is of significance, at least for the aspect of infection control, that ESBL-producing bacteria are widespread among healthy individuals who may serve as reservoir and spread resistant organisms in the community. Molecular epidemiology studies of ESBL-producing clinical isolates in Thailand based on pulsed-field gel electrophoresis often demonstrated that there were no predominant clones, indicating that a large variety of genetically unrelated resistant strains were widely distributed in this country [8]. With this rapidly progressive spread and presence of various genetic derivatives, it may suggest an inadequacy of infection control measures. However, extensive epidemiology study for isolates collected from patients and healthy individuals is needed to better understand how ESBL producers are spread and how to prevent the dissemination of resistant bacteria in the community.

Carbapenem resistance among *Enterobacteriaceae* in Thailand is rare but recognizable. Emergence of *Klebsiella pneumoniae* carbapenemase (KPC)-producing *Enterobacteriaceae* has been reported elsewhere [33]. In a recent Thai study, a small number of *E. coli* and *K. pneumoniae* clinical isolates were identified to have reduced susceptibility to carbapenem in which all isolates were not susceptible to ertapenem and four isolates were not susceptible to imipenem and/or meropenem and/or doripenem [34]. A majority of isolates were recovered from urine and were ESBL positive. Although four isolates had a positive result of modified Hodge test according to the CLSI protocol [10], none of them were detected for bla_{KPC} gene [34]. In fact, KPC-producing *Enterobacteriaceae* has not been reported in Thailand. This indicates that other mechanisms may also play a role in the reduction of carbapenem susceptibility among Thai *Enterobacteriaceae* isolates. The study also demonstrated that use of fosfomycin in a combination regimen with any of carbapenem agent did not yield a synergistic effect against these isolates. Reduced susceptibility to carbapenem is indeed more common among *Enterobacter* spp. A survey among *Enterobacter* spp. clinical isolates during 2007-2009 at a tertiary hospital in Bangkok revealed that up to 32% of isolates were not susceptible to ertapenem but almost all isolates remains susceptible to imipenem and meropenem [13a]. Carbapenemases other than KPC has emerged such as New Delhi metallo-β-lactamase (NDM), a new metallo-β-lactamase conferring carbapenem resistance among *Enterobacteriaceae* first identified in India [35]. Within a short period, NDM-1 producing *Enterobacteriaceae* have been recovered from patients in Europe, North America and Australia in which most patients had a recent history of receiving medical care in India or Pakistan [36]. A number of people from the Indian subcontinent travel to and from Thailand constantly, and thus a close monitoring program is necessary to early recognize and control the spread of this threat. Surveillance at the molecular level is also warranted to detect the emergence of carbapenem non-susceptible isolates in Thailand to better understand the mechanisms underneath the resistance and to explore appropriate measures for infection control.

Resistance is also increasingly recognized among *Salmonella* isolates, particularly among nontyphoidal salmonellae causing extraintestinal infection. *Salmonella* group C, including *S. Choleraesuis* serovar, was reported to be a major group related to bloodstream infection and was found associated with an increase in HIV infection [37]. *S. choleraesuis* isolates from bacteremic patients with resistance to extended-spectrum cephalosporins were shown to be more clonally related than non-resistant strains and carried ESBL gene with an emergence of $bla_{CTX-M-14}$ among several clones [38]. In addition, this epidemiologic study also demonstrated that extended-spectrum cephalosporin-resistant *S. choleraesuis* may also spread to traveler because a strain isolated from a Danish patient who visited Thailand had indistinguishable pulsed-field gel electrophoresis DNA patterns from Thai isolates in this study implicating a concern for public health and travel medicine policies to control resistant bacteria. However, a survey at the university hospital in Thailand revealed that, among blood isolates, *Salmonella* group B most commonly demonstrated MDR phenotype (up to 75%), followed by groups C (40.6%) and D (11.4%) [37]. Overall blood-derived MDR nontyphoidal *Salmonella* from this study was approximately 30% with highly resistant rates against ampicillin, trimethoprim/sulfamethoxazole and chloramphenicol. Reduced susceptibility to fluoroquinolone was also common in *S. Choleraesuis* and *S. virchow* not only in Thailand but also in other Asian countries [39]. On the other hand, *Salmonella* group B was recovered more frequent from fecal sample of patients with diarrhea [40]. Those diarrheal isolates of *Salmonella* group B also demonstrated MDR phenotype while most of them remained susceptible to fluoroquinolone. Therefore, nontyphoidal salmonellae were common in both intestinal and extraintestinal infections in which a high prevalence of MDR isolates should be of concern for both therapeutic options and epidemiologic control.

(A)

% Ciprofloxacin susceptibility

(B)

% Gentamicin susceptibility

(C)

% Ciprofloxacin susceptibility

(D)

% Gentamicin susceptibility

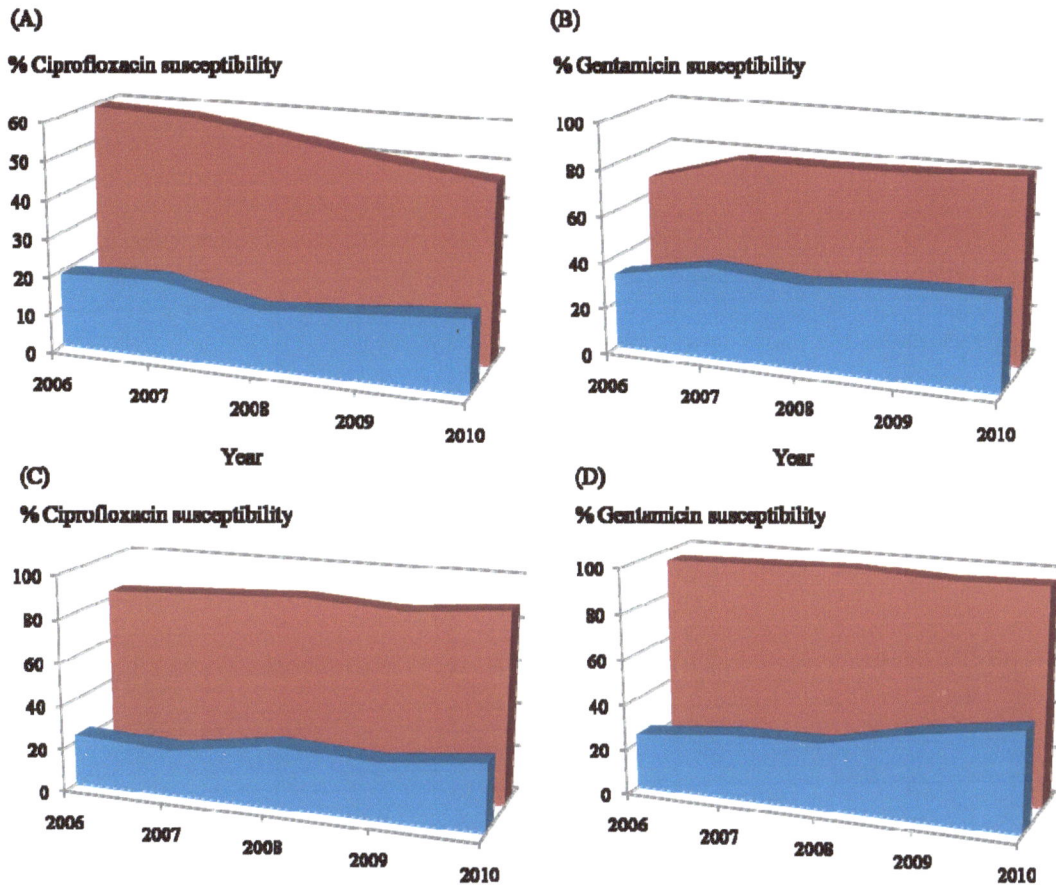

Figure 2: Comparisons of percent susceptibility among ESBL-producing (blue) *vs* non-ESBL-producing (red) *E. coli* to ciprofloxacin **(A)** and gentamicin **(B)** and ESBL-producing (blue) *vs* non-ESBL-producing (red) *K. pneumoniae* to ciprofloxacin **(C)** and gentamicin **(D)** at Siriraj Hospital (Bangkok, Thailand) during 2006-2010.

Pseudomonas aeruginosa

Clinical isolates of *P. aeruginosa* with increasing resistance against anti-pseudomonal penicillins, broad spectrum cephalosporins and carbapenems have become more prevalent in Thailand, especially among patients with hospital-acquired pneumonia, ventilator-associated pneumonia and catheter-related bacteremia, resulting in a high burden of treatment option. *P. aeruginosa* was also reported as a dominant pathogen causing ventilator-associated pneumonia in a Thai neonatal intensive care unit marking its importance to cause invasive infection among highly susceptible, immune-compromised hosts such as newborn [41]. Based on a univariate analysis, risk factors associated with acquiring *P. aeruginosa* bacteremia was analyzed at a large tertiary hospital in Bangkok, which included hospital-acquired infection, hematologic malignancy, neutropenia, chronic obstructive pulmonary disease and patients who received therapy with antimicrobial or cytotoxic agents [42]. Carbapenem-resistant *P. aeruginosa* was common in device-associated infections among Thai patients in medical and surgical intensive care units with the prevalence of approximately 30% [43]. Respiratory tract infection caused by MDR *P. aeruginosa* was also documented to be associated with higher mortality rate or unfavorable outcomes at a Thai tertiary care center [44].

A multi-centered survey by the Thai Ministry of Health during 1998 to 2007 revealed that resistance to ceftazidime among *P. aeruginosa* isolates remained in the range of 23-30% while resistance to imipenem rose from 11% to 30% in this period as shown in Fig. **3** [1]. Another nationwide survey among 28 general hospitals in Thailand during 2000-2005 showed that approximately 25.6%, 14.1% and 12.4% of *P.*

aeruginosa clinical isolates were resistant to ceftazidime, imipenem and meropenem, respectively in which isolates from patients in intensive care units had 1.2- to 2.9-folds higher resistance rates when compared to isolates recovered from non-intensive care patients [45]. A survey at a major 2400-bed tertiary care hospital in Bangkok, Siriraj Hospital, during 2006-2009, however revealed that prevalence of resistance to ceftazidime, imipenem and meropenem *P. aeruginosa* were approximately 32%, 34% and 32%, respectively (Table **2**). The ceftazidime-resistant strains at this hospital were increased from 24% according to data collected during 1999 [46]. Resistance to other classes of antibiotics including aminoglycosides and fluoroquinolone was also noticeable as shown in Table **2**. Interestingly, percent of *P. aeruginosa* isolates resistant to cefoperazone/sulbactam increased at a significant rate from 37% to 67% (1.8 folds) during this four-year period. This suggests that resistance problem among *P. aeruginosa* tends to be seriously increasing and isolates from large referral hospitals are likely to be more resistant, probably related to a heavy use of broad spectrum antibiotics. Drug use evaluation and antimicrobial stewardship programs have been implemented in many tertiary care centers in Thailand to restrict the unnecessary use of broad spectrum antimicrobial agents, especially carbapenems, with an effort to reduce the resistance rates and to prevent the spread of MDR *P. aeruginosa*.

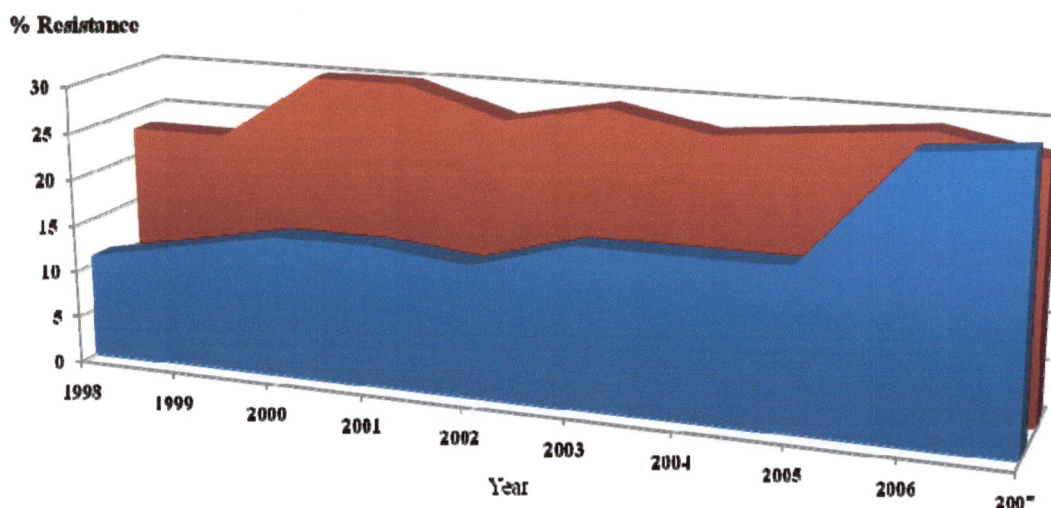

Figure 3: Prevalence (percent) of *P. aeruginosa* isolates resistant to ceftazidime (red) and imipenem (blue) from a Thai national survey during 1998-2007 (modified from reference [1]).

Table 2: Percent Resistance Among *P. Aeruginosa* Isolates at Siriraj Hospital During 2006-2009.

Agents	Year			
	2006	2007	2008	2009
Amikacin	27	25	20	20
Cefepime	34	37	31	33
Cefoperazone/sulbactam	37	47	55	67
Ceftazidime	33	32	32	31
Ciprofloxacin	34	33	29	31
Gentamicin	34	31	27	25
Imipenem	33	30	33	38
Meropenem	32	31	32	34
Piperacillin/tazobactam	23	22	27	22

ESBL-related bla_{VEB} gene was known to be common among *P. aeruginosa* isolates in Thailand and a clonal dissemination of such strains occurred in a university hospital surveillance [20]. Mostly, this gene is integrated as a part of class 1 integron. A study among ceftazidime-resistant *P. aeruginosa* at Siriraj hospital (Bangkok) identified bla_{VEB-1} like genes as the predominant genes [46]. These genes were found as a gene cassette and were associated with other resistance gene cassettes including rifampicin resistance (*arr-2* cassette), aminoglycoside resistance (*aadA1* and *aadB* cassettes) and bla_{OXA-10}-like β-lactamase on class 1 integron. An isolate with plasmid-mediated bla_{VEB-1} like gene was also observed in the mentioned study. Multiple clones and subclones were recognized among these isolates based on pulsed-field gel electrophoresis typing. This indicates that bla_{VEB-1} like gene is associated with MDR phenotype among *P. aeruginosa* isolates and could be easily transferred *via* mobile genetic elements, and various clones of these resistance strains are widely distributed in such hospital setting. bla_{VEB-1} ESBL gene is also not uncommon among *Enterobacteriaceae* isolates with MDR phenotype as described earlier. Therefore, interspecies transfer of resistance genes is likely possible. However, specific insertion sequences such as IS*1999* and IS*2000* were exclusively found preceding bla_{VEB-1} gene on an integron in *P. aeruginosa* isolates, but not in *Enterobacteriaceae* [21, 46]. Such insertion sequences assumedly provide independent promoter for bla_{VEB-1} expression [47].

A combination therapy is often considered in clinical practice when encountering MDR strains. A checkerboard titration study of ceftazidime-resistant *P. aeruginosa* isolated from Thai patients demonstrated that combinations of ceftazidime with gentamicin and fosfomycin with imipenem had a high percentage of synergistic effect (38% and 39% of tested isolates, respectively) [48]. However, antagonistic effect was also observed in combinations of fosfomycin with gentamicin, fosfomycin with ceftazidime and fosfomycin with imipenem at 27%, 22% and 7% of tested isolates, respectively. Therefore, use of an unconventional agent such as fosfomycin as alternative drug or in a combinatory therapy should be cautious of such adversary effect with another agent. Additional information will be required to evaluate an appropriate combination regimen for use against MDR *P. aeruginosa*.

Acinetobacter Baumannii

Highly resistant strains of *A. baumannii* have been emerging as an important causative agent of nosocomial infection in several countries including Thailand. It is of particular concern among critically ill patients in intensive care units which often result in a high mortality rate. *A. baumannii* was identified as the most common pathogen of hospital-acquired pneumonia, ventilator-associated pneumonia, central line-related bacteremia and catheter-related urinary tract infection among patients admitted to intensive care units at various tertiary-care hospitals in Thailand [43, 44]. Interestingly, up to 92.3% of *A. baumannii* isolated from hospital-acquired pneumonia or ventilator-associated pneumonia had MDR or XDR phenotype [44]. Lower respiratory tract was also identified as the most common site of nosocomial infection due to MDR *A. baumannii* which was associated with prolonged hospital stay. A multiple logistic regression analysis revealed that factors associated with MDR *A. baumannii* nosocomial infection included admission longer than a week prior to infection, prolonged catheterization or mechanical ventilation and previous exposure to third- or fourth-generation cephalosporins [49]. A Thai multi-centered survey during 1998-2007 revealed that percent resistance among *A. baumannii* complex to ceftazidime and imipenem had increased 1.2 and 31.5 folds, respectively. As shown in Fig. **4**, it was very striking that, while resistance rates to ceftazidime remained approximately 60-70%, resistance rates to imipenem increased from 2% to 63% within a decade. This is believed to be associated with the use of imipenem that increased quite extensively in Thailand during that period.

Prevalence of MDR *A. baumannii* is usually high at a referral center as demonstrated by the data from Siriraj hospital during 2006 to 2009 that a majority of isolates (range from 72 to 89 percent) were resistant to various classes of antibiotics including aminoglycosides (amikacin and gentamicin), fluoroquinolones (ciprofloxacin), β-lactams (ceftazidime, cefepime, imipenem and meropenem) and trimethoprim/sulfamethoxazole (Table **3**). The resistance rates of ceftazidime and imipenem were obviously higher than what presented from the mentioned national data surveyed at general hospitals. This is also well illustrated that the resistance problem among *A. baumannii* isolates in Thailand becomes a serious issue. Carbapenem-resistant *A. baumannii* (CRAB) was not uncommon and occasionally caused outbreak in Thai medical centers. The SENTRY antimicrobial surveillance program that surveyed the dissemination of class D carbapenemases and metallo-β-lactamases among *Acinetobacter* spp. (94.1% *A. baumannii*) in the Asia-Pacific region including Thailand during 2006-2007 revealed that 42.3% of isolates were not susceptible to imipenem or meropenem while 99.1% remained susceptible to polymyxins [50]. Genes encoding for class D carbapenemase were identified in 70% of these isolates and 95% of which carried bla_{OXA-23} gene. In this surveillance, 59.2% of Thai *A. baumannii* isolates were non-susceptible to imipenem or meropenem and some isolates, in addition to bla_{OXA-23}, also harbored $bla_{OXA-24/40}$ and/or bla_{OXA-58}. Several isolates had more than one class D carbapenemase genes. Another Thai study showed that most CRAB isolates carried bla_{OXA-23} carbapenemase gene in adjacent to the insertion sequence IS*Aba1* structure that may facilitate the spread of this gene [51]. Interestingly, according to molecular typing by ribotyping and pulsed-field gel electrophoresis, a various genetic diversities were shown among isolates carrying only bla_{OXA-23} while clonal dissemination tended to be observed among isolates carrying multiple bla_{OXA} genes. This indicates that isolates with several bla_{OXA} genes, presumably demonstrating a high-level resistance, tended to spread more frequently and successfully than isolates with only bla_{OXA-23} gene. Although additional extensive studies are required, detection of bla_{OXA} gene may be employed as a genetic marker to monitor the clonal spread of this extremely resistant bacterium.

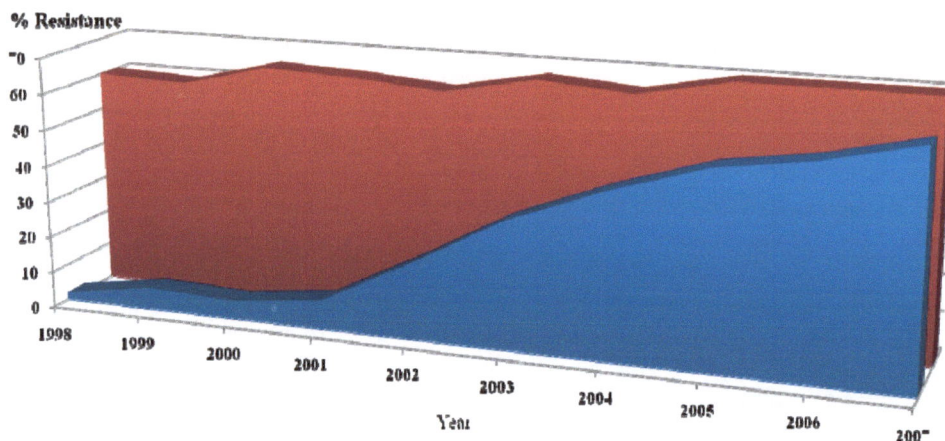

Figure 4: Prevalence (percent) of *A. baumannii* isolates resistant to ceftazidime (red) and imipenem (blue) (modified from reference [1]).

Table 3: Percent Resistance Among *A. baumannii* Isolates at Siriraj Hospital During 2006-2009.

Agents	Year			
	2006	2007	2008	2009
Amikacin	75	72	79	78
Cefepime	89	88	86	85
Ceftazidime	83	89	85	83
Ciprofloxacin	89	83	85	85
Gentamicin	81	77	80	79
Imipenem	84	84	82	84
Meropenem	85	85	83	84
Trimethoprim/sulfamethoxazole	88	88	82	82

Infection due to CRAB resulted in a higher mortality rate when compared to infection due to carbapenem-susceptible strains in many cohort studies. According to multivariable analyses, however, several factors contributed to patient's mortality such as severity of illness and inappropriate empiric treatment whilst resistance to carbapenem of *A. baumannii* may not directly or significantly attribute to the mortality rate [52-54]. Since carbapenems are often used for empirical therapy among serious nosocomial infections,

CRAB infection remains to pose a threat for treatment failure. Based on a case-control study, risk factors that were associated with acquiring CRAB infection included previous admission to intensive care unit and previous exposure to several classes of antibiotics including carbapenem [52].

Colistin (colistimethate sodium or polymyxin E) is usually preferred as an option for salvage therapy against CRAB or XDR *A. baumannii* and also highly resistant strains of *P. aeruginosa*. In a cohort study, it was demonstrated that patients receiving colistin therapy for treatment of *A. baumannii* had better clinical and microbiological responses with lower overall mortality rate when compared to patients receiving non-colistin therapy [55]. However, nephrotoxicity was reported as an adverse effect among patients with colistin treatment in which several patients, however, also had other contributing factors that may impair their renal function. Although colistin efficiently eliminates *A. baumannii* in the initial phase of treatment, prolonged exposure to colistin, specifically if using as a monotherapy, has been experimentally shown *in vitro* according to population analysis profile to induce the emergence of heteroresistance in *A. baumannii* [56]. In addition, lack of pharmacokinetic/phamacodynamic profile of colistin results in a difficulty to justify the optimal dosage for individual patient. Interpretation guideline for colistin susceptibility testing according to CLSI is only available based on dilution method which may not be practical for laboratories serving in an endemic area of highly resistant *A. baumannii* (*e.g.* Thailand). It is noteworthy that colistin-resistant *A. baumannii* has already emerged in Thailand, likely reflecting the rapid increase in colistin use (Kiratisin, unpublished data). Other new agents such as tigecycline may have a potential for use against *A. baumannii* including CRAB, but *in vitro* and clinical data remain inadequate. Therefore, clinicians should be cautious when using these non-traditional agents for treating patients with *A. baumannii* infection.

Combination therapy is often considered for battling MDR or XDR *A. baumannii*. Several *in vitro* studies have demonstrated possibilities of various combination regimens that may have a synergistic effect against *A. baumannii* including regimens containing carbapenem, tigecycline, colistin, sulbactam or fluoroquinolones [57-60]. Most studies demonstrated synergism to some extent dependent on particular combinations and methods. A study of *A. baumannii*, including MDR and XDR isolates, at a Thai medical center based on the E-test® method revealed that a synergy was most observed when using cefoperazone/sulbactam in combination with a carbapenem *i.e.* the synergistic rates were 32.5% for imipenem, 30% for meropenem, and 17.5% for doripenem [61]. In addition, this study demonstrated that each carbapenem had additive effect when used in combination with rifampicin, netilmycin, doxycycline or moxifloxacin whereas antagonistic effect was not recognized in any of the combination. Therefore, carbapenem may have a role in a combination therapy with various agents, especially if colistin usage is not applicable due to its availability or toxicity. However, it should be noted that combination results were strain- and method-dependent. The standard methods for evaluating synergistic activity of two or more antimicrobial agents for a potential use in combination such as time-kill method and checkerboard method are technically laborious and may not be feasible to perform in most clinical laboratories. To date, there is no strong clinical-based evidence to recommend such combinations for empirical therapy and clinical response should be closely monitored when administering the combination therapy.

CONCLUSION

Gram-negative bacteria with MDR phenotype have rapidly spread worldwide and become a serious threat of health care system, particularly of nosocomial infection. This resistance trend has been clearly observed in many countries as a global problem. In Thailand, as a model country with high resistance rate, leading MDR gram-negative organisms include ESBL-producing *Enterobacteriaceae*, *P. aeruginosa* and *A. baumannii*. Prevalence of these resistant bacteria has strikingly increased in the last decade and their broadening spectrum to be resistant to several classes of antimicrobial agents is worrisome. Choices of antibiotics for treating infection due to these MDR organisms are currently very limited, which is reasonably associated with higher mortality rates. Clinical laboratories have an important role to rapidly and accurately identify resistant characteristics, as well as to study epidemiology of resistant isolates to assist physicians in selecting appropriate antimicrobial treatment and implementing measures to prevent further spread of MDR isolates. Several factors, however, should be considered when evaluating resistance problem. For example, in *Burkholderia pseudomallei*, a gram-negative bacterium causing highly fatal melioidosis that is endemic in Thailand, susceptibility to trimethoprim/sulfamethoxazole, a drug of choice for maintenance therapy, is somewhat dependent on testing methods and false-resistance occurs at a high rate when using standard disk diffusion method [62, 63]. Standardized guideline should be carefully followed when performing and interpreting susceptibility results. While new antimicrobial agents with a better spectrum against highly resistant gram-negative bacteria are unlikely to be available in the near future, infection control practice with antimicrobial stewardship program is definitely in need to control the emergence and spread of MDR organisms. Several intervention measures have been shown to be effective in controlling and reducing colonization or infection due to MDR *A. baumannii* including strict isolation, contact precaution, appropriate hand hygiene, relevant surveillance program and efficient hospital environment disinfection (*e.g.* use of 1:100 sodium hypochlorite solution) [64]. Inadequate infection control may result not only in the spread of resistant bacteria, but also the increase of morbidity, mortality and economic loss due to hospital cost. Continuing surveillance program remains to be very beneficial to monitor trends of resistance prevalence and initiate rapid action to control the dissemination of emerging resistant bacteria.

REFERENCES

[1]   National Antimicrobial Resistance Surveillance, Thailand. Department of Medical Sciences. Ministry of Public Health (Thailand). Available from: http://narst.dmsc.moph.go.th/

[2]   Falagas ME, Karageorgopoulos DE. Pandrug resistance (PDR), extensive drug resistance (XDR), and multidrug resistance (MDR) among gram-negative bacilli: need for international harmonization in terminology. Clin Infect Dis 2008; 46: 1121-2.

[3]   Bradford PA. Extended-spectrum β-lactamases in the 21st century: characterization, epidemiology, and detection of this important resistance threat. Clin Microbiol Rev 2001; 14: 933-51.

[4]   Bush K, Jacoby GA, Medeiros AA. A functional classification scheme for β-lactamases and its correlation with molecular structure. Antimicrob Agents Chemother 1995; 39: 1211-33.

[5]   Kiratisin P, Chattammanat S, Sa-Nguansai S, *et al.* A 2-year trend of extended-spectrum beta-lactamase-producing *Escherichia coli* and *Klebsiella pneumoniae* in Thailand: an alert for infection control. Trans R Soc Trop Med Hyg 2008; 102: 460-4.

[6]   Kusum M, Wongwanich S, Dhiraputra C, *et al.* Occurrence of extended-spectrum beta-lactamase in clinical isolates of *Klebsiella pneumoniae* in a University Hospital, Thailand. J Med Assoc Thai 2004; 87: 1029-33.

[7]   Jitsurong S, Yodsawat J. Prevalence of extended-spectrum beta-lactamases (ESBLs) produced in blood isolates of gram-negative bacteria in a teaching hospital in southern Thailand. Southeast Asian J Trop Med Public Health 2006; 37: 131-5.

[8]   Kiratisin P, Apisarnthanarak A, Laesripa C, *et al.* Molecular characterization and epidemiology of extended-spectrum-β-lactamase-producing *Escherichia coli* and *Klebsiella pneumoniae* isolates causing health care-associated infection in Thailand, where the CTX-M family is endemic. Antimicrob Agents Chemother 2008; 52: 2818-24.

[9]   Hawser SP, Bouchillon SK, Hoban DJ, *et al.* Emergence of high levels of extended-spectrum-beta-lactamase-producing gram-negative bacilli in the Asia-Pacific region: data from the Study for Monitoring Antimicrobial Resistance Trends (SMART) program, 2007. Antimicrob Agents Chemother 2009; 53: 3280-4.

[10] Clinical and Laboratory Standards Institute. Performance standards for antimicrobial susceptibility testing. Twentieth informational supplement. Document M100-S20. Wayne, PA: CLSI, 2010.

[11] Jacoby GA, Walsh KE, Walker VJ. Identification of extended-spectrum, AmpC, and carbapenem-hydrolyzing beta-lactamases in *Escherichia coli* and *Klebsiella pneumoniae* by disk tests. J Clin Microbiol 2006; 44: 1971-76.

[12] Bell JM, Chitsaz M, Turnidge JD, *et al.* Prevalence and significance of a negative extended-spectrum beta-lactamase (ESBL) confirmation test result after a positive ESBL screening test result for isolates of *Escherichia coli* and *Klebsiella pneumoniae*: results from the SENTRY Asia-Pacific Surveillance Program. J Clin Microbiol 2007; 45: 1478-82.

[13] Jacoby GA. AmpC β-lactamases. Clin Microbiol Rev 2009; 22: 161-82.
      (a) Kiratisin P. Effect of MIC interpretative breakpoint revision on cephalosporin and carbapenem susceptibility among ESBL-producing Enterobacteriaceae. Asian Biomed (In press).

[14] Bonnet R. Growing group of extended-spectrum beta-lactamases: the CTX-M enzymes. Antimicrob Agents Chemother 2004; 48: 1-14.

[15]   Kiratisin P, Apisarnthanarak A, Saifon P, *et al*. The emergence of a novel ceftazidime-resistant CTX-M extended-spectrum β-lactamase, CTX-M-55, in both community-onset and hospital-acquired infections in Thailand. Diagn Microbiol Infect Dis 2007; 58: 349-55.

[16]   Saladin M, Cao VT, Lambert T, *et al*. Diversity of CTX-M beta-lactamases and their promoter regions from *Enterobacteriaceae* isolated in three Parisian hospitals. FEMS Microbiol Lett 2000; 209: 161-8.

[17]   Poirel L, Lartigue MF, Decousser JW, *et al*. IS*Ecp1B*-mediated transposition of bla$_{CTX-M}$ in *Escherichia coli*. Antimicrob Agents Chemother 2005; 49: 447-50.

[18]   Cao V, Lambert T, Nhu DQ, *et al*. Distribution of extended-spectrum beta-lactamases in clinical isolates of *Enterobacteriaceae* in Vietnam. Antimicrob Agents Chemother 2002; 46: 3739-43.

[19]   Naas T, Benaoudia F, Massuard S, *et al*. Integron-located VEB-1 extended-spectrum beta-lactamase gene in a *Proteus mirabilis* clinical isolate from Vietnam. J Antimicrob Chemother 2000; 46: 703-11.

[20]   Chanawong A, M'Zali FH, Heritage J, *et al*. SHV-12, SHV-5, SHV-2a and VEB-1 extended-spectrum beta-lactamases in Gram-negative bacteria isolated in a university hospital in Thailand. J Antimicrob Chemother 2001; 48: 839-52.

[21]   Girlich D, Poirel L, Leelaporn A, *et al*. Molecular epidemiology of the integron-located VEB-1 extended-spectrum beta-lactamase in nosocomial enterobacterial isolates in Bangkok, Thailand. J Clin Microbiol 2001; 39: 175-82.

[22]   Phongpaichit S, Wuttananupan K, Samasanti W. Class 1 integrons and multidrug resistance among *Escherichia coli* isolates from human stools. Southeast Asian J Trop Med Public Health 2008; 39: 279-87.

[23]   Phongpaichit S, Liamthong S, Mathew AG, *et al*. Prevalence of class 1 integrons in commensal *Escherichia coli* from pigs and pig farmers in Thailand. J Food Prot 2007; 70: 292-9.

[24]   Kiratisin P, Henprasert A. Genotypic analysis of plasmid-mediated β-lactamases among *Enterobacteriaceae* other than *Escherichia* spp. and *Klebsiella* spp. that are non-susceptible to broad-spectrum cephalosporin. Int J Antimicrob Agents 2010; 36: 343-7.

[25]   Perez-Perez FJ, Hanson ND. Detection of plasmid-mediated AmpC β-lactamase genes in clinical isolates by using multiplex PCR. J Clin Microbiol 2002; 40: 2153-62.

[26]   Kiratisin P, Henprasert A. Resistance phenotype-genotype correlation and molecular epidemiology of *Citrobacter, Enterobacter, Proteus, Providencia, Salmonella* and *Serratia* that carry extended-spectrum β-lactamases with or without plasmid-mediated AmpC β-lactamase genes in Thailand. Trans R Soc Trop Med Hyg 2011; 105: 46-51.

[27]   Tenover FC, Emery SL, Spiegel CA, *et al*. Identification of plasmid-mediated AmpC beta- in *Escherichia coli, Klebsiella* spp., and proteus species can potentially improve reporting of cephalosporin susceptibility testing results. J Clin Microbiol 2009; 47: 294-9.

[28]   Apisarnthanarak A, Kiratisin P, Saifon P, *et al*. Risk factors for and outcomes of healthcare-associated infection due to extended-spectrum beta-lactamase-producing *Escherichia coli* or *Klebsiella pneumoniae* in Thailand. Infect Control Hosp Epidemiol 2007; 28: 873-6.

[29]   Apisarnthanarak A, Kiratisin P, Mundy LM. Clinical and molecular epidemiology of healthcare-associated infections due to extended-spectrum beta-lactamase (ESBL)-producing strains of *Escherichia coli* and *Klebsiella pneumoniae* that harbor multiple ESBL genes. Infect Control Hosp Epidemiol 2008; 29: 1026-34.

[30]   Apisarnthanarak A, Kiratisin P, Saifon P, *et al*. Predictors of mortality among patients with community-onset infection due to extended-spectrum beta-lactamase-producing *Escherichia coli* in Thailand. Infect Control Hosp Epidemiol 2008; 29: 80-2.

[31]   Apisarnthanarak A, Kiratisin P, Saifon P, *et al*. Clinical and molecular epidemiology of community-onset, extended-spectrum beta-lactamase-producing *Escherichia coli* infections in Thailand: a case-case-control study. Am J Infect Control 2007; 35: 606-12.

[32]   Sasaki T, Hirai I, Niki M, *et al*. High prevalence of CTX-M beta-lactamase-producing *Enterobacteriaceae* in stool specimens obtained from healthy individuals in Thailand. J Antimicrob Chemother 2010; 65: 666-8.

[33]   Navon-Venezia S, Chmelnitsky I, Leavitt A, *et al*. Plasmid-mediated imipenem-hydrolyzing enzyme KPC-2 among multiple carbapenem-resistant *Escherichia coli* clones in Israel. Antimicrob Agents Chemother 2009; 50: 3098-101.

[34]   Netikul T, Leelaporn A, Leelarasmee A, *et al*. *In vitro* activities of fosfomycin and carbapenem combinations against carbapenem non-susceptible *Escherichia coli* and *Klebsiella pneumoniae*. Int J Antimicrob Agents 2010; 35: 609-10.

[35] Yong D, Toleman MA, Giske CG, *et al.* Characterization of a new metallo-beta-lactamase gene, *bla* (NDM-1), and a novel erythromycin esterase gene carried on a unique genetic structure in *Klebsiella pneumoniae* sequence type 14 from India. Antimicrob Agents Chemother 2009; 53: 5046-54.

[36] Deshpand P, Rodrigues C, Shetty A, *et al.* New Delhi Metallo-*β*-lactamase (NDM-1) in *Enterobacteriaceae*: Treatment options with carbapenems compromised. J Assoc Physicians India 2010; 58: 147-50.

[37] Kiratisin P. Bacteraemia due to nontyphoid *Salmonella* in Thailand: clinical and microbiologic analysis. Trans R Soc Trop Med Hyg 2008; 102: 384-8.

[38] Sirichote P, Hasman H, Pulsrikarn C, *et al.* Molecular characterization of extended spectrum cephalosporinases (ESC) producing *Salmonella* Choleraesuis from patients in Thailand and Denmark. J Clin Microbiol 2010; 48: 883-8.

[39] Lee HY, Su LH, Tsai MH, *et al.* High rate of reduced susceptibility to ciprofloxacin and ceftriaxone among nontyphoid *Salmonella* clinical isolates in Asia. Antimicrob Agents Chemother 2009; 53: 2696-9.

[40] Hanson R, Kaneene JB, Padungtod P, *et al.* Prevalence of *Salmonella* and *E. coli*, and their resistance to antimicrobial agents, in farming communities in northern Thailand. Southeast Asian J Trop Med Public Health. 2002; 33 (Suppl 3): 120-6.

[41] Petdachai W. Ventilator-associated pneumonia in a newborn intensive care unit. Southeast Asian J Trop Med Public Health 2004; 35: 724-9.

[42] Siripassorn K, Santiprasitkul S, Udompanthurak S, *et al.* Risk factors for *Pseudomonas aeruginosa* bacteremia in Thai patients. J Med Assoc Thai 2002; 85: 1095-9.

[43] Thongpiyapoom S, Narong MN, Suwalak N, *et al.* Device-associated infections and patterns of antimicrobial resistance in a medical-surgical intensive care unit in a university hospital in Thailand. J Med Assoc Thai 2004; 87: 819-24.

[44] Weerarak P, Kiratisin P, Thamlikitkul V. Hospital-acquired pneumonia and ventilator-associated pneumonia in adults at Siriraj Hospital: etiology, clinical outcomes, and impact of antimicrobial resistance. J Med Assoc Thai 2010; 93 (Suppl 1): S126-38.

[45] Dejsirirlert S, Suankratay C, Trakulsomboon S, *et al.* National Antimicrobial Resistance Surveillance, Thailand (NARST) data among clinical isolates of *Pseudomonas aeruginosa* in Thailand from 2000 to 2005. J Med Assoc Thai 2009: 92 (Suppl 4); S68-75.

[46] Girlich D, Naas T, Leelaporn A, *et al.* Nosocomial spread of the integron-located veb-1-like cassette encoding an extended-spectrum beta-lactamase in *Pseudomonas aeruginosa* in Thailand. Clin Infect Dis 2002; 34: 603-11.

[47] Naas T, Poirel L, Karim A, *et al.* Molecular characterization of In50, a class 1 integron encoding the gene for the extended-spectrum *β*-lactamase VEB-1 in *Pseudomonas aeruginosa*. FEMS Microbiol Lett 1999; 176: 411-9.

[48] Pruekprasert P, Tunyapanit W. *In vitro* activity of fosfomycin-gentamicin, fosfomycin-ceftazidime, fosfomycin-imipenem and ceftazidime-gentamicin combinations against ceftazidime-resistant *Pseudomonas aeruginosa*. Southeast Asian J Trop Med Public Health 2005; 36: 1239-42.

[49] Surasarang K, Narksawat K, Danchaivijitr S, *et al.* Risk factors for multi-drug resistant *Acinetobacter baumannii* nosocomial infection. J Med Assoc Thai 2007; 90: 1633-9.

[50] Mendes RE, Bell JM, Turnidge JD, *et al.* Emergence and widespread dissemination of OXA-23, -24/40 and -58 carbapenemases among *Acinetobacter* spp. in Asia-Pacific nations: report from the SENTRY Surveillance Program. J Antimicrob Chemother 2009; 63: 55-9.

[51] Niumsup PR, Boonkerd N, Tansawai U, *et al.* Carbapenem-resistant *Acinetobacter baumannii* producing OXA-23 in Thailand. Jpn J Infect Dis 2009; 62: 152-4.

[52] Jamulitrat S, Thongpiyapoom S, Suwalak N. An outbreak of imipenem-resistant *Acinetobacter baumannii* at Songklanagarind Hospital: the risk factors and patient prognosis. J Med Assoc Thai 2007; 90: 2181-91.

[53] Apisarnthanarak A, Mundy LM. Mortality associated with Pandrug-resistant *Acinetobacter baumannii* infections in Thailand. Am J Infect Control 2009; 37: 519-20.

[54] Jamulitrat S, Arunpan P, Phainuphong P. Attributable mortality of imipenem-resistant nosocomial *Acinetobacter baumannii* bloodstream infection. J Med Assoc Thai 2009; 92: 413-9.

[55] Koomanachai P, Tiengrim S, Kiratisin P, *et al.* Efficacy and safety of colistin (colistimethate sodium) for therapy of infections caused by multidrug-resistant *Pseudomonas aeruginosa* and *Acinetobacter baumannii* in Siriraj Hospital, Bangkok, Thailand. Int J Infect Dis 2007; 11: 402-6.

[56] Yau W, Owen RJ, Poudyal, *et al.* Colistin hetero-resistance in multidrug-resistant *Acinetobacter baumannii* clinical isolates from the Western Pacific region in the SENTRY antimicrobial surveillance programme. J Infect 2009; 58: 138-44.

[57] Jung R, Husain M, Choi MK, *et al.* Synergistic activities of moxifloxacin combined with piperacillin-tazobactam or cefepime against *Klebsiella pneumoniae*, *Enterobacter cloacae*, and *Acinetobacter baumannii* clinical isolates. Antimicrob Agents Chemother 2004; 48: 1055-7.

[58] Kiffer CR, Sampaio JL, Sinto S, *et al. In vitro* synergy test of meropenem and sulbactam against clinical isolates of *Acinetobacter baumannii*. Diagn Microbiol Infect Dis 2005; 52: 317-22.

[59] Pankuch GA, Lin G, Seifert H, *et al.* Activity of meropenem with and without ciprofloxacin and colistin against *Pseudomonas aeruginosa* and *Acinetobacter baumannii*. Antimicrob Agents Chemother 2008; 52: 333-63.

[60] Principe L, D'Arezzo S, Capone A, *et al. In vitro* activity of tigecycline in combination with various antimicrobials against multidrug resistant *Acinetobacter baumannii*. Ann Clin Microbiol Antimicrob 2009; 8: 18.

[61] Kiratisin P, Apisarnthanarak A, Kaewdaeng S. Synergistic activities between carbapenems and other antimicrobial agents against *Acinetobacter baumannii* including multidrug resistant and extensive drug resistant isolates Int J Antimicrob Agents 2010; 36: 243-6.

[62] Lumbiganon P, Tattawasatra U, Chetchotisakd P, *et al.* Comparison between the antimicrobial susceptibility of *Burkholderia pseudomallei* to trimethoprim-sulfamethoxazole by standard disk diffusion method and by minimal inhibitory concentration determination. J Med Assoc Thai 2000; 83: 856-60.

[63] Wuthiekanun V, Cheng AC, Chierakul W, *et al.* Trimethoprim/sulfamethoxazole resistance in clinical isolates of *Burkholderia pseudomallei*. J Antimicrob Chemother 2005; 55: 1029-31.

[64] Apisarnthanarak A, Pinitchai U, Thongphubeth K, *et al.* A multifaceted intervention to reduce pandrug-resistant *Acinetobacter baumannii* colonization and infection in 3 intensive care units in a Thai tertiary care center: a 3-year study. Clin Infect Dis 2008; 47: 760-7.

CHAPTER 5

Challenges in Management of Tuberculosis in Developing Countries

Amita Jain[*] and Pratima Dixit

Department of Microbiology, C.S.M. Medical University Lucknow (India), 226003

Abstract: Prevention and control of tuberculosis in middle and low income countries is a great challenge for health care workers as well as funding agencies. Issues which pose challenges in these countries are different from the developed world and hence need to be addressed in a different manner. Key challenges remain; high prevalence of tuberculosis especially drug resistant tuberculosis, Multidrug Resistant Tuberculosis (MDR-TB) and extensively drug resistant tuberculosis (XDR-TB), Human Immunodefiency Virus (HIV) and TB co morbidity, local, social and structural factors (which are different from region to region), economic constrains, poor diagnostic facilities *etc.* To meet these challenges, building a strategy on case management, maintaining high quality of care and preventing drug resistance, building human resource capacity, improving diagnosis and fostering operation research in area of tuberculosis should be the health care priority in these countries. Here, we have focused on each one of the important issues which adversely impact the control and prevention of tuberculosis in economically weaker countries.

Keywords: Multidrug resistant tuberculosis, XDR-TB, HIV, tuberculosis, WHO, TB-associated deaths, HIV-co infected patients, second-line drugs, drug-susceptibility testing.

INTRODUCTION

In 1993, the World Health Organization (WHO) declared tuberculosis (TB) a global public health emergency, recognizing its enormous, rising and far-reaching burden [1]. The magnitude of the global tuberculosis problem is immense, with more than 9 million new cases and nearly 2 million deaths (including 465,000 deaths in HIV-co infected patients) caused by TB reported in 2007 alone [2]. Most of the TB-associated deaths are from low and middle-income countries [3]. Millions of TB cases are either undetected or unnotified or both, and progress in controlling TB is critically constrained by the inadequacy of available means. Moreover, HIV is fuelling the epidemic. The spread of multidrug-resistance tuberculosis (MDR-TB) and extensively drug-resistant TB (XDR-TB) is a major medical and public health concern for the world. MDR-TB is defined as resistant to at least two major anti tuberculosis drugs; rifampicin and isoniazid with or without resistance to other anti-TB drugs whereas XDR-TB is defined as MDR-TB with additional resistance to any fluroquinolones and at least one of three injectable second line drugs *i.e.* amikacin, kanamycin and/or capreomycin. These two forms of highly drug-resistant TB threaten to make TB an untreatable and highly fatal disease, particularly in resource-poor countries with a high prevalence of AIDS [4]. Therapy for multidrug-resistant tuberculosis has been virtually nonexistent [5]. Drug-Susceptibility Testing (DST) and Second-Line Drugs (SLDs) are not cost effective because of limited resources [6]. Rapid and accurate diagnosis is at the core of the international strategy to control TB. Moreover, there is an increasing need for new drugs. There have not been any inventions of new anti TB molecule since 1965 [7]. The highest research priorities for TB management in resource poor countries remain: 1) invention of a new anti-TB drug which can substitute rifampicin, does not interfere with antiretroviral drugs, simplify and shorten treatment and is effective against drug resistant strains, 2) invention and application of a rapid, sensitive, specific, simple and cost effective test which can be used as a point of care test in the field settings of resource poor countries for detection of tuberculosis especially drug resistant TB 3) development of an effective vaccine for TB.

Social and structural issues like poverty, gender discrimination, social stigma associated with disease,

---

*Address correspondence to Amita Jain: Department of Microbiology, C.S.M. Medical University Lucknow (India), 226003; Tel:- +91-9415023928; Fax: +91-522 2287400; E-mail: amita602002@yahoo.com

political indifference *etc.*, leads to the difficulties in TB management like treatment default and non-adherence to treatment. Strict implementation of directly observed treatment short term (DOTS and DOTS plus) for control and prevention of tuberculosis is a big challenge. DOTS stand for "Directly Observed Therapy, Short-course" and is a major plank in the WHO global TB eradication programme [8]. The WHO extended the DOTS programme in 1998 to include the treatment of MDR-TB (called "DOTS-Plus") [9]. Implementation of DOTS-Plus requires the capacity to perform drug-susceptibility testing (not routinely available even in developed countries) and the availability of second-line agents. Regular supply of good quality second line drugs is questionable, in addition to all the requirements for DOTS. DOTS-Plus is therefore much more resource-expensive than DOTS, and requires much greater commitment from countries wishing to implement it. Resource limitations mean that the implementation of DOTS-Plus may lead inadvertently to the diversion of resources from existing DOTS programmes and a consequent decrease in the overall standard of care [10].

HIGH PREVALENCE OF TB AND DRUG RESISTANT TUBERCULOSIS

Globally, there were an estimated 9.27 million incident cases of TB in 2007. This is an increase from 9.24 million cases in 2006, 8.3 million cases in 2000 and 6.6 million cases in 1990. Most of the estimated number of cases in 2007 were in Asia (the South-East Asia and Western Pacific regions) (55%) and Africa (31%), with small proportions of cases in the Eastern Mediterranean Region (6%), the European Region (5%) and the Region of the Americas (3%). The five countries that rank first to fifth in terms of total numbers of cases in 2007 are India (2.0 million), China (1.3 million), Indonesia (0.53 million), Nigeria (0.46 million) and South Africa (0.46 million) [2]. TB is predominantly a disease of poverty with over 80% of cases occurring in Asia or Africa. Greatest numbers of patients live in highly populous countries of Asia and the highest incidence of disease is found in Africa [11]. The estimated numbers of cases in these and other High Burden Countries (HBCs) in 2007 are shown in Table **1**. Among the 15 countries with the highest estimated TB incidence rates, 13 are in Africa, a phenomenon linked to high rates of HIV co infection.

Table 1: Epidemiology Burden of TB (reproduced from WHO, 2009 report).

			Incidence				Prevalence		Mortality				
			All forms		**Smear positive**		**All forms**		**HIV negative**		**HIV positive**		
		Pop. 1000s	No. 1000s	PER 100 000 Pop./ year	No. 1000s	PER 100 000 Pop./ year	No. 1000s	PER 100 000 Pop./ year	No. 1000s	PER 100 000 Pop./ year	No. 1000s	PER 100 000 Pop./ year	HIV pre. in incident TB cases %
1	India	1169016	1962	168	873	75	3305	283	302	26	30	2.5	5.3
2	China	1328630	1306	98	585	44	2582	194	194	15	6.8	0.5	1.9
3	Indonesia	231 627	528	228	236	102	566	244	86	37	5.4	2.4	3.0
4	Nigeria	148 093	460	311	195	131	772	521	79	53	59	40	27
5	South Africa	48 577	461	948	174	358	336	692	18	38	94	193	73
6	Bangladesh	158 665	353	223	159	100	614	387	70	44	0.4	0.3	0.3
7	Ethiopia	83099	314	378	135	163	481	579	53	64	23	28	19
8	Pakistan	163902	297	181	133	81	365	223	46	28	1.4	0.9	2.1
9	Philippines	87960	255	290	115	130	440	500	36	41	0.3	0.3	0.3
10	DR Congo	62636	245	392	109	174	417	666	45	72	6.0	10	5.9
11	Russian Federation	142499	157	110	68	48	164	115	20	14	5.1	3.6	16
12	Viet Nam	87375	150	171	66	76	192	220	18	20	3.1	3.5	8.1
13	Kenya	37538	132	353	53	142	120	319	10	26	15	39	48
14	Brazil	191791	92	48	49	26	114	60	5.9	3.1	2.5	1.3	14

Table 1: cont...

15	UR Tanzania	40454	120	297	49	120	136	337	12	29	20	49	47
16	Uganda	30884	102	330	42	136	132	426	13	41	16	52	39
17	Zimbabwe	13349	104	782	40	298	95	714	6.9	52	28	213	69
18	Thailand	63884	91	142	39	62	123	192	10	15	3.9	6.0	17
19	Mozambique	21397	92	431	37	174	108	504	10	45	17	82	47
20	Myanmar	48798	83	171	37	75	79	162	5.4	11	0.9	1.9	11
21	Cambodia	14444	72	495	32	219	96	664	11	77	1.8	13	7.8
22	Afghanistan	27145	46	168	21	76	65	238	8.2	30	0.0	0	0

Globally, there were 510,545 cases of MDR-TB in 2007. This estimate is based on data from drug resistance surveys or routine surveillance (DRS) for 113 countries reporting new cases and 102 countries reporting re-treatment cases [12]. Cases of MDR-TB are very unevenly distributed; with 27 countries (of which 15 are in Eastern Europe) accounting for 85% of all cases (Table **2**). The countries that rank first to fifth in terms of total numbers of MDR-TB cases are India (131, 000), China (112, 000), the Russian Federation (43, 000), South Africa (16, 000) and Bangladesh (15, 000).

Table 2: Number of MDR-TB Cases Estimated, Notified and Expected to Be Treated, 27 High MDR-TB Burden Countries and WHO Region (reproduced from WHO, 2009 report).

S. No.	Country	Estimated Cases, 2007	
		Percentage of all TB cases with MDR-TB	Number of MDR-TB cases
1	India	5.4	130 526
2	China	7.5	112 34
3	Russian Federation	21	42 969
4	South Africa	2.8	15 914
5	Bangladesh	4.0	14 506
6	Pakistan	4.3	13 218
7	Indonesia	2.3	12 209
8	Philippines	4.6	12 125
9	Nigeria	2.4	11 700
10	Kazakhstan	32	11 102
11	Ukraine	19	9 835
12	Uzbekistan	24	9 450
13	Democratic Republic of the Congo	2.8	7 336
14	Viet Nam	4.0	6 468
15	Ethiopia	1.9	5 979
16	Tajikistan	2.3	4 688
17	Myanmar	4.7	4 181
18	Azerbaijan	36	3 916
19	Republic of Moldova	29	2 231
20	Kyrgyzstan	17	1 290
21	Belarus	16	1 101
22	Georgia	13	728
23	Armenia	17	486
24	Lithuania	17	464
25	Bulgaria	12	371
26	Latvia	14	202
27	Estonia	20	123
Total	**High MDR-TB burden countries**	**5.7**	**435 470**

By the end of 2008, 55 countries and territories had reported at least one case of XDR-TB. Reported overall prevalence of XDR-TB among all multi-drug resistant tuberculosis isolates was 6.6% worldwide, 6.5% in industrialized countries (*e.g.* United States, United Kingdom, Ireland, Germany, France, Belgium, Spain, Japan and Australia) and 13.6% in Russia and Eastern Europe (*e.g.* Republic of Georgia, Czech Republic, Armenia and Azerbaijan). However, reported XDR prevalence is around 1.5% in Asia (Bangladesh, Indonesia, Papua New Guinea, Thailand and East Timor) and only 0.6% in Africa and Middle East. Republic of Korea represents maximum numbers of XDR-TB cases that is 15.4% XDR-TB cases among all multi-drug resistant tuberculosis patients [13]. In the USA, 4% of the MDR-TB strains isolated between 1993 and 2004 were XDR-TB. In Europe, data from Latvia shows that 19% of the MDR strains isolated during 2000-2002 were XDR.

HIV-TB CO- MORBIDITY

Among the 9.27 million incident cases of TB in 2007, an estimated 1.37 million (14.8%) were HIV-positive (15% of the total global TB burden) and 0.46 million TB deaths occurred in HIV-positive people (23% of global HIV/AIDS mortality) [2]. The global number of incident HIV-positive TB cases is estimated to have peaked in 2005, at 1.39 million. India has the second largest HIV infected population in the world after Africa, with over five million Indians infected with HIV. Approximately 3% of TB cases in India are infected with HIV [12].

The relationship of HIV infection and MDR-TB is not yet fully understood. HIV infection has been associated with MDR-TB outbreaks in institutional settings, such as hospitals and prisons [14]. It remains less clear whether HIV infection is also associated with MDR-TB in community settings. With increasing prevalence of drug resistance globally, a higher percentage of recent infections are likely to be multi-drug resistant, resulting in higher rates of MDR-TB in HIV-positive individuals [15].

First report of XDR-TB with HIV came from Kwazulu Natal, South Africa (KZN) province [16]. Of 544 TB patients at Church of Scotland Hospital of KZN, which serves a rural area with high HIV rates, 221 were found to have MDR, of these, 53 were diagnosed with XDR-TB. Fifty-two of these patients died, most within 25 days. Of 53 patients, 44 were tested for HIV and all 44 were HIV-positive. In KZN two health care workers died from XDR-TB with HIV. A study from India with 54 full-blown AIDS patients, suspected of having HIV- TB co-infection showed that 12 (22.2%) were MDR-TB cases and among them, 4 (33.3%) were XDR-TB cases. All 4 patients, in whom XDR-TB was confirmed, died within 2.6 months of diagnosis [17].

LACK OF ACCURATE, RAPID AND COST-EFFECTIVE DIAGNOSTIC TOOLS

The laboratory plays a critical role in the diagnosis and management of tuberculosis more so of drug-resistant TB. The routine diagnostic methods that are used in various parts of the world, (Acid Fast Bacilli (AFB) smear examination and X-ray chest) are still very similar to those used 100 years ago [18]. Under field conditions sputum smear microscopy shows a sensitivity of only 40-60%. Poor sensitivity is exacerbated in the presence of HIV co-infection because HIV-associated TB is more commonly paucibacillary. Currently, only small fractions (16%) of TB patients are reported with a laboratory-confirmed diagnosis.

Culture and drug susceptibility tests for *M. tuberculosis* are considered the gold standard for diagnosis, treatment and surveillance of drug resistance. TB culture is more sensitive but is only performed in reference centers, takes from four to ten weeks for results and thus comes mostly too late to impact patient management and outcome. Using standardized DST procedures with conventional methods, eight to twelve weeks are required to identify drug-resistant microorganisms on solid media (*i.e.*, Lowenstein-Jensen medium) [19]. Unlike testing of first line TB drugs, susceptibility testing of Second Line Drugs (SLDs) has poor reproducibility and is not standardized throughout the world, even among national reference laboratories [20]. Critical concentrations used for testing SLDs vary greatly among laboratories [20] despite published recommendations [21] and validation of SLD susceptibility testing by several groups [22, 23].

There is also limited quality control of SLD testing [24]. Finally, the association between the *in vitro* efficacy of a SLD and the clinical outcome is not well established [21].

Rapid phenotypic methods, such as TK Medium (Salubris Inc, USA), Microscopic-Observation Drug-Susceptibility assay (MODS) and FAST Plaque-Response bacteriophage assay (Biotech Laboratories Ltd, UK) are cheaper but not always simple to perform, with some requiring high standards of biosafety and quality control [25]. MODS are technically more difficult and cannot distinguish between *M. tuberculosis* and non-tuberculous mycobacteria. Automated liquid culture systems are more sensitive than solid media cultures, and they significantly reduce turnaround time. However, even with liquid cultures, two to four weeks are still needed to obtain results, and their substantially higher cost is an issue for resource-limited countries. The BACTEC 460 TB radiometric system (Becton Dickinson, USA) was considered to be a major advancement, but has been replaced by the Mycobacteria Growth Indicator Tube system (Becton Dickinson, USA). Several published studies have shown the excellent performance of the Mycobacteria Growth Indicator Tube system for the rapid detection of resistance to first- and second-line anti-TB drugs [23]. Detection of drug resistance can be accomplished in days rather than weeks, although still constrained by high cost (equipment and consumables).

Molecular approaches for detection of drug resistant tuberculosis are still insensitive for many of the mutations. All genotypic tests require DNA extraction, gene amplification and detection of mutation and are, therefore, relatively expensive and demand resources and skills that are usually unavailable in most regions where rates of MDR-TB and XDR-TB are high. Molecular tools are based on nucleic acid amplification in conjunction with electrophoresis, sequencing or hybridization. Direct sequencing is another approach to detecting mutations, but it is an expensive and time-consuming process. Techniques, such as real-time polymerase chain reaction, that make use of wild-type primer sequences to amplify genes and enable the use of specific probes (*i.e.* molecular beacons) to identify mutations are expensive and complicated [21].

Effective control of MDR-TB and XDR-TB will require massive scaling-up of culture and DST capacity, and the expanded use of novel and rapid assays for drug resistance. Laboratory methods and reporting, especially for susceptibility to second-line drugs, should be standardized through expert consensus. Internationally, competent, high-quality reference laboratory services with capacity to perform required testing of samples and to report results in a prompt manner to providers and health officials must be available [20]. The WHO and the International Union against Tuberculosis and Lung Disease plan on setting up a network of supranational reference laboratories, to determine the quality control and standardization of susceptibility testing, needed for international comparison. The WHO is also planning on supporting national reference laboratories in developing countries. Therefore, many new diagnostic tools are being evaluated for performance, feasibility of implementation, and sustainability in resource-limited settings [26]. The WHO has recently endorsed the use of advanced diagnostic technologies (liquid culture and molecular line probe assay) for laboratory diagnosis of TB and MDR-TB in developing countries [27]. The challenge, therefore, is to not only develop new tools, but to also make sure that benefits of promising new tools actually reach the populations that need it most, but can least afford them [28].

POOR IMPLEMENTATION OF DOTS

Effective implementation of the DOTS strategy saves lives through decreased risk for individual TB patients of treatment failure, TB relapse, and death. The WHO extended the DOTS programme in 1998 to include the treatment of MDR-TB (called "DOTS-Plus") [9]. Constraints which affect this strategy are: lack of qualified staff, poor monitoring and evaluation, private sector involvement, weak laboratories, wavering political commitment. increasing TB/HIV co- infection, limited access to DOTS, low public awareness, administrative constraints and adverse policy, unreliable drug supply or undeveloped drug policy and insufficient funds.

NO NEW ANTI- TUBERCULAR DRUG AND VACCINE

The introduction of anti-tuberculosis drugs in the 1950s and the development of the various drug regimens by the 1980s meant that there was a 98% chance of TB cure. Resistance to either INH or R may be managed with other first line drugs but MDR-TB demands treatment with second line drugs that have limited sterilizing capacity, are costly and are more toxic [29]. Unfortunately, no new drug except rifabutin and rifapentine has been marketed for TB during the last forty years after release of Rifampicin. There are a number of constraints that companies have from investing in new anti-TB drugs. The research is expensive, slow and difficult and requires specialized facilities for handling *M. tuberculosis*. There are few animal models that closely mimic the human TB disease. Development time of any anti-TB drug will be long. In fact minimum six month therapy will require a follow up period of one year or more [30]. Of the most urgent goal of chemotherapy of tuberculosis especially that associated with HIV infection is to develop highly active, low cost drugs which can be used not only in industrialized countries but also in developing countries, since the incidence of AIDS associated intractable tuberculosis is rapidly increasing in the latter [31]. Development of new drugs is very costly and not seen as a priority in the market orientated economics of the pharmaceutical industry.

Fundamental and applied research in TB diagnostics is needed for (i) rapid identification of *M. tuberculosis*, (ii) determination of its drug resistance profile, (iii) rapid diagnosis or ruling out of TB in patients and their contacts [32]. In addition to sputum smear and culture, amplification techniques are already used to diagnose tuberculosis and antigen-detection tests for this purpose are being developed. Molecular typing and DNA microarrays provide new insights in the natural history and transmission of tuberculosis [33]. Knowledge gaps remain regarding the genetics and growth characteristics of *M. tuberculosis* and the physiology and biochemistry of both the host and pathogen during infection.

Factors hampering the development and evaluation of new vaccines include problems with extrapolation from animal models, incomplete natural immunity, and limited knowledge about protective immunity [33]. In those parts of the world where the disease is common, the World Health Organization recommends that infants receive BCG (Bacille Calmette Guerin). BCG has its own drawbacks; it does not protect adults very well against TB. BCG may interfere with the TB skin test, showing a positive skin test reaction. This confers incomplete protection against tuberculosis, and is not safe in infants infected with the human immunodeficiency virus. In countries where BCG vaccine is used, the ability of the skin test to identify people infected with *M. tuberculosis* is limited. A new, safe vaccine regimen, which better protects against lung disease, is urgently needed to control TB in high-burden countries. Identifying new candidate TB vaccines and immune-boosting vaccine adjuvant to prevent infection or disease and evaluation of the potential of synthetic vaccines to help shorten TB drug treatment regimens is being tried at some institutes.

SOCIAL ISSUES

Some of the resource poor countries have unique social and structural factors which usually have negative influence (mainly non adherence to treatment) on the management and prevention of tuberculosis. These factors have been defined as barriers or facilitators that relate to economic, social, policy, organizational, or other aspects of the environment [34]. Usually patients have no personal control over most of these issues. The developing world is most vulnerable, with factors like poverty, gender discrimination, malnutrition, overcrowding and poor access to healthcare services. Structural factors are discussed in various ways with poverty remaining one of the most important of these for treatment taking, especially when linked to health care service factors, such as poorly accessible, poorly equipped, and distant clinics [35].

Personal and social factors, including poverty and social marginalization, may be used to identify patients at risk of nonadherence to their medication regimen. However, it cannot be assumed that all individuals sharing a particular characteristic face the same barriers to adherence. Nonadherence can also be a product of programme failures, such as an inadequate supply of drugs, rather than patient-related problems or failures [36]. Lack of motivation and knowledge, local beliefs and attitudes are important factors related to non adherence to treatment. These factors influenced patients' understanding of treatment, including its duration and the consequences of defaulting, on adherence to treatment [37]. The long treatment period is poorly understood by patients [38].

Patients' interpretation of illness and wellness is also an important factors due to which patients stop treatment as they felt better and think that they are cured [39]. Patients whose symptoms abated might be more likely to interrupt treatment [40]. Patients who felt worse than before treatment [36, 41] or saw no improvement in their condition might be more likely to interrupt treatment. Patient motivation and willingness, and the effect of incentives on treatment taking, have received some attention [42]. Reasons for defaulting from TB and MDR-TB treatment include patients' perceptions of negative attitudes among health-care workers, substance abuse and employment concerns, unemployment rates of up to 40%, as well as the resultant migration [42].

Table 3: List of Important Social and Structural Factors Impacting the Disease Outcome in Low And Middle Income Countries.

Factors	Comments
Poverty	High cost of ATT, in some countries leads to nonadherence
Malnutrition	Drug intolerance in these patients is common, so they stop the treatment
Overcrowding	Transmission of disease is more common in places like jails which are overcrowded
Gender discrimination	Women are not usually bread earners so their treatment is not a priority
Alcoholism and drug abuse	Are seen as common cause of nonadherence
Homelessness	Nonadherence is common because homeless people are difficult to trace
Frequent migration	Daily wagers and people absconding from law are frequently migrating, hence do not adhere to treatment
Stigma associated with TB	Usually keeps people away from TB clinics, as they do not want to attend these facilities
Unemployment	Economic reasons are important for this population
Lack of knowledge and motivation	They are unable to figure out the importance of the duration of treatment.
Interpretation of illness and wellness	As soon as the symptoms are relieved they stop the treatment
Beliefs and attitude	Local beliefs of cause of disease and treatment by quacks does lot of damage

Patients' ability to manage TB treatment is a product of dynamic processes, in which social and economic costs and other burdens change and interplay over time. Interventions to facilitate adherence to TB treatment needs to address both time-specific and local factors. Management of early tuberculosis symptoms and adherence to medical treatment are main challenges in controlling TB. Social context (Family, Community, and Household) also influences the management of Tuberculosis. TB patients may hide their diagnosis [43], and feel guilt and shame because of the disease. Stigma may also make patients afraid to ask for support from their employer to purchase medication, thereby reducing adherence. Sometimes a patient's role and responsibilities in the family could motivate them to adhere to treatment in order to recover and resume those duties [44]. But responsibilities in the home, such as providing income and caring for children also reduced the likelihood of adherence for some [41]. Family support, including financial assistance, collecting medication, and emotional support, appeared to be a strong influence on patient adherence to treatment [45].

Health care service factors, such as long waiting times, lack of privacy and inconvenient opening times in clinics [46] add to economic discomfort and social disruption for patients and negatively influence adherence. The patients often face a choice between employment and taking medication for TB; and there is evidence that patients consciously estimate the opportunity costs of taking treatment. Treatment side effects and adherence is also associated with Health care service of patients. Some patients stopping medication because of adverse effects [38], while others say that they were not informed about side effects and what to do to counter them [44, 47]. In some cases, patients had not communicated side effects to providers. Only few patients acknowledged that side effects had influenced their decision to abandon treatment [48].

Prevention and control of TB in the low and middle income countries require a robust public health infrastructure that includes a workforce trained in TB prevention, diagnosis, treatment, and case management. Tuberculosis can be controlled if appropriate policies are followed, effective clinical and public health management is ensured, and there are committed and coordinated efforts from within and outside the health sector. Apart from a strong tuberculosis control programme, there is also a need for a continuous and periodic survey of drug resistance, which will provide information on the type of chemotherapy to be used for the treatment of patients and also to serve as a useful parameter in evaluation of current and past chemotherapy programmes. There is a need for revision of guidelines of national programmers based on levels of resistance, training of professionals in private sector, strengthening of existing National Tuberculosis Control Programme, restricting use of Rifampicin, taking logistic measures to ensure regular supply of drugs at all levels of National Tuberculosis Control Programme and by ensuring compliance enhancing measures like providing free antitubercular drugs, supervised treatment and health education. Key challenges that remain, are overcoming the weakness of a strategy built on case management, sustaining commitment, competing priorities, the threat of HIV, maintaining high quality of care and preventing drug resistance, building human resource capacity, improving diagnosis and fostering operations research.

REFERENCES

[1]   Murali MS, Sajjan BS. DOTS Strategy for control of tuberculosis epidemic Indian. J Med Sci. 2002; 56(1): 16-18.

[2]   WHO. Global tuberculosis control: epidemiology, strategy, financing: WHO Report WHO/HTM/TB/2009. 411.WHO, Geneva, Switzerland 2009; 1-303.

[3]   Lopez AD, Mathers CD (Eds.). Global burden of disease and risk factors. Oxford University Press, NY, USA 2006.

[4]   Chan ED, Iseman MD. Multidrug-resistant and extensively drug-resistant tuberculosis: a review. Curr Opin Infect Dis. Dec 2008; 21(6): 587-95.

[5]   Mitnick, C., J Bayona, J . *et al.* Community-based therapy for multidrug resistant tuberculosis in lima, Peru. The New England Journal of Medicine 2003; 348(2): 119-28.

[6]   Dye C, Williams BG, Espinal MA, *et al.* Erasing the world's slow stain: strategies to beat multidrug-resistant tuberculosis. Science Mar 2002; 15 (5562): 2042-46.

[7]   Schwalbe N, Ignatius H. New drugs for TB past time to deliver. TB Alliance Newsletter 9 September 2006. Available at: http://new tballiance.org/newscenter/view-innews.php? idp624.

[8]   Elzinga G, Raviglione MC, Maher D. Scale up: meeting targets in global tuberculosis control. Lancet 2004; 363(9411): 814-19.

[9]   Iseman MD. MDR-TB and the developing world-a problem no longer to be ignored: the WHO announces 'DOTS-Plus' strategy. Int J Tuberc Lung Dis 1998; 2(11): 867.

[10]   Sterling TR, Lehmann HP, Frieden TR. Impact of DOTS compared with DOTS-plus on multidrug-resistant tuberculosis and tuberculosis deaths: decision analysis. BMJ 2003; 326(7389): 574.

[11]   Corbett EL, Marston B, Churchyard GJ, *et al.* Tuberculosis in sub-Saharan Africa: opportunities, challenges, and change in the era of antiretroviral treatment. Lancet 2006; 367:926-37.

[12]   WHO/IUATLD Global Project on Anti-tuberculosis Drug Resistance Surveillance.WHO Report (WHO/HTM/TB/2008.394), WHO, Geneva 2008; 1-142.

[13]   Shah SN, Wright, A, Bai HG, *et al.* Worldwide emergence of extensively drug-resistant tuberculosis. Emer Infect Dis 2007; 13: 380-87.

[14]   Valway SE, Greifinger RB, Papania M, *et al.* Multidrug-resistant tuberculosis in the New York State prison system, 1990-1991. J Infect Dis 1994; 170: 151-56.

[15]   Espinal MA, Laszlo A, Simonsen L, *et al.* Global trends in resistance to antituberculosis drugs. World Health Organization-International Union against Tuberculosis and Lung Disease Working Group on Anti-Tuberculosis Drug Resistance Surveillance. N Engl J Med 2001; 344: 1294-303.

[16]   Gandhi NR, Moll A, Sturm AW. Extensively drug resistant tuberculosis as a cause of death in patients co-infected with tuberculosis and HIV in a rural area of South Africa. Lancet 2006; 368: 1575-80.

[17]   Singh S, Sankar MM, Gopinath K. High rate of extensively drug-resistant tuberculosis in Indian AIDS patients. AIDS 2008; 21: 2345-47.

[18] LoBue, P., Sizemore, C. *et al.* Plan to combat extensively drug-resistant tuberculosis recommendations of the federal tuberculosis task force. Recommendations and reports 2009; 58: 1-43.

[19] Migliori, GB. And Matteelli, A. Diagnosis of multidrug-resistant tuberculosis and extensively drug-resistant tuberculosis: Current standards and challenges. Can J Infect Dis Med Microbiol 2008; 19(2): 169-72.

[20] Kim SJ, Espinal MA, Abe C, *et al.* Is second-line anti-tuberculosis drug susceptibility testing reliable? Int J Tuberc Lung Dis 2004; 8: 1157-58.

[21] World Health Organization. Guidelines for drug susceptibility testing for second-line anti-tuberculosis drugs for DOTS-plus. WHO/CDS/TB/2001.288. 2001.

[22] Kruuner A, Yates MD, Drobniewski FA. Evaluation of MGIT 960-based antimicrobial testing and determination of critical concentrations of first and second- line antimicrobial drugs with drug- resistant clinical strains of *M. tuberculosis*. J Clin Microbial 2006; 44: 811-18.

[23] Rusch-Gerdes S, Pfyffer GE, Casal M, *et al.* Multicenter laboratory validation of the BACTEC MGIT 960 technique for testing susceptibilities of *Mycobacterium tuberculosis* to classical second-line drugs and newer antimicrobials. J Clin Microbiol 2006; 44: 688-92.

[24] Fattorini L, Iona E, Cirillo D, *et al.* External quality control of *Mycobacterium tuberculosis* drug susceptibility testing: results of two rounds in epidemic countries. Int J Tubec Lung Dis 2008; 12: 214-17.

[25] Pai M, Kalantri S, Dheda K. New tools and emerging technologies for the diagnosis of tuberculosis: Part II. Active tuberculosis and drug resistance. Expert Rev Mol Diagn 2006; 6: 423-32.

[26] Pai M, Ramsay A, O Brien R. Evidence based tuberculosis diagnosis. PLoS Med 2008; 5(7): e156.

[27] World Health Organization 2007. The use of liquid medium for culture and DST.Available:http://www.who.int/tb/dots/laboratory/policy/en/index3.html

[28] Perkins MD, Roscigno G, Zumla A. Progress towards improved tuberculosis diagnostics for developing countries. Lancet 2006; 367: 942-43.

[29] Ormerod LP. Multidrug-resistant tuberculosis (MDR-TB): epidemiology, prevention and treatment. Br Med Bull 2005; 73-74: 17-24.

[30] Tomioka H, Namba K. Development of antituberculous drugs: current status and future prospects. Kekkaku 2006; 81(12): 753-74.

[31] Tomioka H. Prospects for development of new antituberculous drug. Kekkaku 2002; 77(8): 573-84.

[32] Fauci, AS. and the NIAID Tuberculosis Working Group Multidrug-Resistant and Extensively Drug-Resistant Tuberculosis: The National Institute of Allergy and Infectious Diseases Research Agenda and Recommendations for Priority Research. The Journal of Infectious Diseases 2008; 197: 1493-98.

[33] Borgdorff MW, Kolk A, van Soolingen D, *et al.* Research into new methods for diagnosing, treating and preventing tuberculosis. Ned Tijdschr Geneeskd 2003; 147(38): 1838-41.

[34] Sumartojo E. Structural factors in HIV prevention: Concepts, examples and implications for research. AIDS 2000; 14: S3-S10.

[35] Sumartojo E. When tuberculosis treatment fails: A social behavioural account of patient adherence. Am Rev Respir Dis 1993; 147: 1311-20.

[36] Jaiswal A, Singh V, Ogden JA, *et al.* Adherence to tuberculosis treatment: Lessons from the urban setting of Delhi, India. Trop Med Int Health 2003; 8: 625-33.

[37] Demissie M, GetahunH, Lindtjorn B. Community tuberculosis care through 'TB clubs' in rural north Ethiopia. Soc Sci Med 2003; 56: 2009-18.

[38] Watkins RE, Rouse CR, Plant AJ. Tuberculosis treatment delivery in Bali: A qualitative study of clinic staff perceptions. Int J Tuberc Lung Dis 2004; 8: 218-25.

[39] Rowe KA, Makhubele B, Hargreaves JR, *et al.* Adherence to TB preventive therapy for HIV-positive patients in rural South Africa: implications for antiretroviral delivery in resource-poor settings? Int J Tuberc Lung Dis 2005; 9: 263-69.

[40] Pushpananthan S, Walley JD, Wright J. Tuberculosis in Swaziland: A health needs assessment in preparation for a community-based programme. Trop Doc 2000; 30: 216-20.

[41] Greene JA. An ethnography of non-adherence: Culture, poverty, and tuberculosis in urban Bolivia. Cult Med Psychiatry 2004; 28: 401-25.

[42] Tulsky JP, Hahn JA, Long HL, *et al.* Can the poor adhere? Incentives for adherence to TB prevention in homeless adults. Int J Tuberc Lung Dis 2004; 8: 83-91.

[43] Harper M, Ahmadu FA, Ogden JA, *et al.* Identifying the determinants of tuberculosis control in resource-poor countries: Insights from a qualitative study in The Gambia. Trans R Soc Trop Med Hyg 2003; 97: 506-10.

[44]   Wares DF, Singh S, Acharya AK, *et al.* Non-adherence to tuberculosis treatment in the eastern Tarai of Nepal. Int J Tuberc Lung Dis 2003; 7: 327-35.

[45]   Khan MA, Walley JD, Witter SN, *et al.* Tuberculosis patient adherence to direct observation: Results of a social study in Pakistan. Health Policy Plan 2005; 20: 354-65.

[46]   Joseph HA, Shrestha-Kuwahara R, Lowry D, *et al.* Factors influencing health care workers' adherence to work site tuberculosis screening and policies. Am J Infect Control 2004; 32: 456-61.

[47]   Edginton ME, Sekatane CS, Goldstein SJ. Patients' beliefs: Do they affect tuberculosis control? A study in a rural district of South Africa. Int J Tuberc Lung Dis 2002; 6: 1075-82.

[48]   Rowe KA, Makhubele B, Hargreaves JR, *et al.* Adherence to TB preventive therapy for HIV-positive patients in rural South Africa: implications for antiretroviral delivery in resource-poor settings? Int J Tuberc Lung Dis 2005; 9:263-69.

CHAPTER 6

Drug Resistance in Tuberculosis

UD Gupta[*] and Anuj Kumar Gupta

National JALMA Institute for Leprosy & Other Mycobacterial Diseases (ICMR), Tajganj, Agra- 282001, India

Abstract: Drug resistance in tuberculosis (TB) is known since the start of anti-tubercular therapy to treat tuberculosis. It arises as a result of inadequate treatment procedures or poor compliance to drugs by the patients, which result in selection and spread of resistant tubercle bacilli in the population. Multidrug resistance (MDR), and recently extensive drug resistance (XDR), have become a great challenge to our fight against TB. The resistant forms of tuberculosis are difficult to treat and the treatment is lengthy, more toxic and costlier than for drug sensitive form. The accumulation of mutations in the genes targeted by anti-TB drug is the primary mechanism behind the development of resistance. However, other mechanisms such as impermeability of bacterial cell to drugs and activation of efflux mechanisms also contribute significantly to drug resistance. Current tests to diagnose resistant TB are either lengthy, less sensitive or less specific or are expensive enough to be used in low financial clinical settings. The drugs being used to treat drug resistant TB are again costly, have side effects and still are less effective. To develop suitable and effective diagnostic tools and cheaper and less toxic effective drugs against resistant tuberculosis, a comprehensive understanding of its molecular mechanisms is needed.

Keywords: Tuberculosis, anti-TB drugs, MDR, XDR, drug sensitivity, molecular mechanisms.

INTRODUCTION

Drug resistance is a phenomenon whereby an organism becomes fully or partially resistant to drugs or antibiotics being used against it. In other terms it can be defined as temporary or permanent capacity of the organism to remain viable or to multiply in the presence of the drug concentration that would normally destroy or inhibit the growth of their cells [1]. Drug resistance is a man-made condition, which develops either by poor compliance of patients to drugs or by poor drug administration by health care workers. This is also important in other non-tuberculous mycobacterial infections, which tend to be intrinsically resistant to most of the conventional anti-TB drugs and many other common antibiotics. The rapid spread of drug resistant forms of TB was the reason behind the declaration of tuberculosis as 'Global Emergency' by World Health Organization (WHO) in 1993 [2]. Multidrug Resistance (MDR) in tuberculosis (TB) is characterized by the presence of *M.tuberculosis* strains simultaneously resistant to isoniazid and rifampicin, two of the major first line anti-tubercular drugs. Recently, its more severe form, extensive drug resistance (XDR) has emerged and caused a virtual scare globally. WHO is concerned over emergence of XDR-TB strains that are virtually untreatable. XDR is defined as occurrence of TB in persons whose *M.tuberculosis* isolates are resistant to isoniazid and rifampicin plus resistant to any fluoroquinolone and at least one of three injectable second-line drugs *i.e.* amikacin, kanamycin, or capreomycin [3].

These resistant forms of TB are difficult to treat and the treatment is very expensive as compared to drug regimen for the treatment of sensitive TB, which is cheaper, easy to afford and less toxic. The elevated cost and poor availability of drugs used to treat MDR-TB is the main accused of its spread among population with limited financial strength in developing countries.

ANTI-TB DRUGS

Treatment for TB uses antibiotics to kill the bacteria. However, instead of the short duration of antibiotics

*Address correspondence UD Gupta: National JALMA Institute for Leprosy & Other Mycobacterial Diseases (ICMR), Tajganj, Agra- 282001, India; Tel: 0562-2331751-54; Ext.266; Fax: 0562-233175; E-mail: gupta.umesh95@gmail.com

administration used to treat other bacterial infections, TB requires much longer periods of treatment (around 6 to 12 months, sometimes may be more). Keeping in view the usage, toxicity and effectiveness, anti-TB drugs are classified as:

(a) First Line Drugs (Primary Agents)

First line anti-TB drugs are those, which are given to new cases supposed to possess susceptible forms of TB. These include Isoniazid, Rifampicin, Ethambutol, Pyrazinamide, and Streptomycin. First line drugs are most effective against the tubercle bacterium and are less toxic to humans. These are the essential component of anti-TB therapeutic regimen with and without the use of second and third line drugs. However multiple forms of drug resistance to first line drugs are encountered among cases and Streptomycin is no longer considered as first line drug due to its high incidence of resistance.

(b) Second Line Drugs (Retreatment Agents)

Second line anti-TB drugs are generally given to patients with treatment failure or known forms of drug-resistant tuberculosis. There are six classes of second-line drugs used for the treatment of TB. A drug may be grouped into this catagory for one of three possible reasons: it may be less effective than the first-line drugs (*e.g.,*, p-aminosalicylic acid); or, it may have toxic side-effects (*e.g.,* cycloserine); or it may be unavailable in many developing countries (*e.g.,*, fluoroquinolones). These include aminoglycosides (*e.g.,* kanamycin, KAN; amikacin, AMI and streptomycin, SM), the polypeptides (*e.g.,* capreomycin, CAP and viomycin, VIO, enviomycin, ENV), the thioamides (*e.g.,* ethionamide, ETH and prothionamide, PTH), several fluoroquinolones (FQs) (*e.g.,* ofloxacin, OFX; levofloxacin, LFX; moxifloxacin, MFX; and gatifloxacin, GFX), para-amino salicylic acid (PAS) and D- cycloserine (CS). Second line drugs are mostly used in the treatment of MDR-TB and as a result prolong the total treatment time from 6 to 9 months [4].

(c) Third Line Drugs

Third line drugs are usually prescribed to patients with TB resistant to even second-line anti-TB drugs. These drugs may be considered "third-line drugs" either because they are not very effective (*e.g.,*, clarithromycin) or because their efficacy in treatment of TB has not been proven (*e.g.,*, linezolid, R207910). For example, Rifabutin, being effective, not included in the WHO list because for most developing countries, it is impractically expensive. Following drugs can be kept in the category of third-line drugs. Rifabutin, macrolides: *e.g.,*, clarithromycin (CLR), linezolid (LZD), thioacetazone (T), thioridazine, arginine, vitamin D, R207910.

TYPES OF DRUG RESISTANCE

(a) **Primary Resistance:** It is defined as the presence of drug resistance in a tuberculosis patient who has never received prior treatment with anti-TB drug. Primary resistance to anti-TB drugs occurs when a patient is infected with wild type *M.tuberculosis* which is resistant to anti-TB drugs. Much higher rates of primary resistance have been observed in HIV-infected patients [5]. Simultaneous treatment of HIV-TB coinfection may lead to malabsorption and suboptimal therapeutic blood levels of RIF and INH (despite adherence to therapy) that facilitate the development of drug-resistant TB and MDR-TB [6, 7]. The prevalence of primary resistance to anti-TB drugs shows marked geographical differences and several reports are available worldwide investigating separately the prevalence of drug resistance in tuberculosis.

(b) **Secondary or Acquired Drug Resistance:** It is defined as the resistance that arises during or after a course of treatment, usually as a result of non-adherence to the recommended drug regimen or faulty prescription. Acquired resistance to anti-TB drugs occurs when a patient is infected with susceptible forms of *M. tuberculosis* which become resistant during treatment. While primary drug resistance is an indicative of presence of drug resistant bacilli in the population, from which healthy individuals receive infection, acquired drug resistance describes poor management of tuberculosis either by improperly trained medical health care workers or by poor patient compliance. Serious consequences of this poor management result in selection and spread of drug resistant *M. tuberculosis* strains within the population. As it is difficult to trace out and confirm the history of the patients, it is more appropriate to use the terms resistance among new cases and previously treated case in place of the terms, primary resistance and acquired resistance.

(c) **Initial or Transitional Drug Resistance:** This type of drug resistance is found during treatment where occasionally a few colonies of resistant culture are obtained just before sputum conversion. These organisms do not multiply, nor does their presence influences treatment response.

(d) **Multidrug Resistance (MDR):** Multidrug resistance is defined as resistance to isoniazid & rifampicin, with or without resistance to other drugs. The WHO/IUATLD Global Project on Drug Resistance surveillance has produced reliable and accurate data on multidrug resistance. Hot spots for MDR include states of the former Soviet Union and China but also has been reported in several other countries [8-10].

(e) **Extensive Drug Resistance (XDR):** XDR is defined as occurrence of TB in persons whose *M. tuberculosis* isolates are resistant to isoniazid and rifampicin plus resistant to any fluoroquinolone and at least one of three injectable second-line drugs *i.e.*, amikacin, kanamycin, or capreomycin [3]. Overburdened public-health systems with inadequate resources for case detection and management and high HIV co-infection rates in many regions have contributed to the emergence of XDR-TB [11]. It generally takes several weeks to detect XDR-TB using conventional culture-based methods, although some progress is being made in developing rapid molecular tests. Treatment for XDR-TB is difficult, usually requiring at least 18-24 months of four to six second-line anti-TB drugs. Treatment success rates are generally 30-50%, with very poor outcomes in HIV-infected patients [12]. Although few studies report that the use of anti-retroviral therapy for treating HIV infection also results in declining prevalence of drug resistant tuberculosis in HIV-TB co-infected patients [13].

WORLDWIDE SCENARIO OF DRUG RESISTANT TB

MDR-TB and XDR-TB have been areas of growing medical concern globally and is posing threat to the control of tuberculosis. The level of primary resistance to isoniazid (INH) as single agent ranged from 0-16.9%. The rate of primary resistance to streptomycin (SM) ranges from 0.1-23.5%. Primary resistance to rifampicin (RIF) was unusual with a rate ranging from 0-3% and the rate of resistance to ethambutol (EMB) was similarly low ranging from 0-4.2%. The rates of acquired resistance to INH ranged from 4-53.7%, to SM from 0-19.4%, to RIF ranged from 0-14.5% and to EMB from 0-13.7%. The rate of MDR-TB was very low from 0-10.8% in case of primary resistance and from 0-48% for acquired resistance [14].

Through the WHO/IUATLD Global Project on Drug-Resistance Surveillance launched in 1994, a large number of reliable and accurate data increased our understanding about the extent of the problem of MDR-TB. The data available suggest that globally MDR-TB is not a problem (around 1% in 64 countries). However, it is critical in specific regions of the world. Hot spots for MDR-TB worldwide include Estonia, Latvia, the Oblasts of Ivanovo and Tomsk in Russia, and the provinces of Henan and Zhejiang Provinces in China [5]. Most of the studies conducted between 1970 and 1990 were not able to estimate the real magnitude of drug resistance due to problems related to the representativeness and size of the population sampled, and lack of standardized laboratory methods. Cohn *et al.* [15] in a review of 63 surveys conducted between 1985 and 1994 suggested that primary MDR-TB was between 0% and 10.8%. Four successive reports of Global Projects on antitubercular drug resistance surveillance sponsored by WHO were published in 1997, 2001, 2006 and 2008. The latest report collected Drug Susceptibility Testing (DST) data for INH, RIF, SM and EMB from 93 settings in 81 countries during 2002-2007 and showed that resistance to at least one anti-TB drug (any resistance) among new TB cases was lower (varying from 0% to 56%)

than in previously treated TB patients (varying from 0% to 86%). The worldwide average for any resistance; INH resistance and MDR among all TB cases were estimated to be 20%, 13.3% and 5.3%, respectively. The rates of resistance for any drug, INH and MDR were higher in retreatment *vs* new TB cases. The data showed that 489139 cases of MDR-TB occurred in 2006 representing 4.8% of all TB cases. The highest percentage of MDR-TB cases were estimated for countries of Eastern Europe (19.2%) followed by Western Pacific region (7%) and Southeast Asia (4.3%) [7, 16]. According to the fourth report of IUATLD on global anti-TB drug resistance, the median prevalence of multi-drug-resistant TB (MDR-TB) in new TB cases was 1.6%, and in previously treated TB cases 11.7%. Of the half a million MDR-TB cases estimated to have emerged in 2006, 50% were in China and India. High prevalence of drug resistance among previously treated cases was found in many of the countries surveyed. The median prevalence of resistance to at least one drug was 36% (range: 5-100%) and MDR-TB was 13% (range: 0-54%). Prevalence of resistance to at least one drug among new cases was 10.7% (range: 2-36%) and MDR-TB was 1% (range: 0-14%) (Table 1).

Table 1: Global population weighted proportion of resistance.

	Any Resistance	**Isoniazid Resistance**	**MDR**
New cases	17.0%	10.3%	2.9%
Previously treated cases	35.0%	27.7%	15.3%
All cases	20.0%	13.3%	5.3%

Adapted from reference [7].

Indian Situation of Drug Resistant TB

India is the highest TB burden country in the world, accounting for one fifth of the global incidence - an estimated 1.9 million cases annually, and an estimated prevalence of 299 / lakh, with a mortality of 28 / lakh according to WHO 2008 (RNTCP 2009). Though the development of drug resistance in India was noted since the beginning of the chemotherapeutic era, it was based on clinical perception and several isolated reports, which were unable to give the exact national situation as a whole. a study conducted by TRC, Chennai in collaboration with the National Tuberculosis Institute Bangalore using WHO/IUATLD guidelines between 1999 and 2002 including 6 districts in India showed that incidence of primary MDR ranged from 0.7-2.8%. According to third Global Report of WHO total prevalence of drug resistance among new cases in India (Wardha) is 19.8% and MDR is 0.5% [17].

In a study from Gujrat, India, of 1571 isolates from new patients, MDR-TB was found in 37 (2.4%). Of 1047 isolates from previously treated patients, MDR-TB was found in 182 (17.4%). Among 216 MDR-TB isolates, seven cases of extensively drug-resistant TB (XDR-TB) were found, all of whom were previously treated cases [18]. In another recent study reported from India, 2816 tuberculosis patients who had failed repeated treatments from 2001 to 2004 were retrospectively analysed. Whereas 1498 (53%) were identified as having multidrug-resistant TB (MDR-TB), 69 (4.6%) were extensively drug-resistant TB (XDR-TB). 671 (44.8%) were resistant to > or =1 second-line drugs (SLDs): 490 (32.7%) to ethionamide, 245 (16.4%) to ofloxacin and 169 (11.3%) to kanamycin (Paramasivan *et al.* 2010). Separately, from 194 referred cases, 47 patients of XDR-TB and 30 of MDR-TB have also been reported from India [19]. The magnitude of drug resistance, which has been reported in these studies relied upon the number and type of samples included, the region of sample inclusion selected and the method of testing applied. However, in almost all the cases the percentage of primary MDR has not been observed beyond 3%.

MOLECULAR MECHANISMS OF DRUG RESISTANCE

In order to control the drug resistance epidemic it is necessary to gain insight into how *M.tuberculosis* develops drug resistance. This knowledge will help us to understand how to prevent the occurrence of drug resistance as well as identifying genes associated with resistance to new drugs.

There are four primary ways, which a microorganism develops to resist the toxic effects of antibiotics & other drugs. These include:

(a) **Drug Inactivation:** Microorganisms may produce certain enzymes that inactivate antibiotics by hydrolysis or the formation of inactive derivatives [20]. Well-known examples are Beta-lactamases & enzymes that phosphorylate, adenylate or acetylate aminoglycoside antibiotics (Fig. 1a).

(b) **Target Alteration:** In this mechanism, cellular target can be altered by mutation or enzymatic modification in such a way that the affinity of the antibiotic for the target is reduced (Fig. 1b).

(c) **Prevention of Drug Influx:** The third mechanism of drug resistance is the inhibition of drug entry into the cell due to the low permeability of the outer membrane of gram negative bacteria [21] and exceptionally efficient barrier of the gram positive mycobacteria by which drug diffusion across the cell wall is reduced (Fig. 1c).

(d) **Active Efflux of Drug:** Once the drug has entered the cell, these can be actively effluxed out by the help of active proteins [22]. These efflux pumps are energy dependent and may utilize the transmembrane electrochemical gradient of protons or ATP to drive the extrusion of drug from the cell (Fig. 1d).

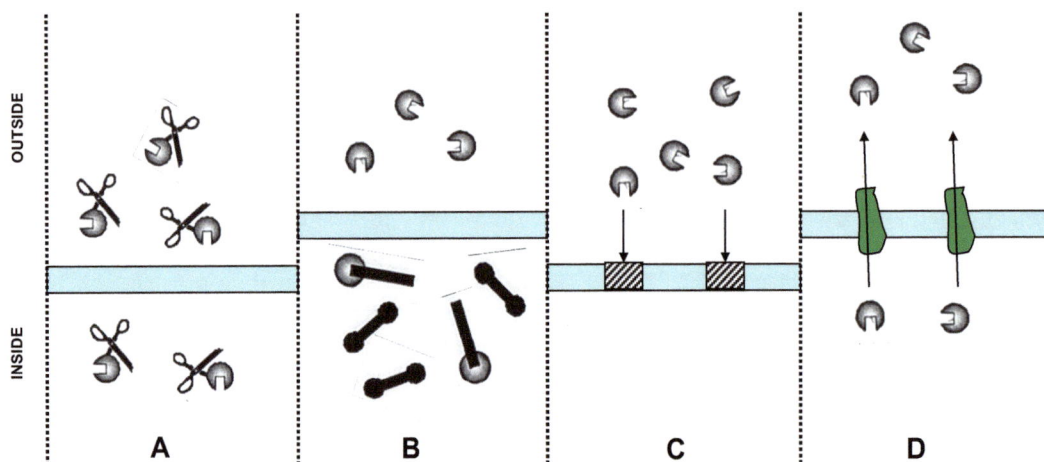

Figure 1: Resistance Mechanisms in Bacteria (A) Drug inactivation, **(B)** Target alteration, **(C)** Prevention of drug influx and **(D)** Activation of efflux.

Mutations in the genome of *M. tuberculosis* that can confer resistance to anti-TB drugs occur spontaneously with an estimated frequency of 3.5×10^{-6} for INH and 3.1×10^{-8} for RIF. Because the chromosomal loci responsible for resistance to various drugs are not linked, the risk of a double spontaneous mutation is extremely low: 9×10^{-14} for both INH and RIF [23]. MDR-TB defined as resistance to at least INH and RIF will thus occur mainly in circumstances where sequential drug resistance follows sustained treatment failure.

Resistance to Rifampicin

Rifampicin (RIF) is an important first line anti-tubercular drug that kills log phase and also to a great extent stationary phase tubercle bacilli. Rifampicin easily diffuses through the cell membrane due to its lipophilic nature, where it acts by binding to the bacterial RNA polymerase thereby inhibiting RNA synthesis. Various studies have shown that resistance to RIF in *M. tuberculosis* is mainly due to a single mutation in an 81 base pair region in the *rpoB* gene, a gene encoding the DNA dependent RNA polymerase beta subunit, mainly involving rpoB codons 531, 526 and 516 [24-27]. Mutations in this gene result in high level resistance to RIF. Monoresistance to RIF is rare except in HIV-coinfected patients and RIF resistance is often a surrogate marker for MDR-TB since approx. 85-90% RIF resistant strains are also resistant to INH [28-30]. Missense mutations at rpoB codon 511, 518 or 522 cause low-level while those at codon 516, 526 or 531 cause high-level RIF resistance [31, 32].

Resistance to Isoniazid

Isoniazid is another important first line antituberculosis drug responsible for the dramatic decrease in actively metabolizing bacilli during treatment of TB. INH is a prodrug that requires activation by *M. tuberculosis* catalase-peroxidase enzyme (KatG) to its active form. Isoniazid exhibits inhibitory effect on mycolic acid biosynthesis in mycobacteria. In *M. tuberculosis*, resistance to INH has been discussed to be due to mutations or deletions in the *katG* gene [33]. Various mutations in the *katG* gene have been reported among INH-resistant isolates [34, 35]. The katG gene mutations occur frequently between codons 138 and 328, particularly at codon 315 (katG315). Mutation in the Ser 315 Thr, which is present in approximately 50% of all INH resistant isolates results in high level resistance to INH. However, *katG* gene does not account for all INH-resistant strains. The gene *inhA*, encoding an NADH-dependent enoyl Acyl Carrier Protein (ACP) reductase has also been shown to be involved in INH resistance. Mutations in the *inhA* region appear to be responsible in approximately 25% clinical isolates and are generally associated with low level isoniazid resistance. Mutations in another gene *aphC* were identified in approximately 10-15% of clinical isolates.

Resistance to Streptomycin

Streptomycin (SM) inhibits protein synthesis by binding to the 30S subunit of the bacterial ribosome causing misreading of the mRNA message during translation. Globally, highest level of resistance to an anti-TB drug is also observed for SM [7, 36]. The site of action of the aminoglyoside SM is typically through mutation in S12 (*rpsL*) and 16S rRNA (*rrs*). The most common mutations in *rpsL* is a substitution in codon 43 from lysine to arginine causing high level resistance to SM. Mutation in the rrs gene usually account for low level resistance. Since *M. tuberculosis* genome contains a single rrs gene, nearly 30% of SM-resistant *M. tuberculosis* isolates contain mutations in the rrs gene. The remaining SM resistant *M. tuberculosis* strains either contain mutations in rpsL (at rpsL43 or rpsL88) or in other genes [37, 38]. Together, mutations in the *rpsL* and rrs genes account for approximately 75% of all SM-resistant isolates. Another possible mechanism may be alterations in drug uptake, which have been thought to contribute to drug resistance [38]. Other aminoglycosides used as second-line anti-TB injectable drugs are kanamycin (KAM) and amikacin (AMI). Although cross-resistance between KAN and AMI has been reported, cross-resistance between SM and either KAN or AMI is not reported, hence KAN/AMI may be used for SM resistant strains [39].

Resistance to Ethambutol

Ethambutol (EMB) inhibits synthesis of arabinogalactan, a major cell wall component of mycobacteria [40]. Ethambutol is now used in place of streptomycin (SM) in combination therapy with INH, RIF and PZA since resistance of *M. tuberculosis* strains to EMB is much less compared to SM [7]. Mechanism of resistance to this anti-tuberculosis agent is primarily associated with point mutations in the *embCAB* operon [41] encoding various arabinosyl transferase enzymes necessary for cell wall biosynthesis. Mutations in embB, particularly at embB306, embB406 and embB497 occur more frequently and confer resistance to EMB [42, 43]. One of the most common mutations (20-70 %) in this operon is associated with amino acid substitutions at codon Met 306 of the *embB* gene [44, 45].

Resistance to Pyrazinamide

Pyrazinamide (PZA) is a structural analogue of nicotinamide that is used as a first line anti-TB drug. PZA kills semi-dormant tubercle bacilli under acidic conditions. It is believed that in the acidic environment of phagolysosomes the tubercle bacilli produce pyrazinamidase, an enzyme that converts PZA to pyrazinoic acid, the active derivative of this compound. Wide diversity of *pncA* mutations scattered along the entire length of the gene and its upstream region conferred PZA resistance. Lack of *pncA* mutations in 10-28 % of PZA resistant isolates suggested the existence of at least one additional gene participating in resistance [41, 46]. The PZA is highly specific against *M. tuberculosis*, other mycobacteria are intrinsically resistant to PZA due to lack of an efficient pyrazinamidase. Nearly 20-30% of PZA-resistant *M. tuberculosis* strains contain wild-type pncA, suggesting the existence of other resistance conferring mechanisms [26, 47].

Resistance to Fluoroquinolones

In *M. tuberculosis* resistance to fluoroquinolones such as ciprofloxacin or ofloxacin is associated with mutations in a 40 amino acid region in *gyrA* [48, 49] which accounts for 40-70% of fluoroquinolone resistance isolates. Resistance does occur in strains lacking mutations in these codons suggesting alternative mechanism of resistance. Higher levels of resistance can have mutations in both *gyrA* and *gyrB* [49]. In *M. smegmatis* increased expression of LfrA efflux pump has been shown to cause resistance to fluoroquinolones EtBr, rhodamine and acriflavine [50, 51]. The new-generation FQs (Levofloxacin, LFX, moxifloxacin, MFX and gatifloxacin, GFX) have excellent bactericidal activity against *M. tuberculosis*. Important loci associated with the resistance to anti-TB drugs are summarized in Table **2**, taken from [16].

Table 2: Important Genes (and their encoded products) of *M. tuberculosis* Conferring Resistance to First-Line and Some Second-Line Anti-TB Drugs [16].

Anti-TB Drug(s)	Genomic Target	Encoded Protein or RNA Product	Major Target Region in Encoded Product	Level of Resistance
RIF	*rpoB*	β-Subunit of RNA polymerase	81-bp HSR	High
INH	*katG*	Catalase/peroxidase	Entire gene	High
INH/ETH	*inhA*	Enoyl-acyl carrier protein reductase	Upstream regulatory region	Low
PZA	*pncA*	Pyrazinamidase	Several codons	High
EMB	*embB*	Arabinosyltransferase	Several codons	High
EMB	*embA*	Arabinosyltransferase	Several codons	High
EMB	*iniA*	Isoniazid-inducible gene	Few codons	High
SM	*rrs*	16S rRNA	Several nucleotides	Low
SM	*rpsL*	Ribosomal Protein S12	Codons 43 and 48	High
FQs	*gyrA*	A subunit of DNA gyrase	Few codons	High
FQs	*gyrB*	B subunit of DNA gyrase	Few codons	High
KAN/AMI	*rrs*	16S rRNA	Position 1401 or 1484	High
CAP/VIO	*rrs*	16S rRNA	Position 1401 or 1484	High
CAP/VIO	*tlyA*	Cytotoxin/haemolysin homologue	Several codons	High

RIF, rifampin; INH, isoniazid; ETH, ethionamide; PZA, pyrazinamide; EMB, ethambutol; SM, streptomycin; FQs, fluoroquinolones (ciprofloxacin, ofloxacin, levofloxacin); KAN, kanamycin; AMI, amikacin; CAP, capreomycin; VIO, viomycin; and HSR, hot-spot region. Table taken from [16].

THE ROLE OF MICROARRAY IN IDENTIFYING MECHANISMS OF DRUG RESISTANCE

Few important contributions of microarray technology in identifying genes related to drug resistance in *M. tuberculosis* include that of Wilson *et al.* [52], who in their initial experiments of drug-induced transcriptome analysis, analyzed altered expression of a number of genes in response to the anti-tuberculous drug Isoniazid (INH). Several genes related to the mode of action of the drug including operonic cluster encoding type II fatty acid synthase and trehalose dimycosyl transferase have been found to be induced by INH. Fu & Shinnick [53] explored the mechanism of INH resistance in resistant and sensitive isolates at low as well as high INH concentrations using Affymetrix oligonucleotide GeneChip. They found that resistant strains show the characteristic signature of fatty acid synthase (FAS-II) inhibition only at higher INH concentration, although the response was less relative to that of susceptible strains. In another study Fu [54] identified 42 genes up-regulated and 21 down-regulated two or more than two fold in case of INH treatment.

Fu & Shinnick [55] also conducted a study on the mechanism of another important drug capreomycin in *M. tuberculosis* using Affymetrix oligonucleotide GeneChip and suggested that capreomycin primerily acts on information pathways, cell wall, cell processes, intermediate metabolism and respiration. Besides its specific molecular target 16S rRNA, they have suggested some new targets for capreomycin including Rv0054, Rv3715c and Rv3260c. Manjunatha *et al.* [56] have performed microarray experiments to unravel the mechanism behind PA-824 (a nitroimidazo-oxazine) resistance. Besides confirmation of the known mechanisms of PA-824 resistance, new, previously unidentified, protein Rv3547 has also been found to be associated with PA-824 resistance. Microarray has been successfully used to detect >95% of rifampicin resistant isolates and 80% of isoniazid resistant isolates of *M. tuberculosis* within 12 hours in a study conducted on 220 drug resistant isolates and 131 clinical samples of *M. tuberculosis* [57].

Recently we have published a study involving expression profiling of drug efflux pump genes of *M. tuberculosis*. We monitored changes in the expression of these genes on exposure of common anti-TB drugs in multidrug resistant isolates. Ten efflux pump genes were identified to be overexpressed following exposure to various anti-TB drugs, out of which increased activity of eight genes have been reported for the first time by us. It was observed that a simultaneous overexpression of efflux pump genes Rv2459, Rv3728, and Rv3065 was associated with resistance to the combination of isoniazid and ethambutol, but No comparable differences in expression were observed simultaneously in rifampicin and isoniazid drug stress combinations, that is, classical multidrug resistance as compared with the other drugs [58].

DETECTION OF DRUG RESISTANCE

Successful detection of drug resistance in tuberculosis helps in effective treatment of patients and further spread of resistant *M. tuberculosis* strains in the population. Although the efforts to develop rapid, easy and cost effective molecular methods to detect the presence of drug resistance in *M. tuberculosis* are being taken continuously, determination of Minimum Inhibitory Concentration (MIC) in the presence of anti-TB drug is still the primary way to report drug resistance in TB patients. Various methods for detection of drug resistance in tuberculosis are summarized below.

(A) CONVENTIONAL METHODS

Conventional methods for detection of drug resistance in tuberculosis involve determination of MIC of *M. tuberculosis* culture in liquid medium in the presence of anti-TB drugs by one of the following means.

Absolute Concentration Method

In this method, standard bacterial suspension is inoculated on the drug containing as well as drug free media slopes. The resistance is expressed in terms of Minimal Inhibitory Concentration (MIC), which is the lowest concentration of the drug inhibiting the growth of the bacteria [59].

Resistance Ratio (RR) Method

This method compares the resistance of test strains with the standard laboratory strain & resistance is expressed in terms of the standard of the ratio of MIC of test strain to MIC of standard strain in the same experimental settings [59].

Proportion Method

This method consists of inoculating equal quantities of several 10 fold dilutions of roughly measured inoculum on both control and drug containing medium. Resistance is then determined by comparing the number of colonies that grow on drug containing media with the number of colonies on drug free media slopes and expressing as percentage proportion of the total population [59]. Proportion method is used as a Gold Standard in the evaluation of other methods of drug susceptibility testing in *M. tuberculosis*.

(B) ALTERNATIVE METHODS

Alternative methods have been developed and tested in order to determine MIC in a easier and rapid way. As the conventional method require longer time for reporting results to the patient, rapid methods are useful but hold different sensitivities and specificities. Alternative methods used for Drug Susceptibility Testing (DST) of *M. tuberculosis* are:

BACTEC System

It is the most reliable & sensitive medium used for the early detection of growth of mycobacteria. This method utilizes radiolabelled palmitic acid (C^{14}) as a substrate. As mycobacteria metabolize, labelled CO_2 is released & is detected by the BACTEC-460 instrument [60, 61]. Susceptibility testing of *M. tuberculosis* by BACTEC 460 TB system is based on the modified proportion method and the method is FDA approved for first-line anti-TB drug susceptibility testing [61]. BACTEC system reports DST results within 4-12 days from primary cultures, while solid media-based methods require nearly 3 weeks.

BacT/ALERT 3D System

Colorimetric BacT/ALERT 3D system (bioMérieux Inc., Durham, NC), previously designated MB/BACT (Organon Teknika, Boxtels, The Netherlands) [62], has been reported to be useful for rapid and reliable susceptibility testing of *M. tuberculosis* isolates [63].

Mycobacteria Growth Indicator Tube (MGIT)

This technique detects growth of bacteria with the help of oxygen sensitive fluorescent sensors [64, 65]. The activity of growing bacteria deletes the dissolved O_2 of broth and allows sensors to fluoresce in a 36 nm UV light. The positive result emits a vivid orange fluorescent glow. The time of growth of *M. tuberculosis* varies from 4 to 14 days [66, 67].

Microwell Alamar Blue Assay and Nitroblue Tetrazolium Reduction Assay

These test are colorimetric based on the oxidation-reduction of the dye Alamar Blue or MTT 3-(4,5-dimethylthiazol-2yl)-2,-5 diphenyl tetrazolium bromide). Bacterial growth is detected by the reduction of the dye from blue to pink due to oxidation reduction metabolism of viable *M. tuberculosis* [68].

Luciferase Reporter Phage Assay

This test uses Mycobacteriophage, a virus that infects *M.tuberculosis* and has a cloned gene for production of luciferase reporter enzyme. The phage when mixed with culture of bacterial cells result in production of light. If drug kills the bacteria no light is produced, revealing sensitivity of the organism to the drug. If mycobacterium is resistant to the drug, the cell remains unaffected and light will be produced [69].

Slide Culture

It is also called Microscopic observation drug susceptibility assay [70]. Mycobacteria are fixed on slide and then transferred to the liquid medium containing drug. This is incubated at 37°C for one week and growth is examined microscopically. It gives sensitivity results within 8-10 days.

E-Test

The E-test is a strip based method, which gives MIC values in a very simple, yet accurate way and thus may be applicable to second line and some experimental drugs [71]. It gives results in 7-10 days. E test has also been shown to be a promising method for the susceptibility testing of more slowly growing and even the rapidly growing mycobacteria [72].

Flow Cytometric Assay

Comparing the intensity of fluorescence of Mycobacterium cells incubated with antimycobacterial drugs with that of drug-free cells, after staining with SYTO 16, it is possible to distinguish between sensitive, intermediate and resistant phenotypes. The Flow cytometric assay is reported to be a simple, fast, safe and accurate way to determine susceptibility of *M. tuberculosis.* [73].

REMA

Resazurin microplate assay (REMA), described by Palomino *et al.* [74] and Martin *et al.* [75] for Drug Susceptibility Testing (DST) of *M. tuberculosis* isolates has shown good concordance with proportion method of DST of *M. tuberculosis* [76, 77]. This is a rapid and inexpensive 96-well plate based system using liquid medium.

(C) MOLECULAR METHODS

Molecular methods, also called genotypic methods, are developed to detect drug resistance in tuberculosis in a rapid way. Whereas conventional methods require bacteria to grow in different culture medium, which takes several days to several weeks, molecular methods target nucleic acids and employed by means of gene specific or mutation specific probes and primers. The aim of these molecular methods is to detect mutations in the genes, which are associated with resistance to antituberculosis drugs by sequencing or nucleic acid hybridization. The best advantages of molecular methods are rapid results (within 1-2 days) and direct applicability on clinical samples. Molecular methods are primarily developed targeting a particular mutation in a particular gene or locus. Thus, detection of RIF resistance by molecular method is more practical, since 90-95% RIF resistant strains contain mutations in a small 81-bp region of a single (*rpoB*) gene and is important as RIF resistance is a surrogate marker for MDR-TB. For other anti-TB drugs, the sensitivity of resistance detection varies more widely due to the number of gene loci involved and the sheer diversity of mutations [16]. Several methods have been developed and evaluated for the detection of resistance conferring mutations in MDR-TB strains.

DNA Sequencing

DNA sequencing is the gold standard of all the molecular methods targeting detection of mutation(s). Other methods need to be confirmed and validated by sequencing prior to be used clinically for the detection of drug resistance. However, due to multiple loci involved in resistance to some drugs such as INH, it is not practical to sequence all possible loci for deception of drug resistance in each isolate. Sequencing is particularly suitable for RIF, where >90% RIF-resistant strains contain mutations in a 81 bp region of rpoB gene and PZA, due to small size of pncA gene [78, 79].

PCR-RFLP

The PCR-Restriction Fragment Length Polymorphism (PCR-RFLP) analysis is a simple, rapid and inexpensive method to detect polymorphism at a single or few codons that are mutated in drug-resistant strains. The PCR-RFLP has been mostly used for the detection of katG315 and embB306 mutations for rapid detection of INH and EMB resistance, respectively [79, 80].

Real Time PCR

Detection of drug resistance by Real Time PCR employs the use of primers and probes specific to the mutation in the targeted loci. Whereas mostly it is developed to detect one mutation in a single locus at a time, multiplexing is also possible, which facilitates simultaneous detection of multiple mutations in different genes by means of melting curve analysis. Real Time PCR assays for detection of drug resistance has been mainly used for rpoB, katG and inhA mutations [81, 82].

INNO-LiPA

INNO-LiPA test developed by Beenhouwer *et al.* [83] based on reverse blot hybridization has been reported to be useful in identification of mutations in rpoB gene and holds promise in clinical practice [84, 85].

MANAGEMENT OF DRUG RESISTANCE IN TUBERCULOSIS

The principles of treatment for MDR-TB and for XDR-TB are the same. The main difference is that XDR-TB is associated with a much higher death rate than MDR-TB, because of a reduced number of effective treatment options. Treatment courses are lengthy, a minimum of 18 months and may last years; still death rates remain high. In the treatment of drug resistant tuberculosis, second line drugs are included alongwith the continuation of first line drugs according to the sensitivity of the drugs. However, second-line drugs are more toxic, more expensive and still less effective. Wide spectrum antibiotics like fluoroquinolones (FQs) show excellent response against drug resistant form of TB. Some of the most effective FQs are moxifloxacin and gatifloxacin (MFX and GFX). Medical supervisors also do prescribe some other drugs in combination for the treatment of drug resistant TB, that are not *M.tuberculosis* specific but exhibit significant activity against *M. tuberculosis*. These include clarithromycin (CLR), clofazimine (CFZ), amoxicillin-clavulanic acid (AMX-CLV) and linezolid (LZD) [86-88].

Treatment of MDR-TB must be done on the basis of sensitivity testing: it is impossible to treat such patients without this information. If treating a patient with suspected MDR-TB, the patient should be started on SHREZ + MFX + cycloserine pending the result of laboratory sensitivity testing.

PROVISION OF TREATING MDR IN DOTS

DOTS stands for "Directly Observed Treatment, Short-course" and is a major plank in the WHO global TB eradication programme. This means an independent observer watching tuberculosis patients swallow their anti-TB therapy. DOTS is used with intermittent dosing (thrice weekly or $2HREZ/4HR_3$). Treatment with properly implemented DOTS has a success rate exceeding 95% and prevents the emergence of further multi-drug resistant strains of tuberculosis and hence advertised by a slogan "DOTS- sure cure for TB". The WHO extended the DOTS programme in 1998 to include the treatment of MDR-TB, called "DOTS-Plus" [89]. Implementation of DOTS-Plus requires the capacity to perform drug-susceptibility testing (not routinely available even in developed countries) and the availability of second-line agents, in addition to all the requirements for DOTS. DOTS-Plus is therefore much more resource-expensive than DOTS, and requires much greater commitment from countries wishing to implement it. DOTS-Plus is a comprehensive management strategy, which takes into account specific issues (such as the use of second-line anti-TB drugs) that need to be addressed in areas where there is high prevalence of MDR-TB. Thus, DOTS-Plus works as a supplement to the standard DOTS strategy.

HOPE FOR FUTURE

For treatment for multidrug resistant and extensive drug resistant tuberculosis, combinations therapy including second and third line drugs along with effective first-line anti-TB agents is prescribed based on drug susceptibility pattern of *M. tuberculosis* isolated from patient. Despite being expensive the treatment has very low success rate. Hence monitoring of TB treatment, adherence to treatment guidelines and good patient compliance to the therapy is the ultimate solution to prevent drug resistant form of tuberculosis from spreading in the population. Although a number of synthetic compounds have been reported to be effective against drug resistant tuberculosis and are under various stages of testing [16], their efficacy and safety need to be proven for their ultimate use in clinical settings. There are however, possibilities of identification of more new compounds with anti-bacterial property, molecular modeling and docking strategies can be seen as hope for future, by which newer drugs with effective anti-TB property can be designed/developed.

REFERENCES

[1]   Ghosh SC. Cost effective management of drug resistance in pulmonary medicine. Pulmon 2001; 3: 49-52

[2]   World Health Organization. 1993. Tuberculosis: a global emergency. World Health Forum 14: 438.

[3]   Centers for Disease Control and Prevention, CDC (2006). Notice to readers: Revised definition of extensively drug resistant tuberculosis. MMWR 55: 1176. http://www.cdc.gov/MMWR/preview/mmwrhtml/mm5543a4.htm.

[4]   Cheng AF, Yew WW, Chan EW, *et al.* Multiplex PCR amplimer conformation analysis for rapid detection of gyrA mutations in fluoroquinolone-resistant *Mycobacterium tuberculosis* clinical isolates. Antimicrob. Agents Chemother 2004; 48: 596-601.

[5]   Espinal MA. The global situation of MDR-TB. *Tuberculosis (Edinb)* 2003; 83: 44-51.

[6]   Wells CD, Cegielski JP, Nelson LJ, *et al.* HIV infection and multidrug-resistant tuberculosis - the perfect storm. J Infect Dis 2007; 196: S86-107.

[7]   World Health Organization. Anti-tuberculosis drug resistance in the world: fourth Global report. WHO/HTM/TB/2008.394. Geneva, Switzerland: WHO; 2008.

[8]   Aziz MA, Wright A. The World Health Organization/International Union Against Tuberculosis and Lung Disease. Global project on surveillance for anti-tuberculosis drug resistance: a model for other infectious diseases. Clin Infect Dis 2005; 15: S258-62.

[9]   WHO. Anti-tuberculosis drug resistance in the world report no. 4. The WHO/IUATLD global project on anti-tuberculosis surveillance 2002-07.

[10]   Mokrousov I, Ly HM, Otten T, *et al.* Origin and primary dispersal of the *Mycobacterium tuberculosis* Beijing genotype: clues from human phylogeography. Genome Res. 2005; 15: 1357-64.

[11]   Banerjee R, Schecter GF, Flood J, *et al.* Extensively drug-resistant tuberculosis: new strains, new challenges. Expert Rev Anti Infect Ther 2008 6: 713-24.

[12]   LoBue P. Extensively drug-resistant tuberculosis. Curr Opin Infect Dis 2009; 22: 167-73.

[13]   Sungkanuparph S, Eampokalap B, Chottanapund S, *et al.* Declining prevalence of drug-resistant tuberculosis among HIV/tuberculosis co-infected patients receiving antiretroviral therapy. J Med Assoc Thai 2007; 90: 884-88.

[14]   World Health Organization. (2006). Global tuberculosis control: surveillance, planning, financing. WHO report 2006. Geneva, World Health Organization (WHO/HTM/TB/2006.362).

[15]   Cohn DL, Bustreo F, Raviglione MC. Drug-resistant tuberculosis: review of the worldwide situation and the WHO/IUATLD Global Surveillance Project. International Union Against Tuberculosis and Lung Disease. Clin Infect Dis 1997; 24: S121-130.

[16]   Ahmad S, Mokaddas E. Recent advances in the diagnosis and treatment of multidrug-resistant tuberculosis. Respiratory Medicine 2009; 103: 1777-90.

[17]   Paramasivan CN, Venkataraman P. Drug resistance in tuberculosis in India. Indian J Med Res 2004; 120: 377-86.

[18]   Ramachandran R, Nalini S, Chandrasekar V, *et al.* Surveillance of drug-resistant tuberculosis in the state of Gujarat, India. Int J Tuberc Lung Dis. 2009; 13: 1154-60.

[19]   Balaji V, Daley P, Anand AA, *et al.* Risk Factors for MDR and XDR-TB in a Tertiary Referral Hospital in India. PLoS One 2010; 5: e9527.

[20]   Davies J. Inactivation of antibiotics and the dissemination of resistance genes. Science 1994; 264: 375-82.

[21]   Nikaido H. Role of permeability barrier in resistance to B lactame antibiotics. Pharmacol Ther 1985; 27: 197-31.

[22]   Levy S. Active efflux mechanisms for antibiotic resistance. Antimicrob Agents Chemother 1992; 36: 695-703.

[23]   Dooley SW, Simone PM. The extent and management of drug-resistant tuberculosis: the American experience. Clinical tuberculosis. London: Chapman & Hall 1994; 171-89.

[24]   Telenti A, Imboden P, Marchesi F, *et al.* Detection of rifampicin-resistance mutations in *Mycobacterium tuberculosis*. Lancet 1993; 341: 647-50.

[25]   Ahmad S, Mokaddas E, Fares E. Characterization of rpoB mutations in rifampin-resistant clinical *Mycobacterium tuberculosis* isolates from Kuwait and Dubai. Diagn Microbiol Infect Dis 2002; 44: 245-52.

[26]   Johnson R, Streicher E, Louw G, *et al.* Drug resistance in *Mycobacterium tuberculosis*. Curr Issues Mol Biol 2006; 8: 97-111.

[27]   Sheng J, Li J, Sheng G, *et al.* Characterization of rpoB mutations associated with rifampin resistance in *Mycobacterium tuberculosis* from eastern China. J Appl Microbiol 2008; 105: 904-11.

[28]   Van Rie A, Warren R, Mshanga I, *et al.* Analysis for a limited number of gene codons can predict drug resistance of *Mycobacterium tuberculosis* in a high-incidence community. J Clin Microbiol 2001; 39: 636-41.

[29]   Siddiqi N, Shamim M, Hussain S, *et al.* Molecular characterization of multidrug-resistant isolates of *Mycobacterium tuberculosis* from patients in North India. Antimicrob Agents Chemother 2002; 46: 443-50.

[30]   Mokaddas E, Ahmad S, Abal AT, *et al.* Molecular fingerprinting reveals familial transmission of rifampin-resistant tuberculosis in Kuwait. Ann Saudi Med 2005; 25: 150-53.

[31] Yang B, Koga H, Ohno H, *et al.* Relationship between antimycobacterial activities of rifampicin, rifabutin and KRM-1648 and rpoB mutations of *Mycobacterium tuberculosis.* J Antimicrob Chemother 1998; 42: 621-28.

[32] Heep M, Brandstatter B, Rieger U, *et al.* Frequency of rpoB mutations inside and outside the cluster I region in rifampin resistant clinical *Mycobacterium tuberculosis* isolates. J Clin Microbiol 2001; 39: 107-10.

[33] Zhang Y, Heym B, Allen B, *et al.* The catalase-peroxidase gene and isoniazid resistance of *Mycobacterium tuberculosis.* Nature 1992; 358: 591-93.

[34] Siddiqi N, Shamim M, Hussain S, *et al.* Molecular characterization of multidrug-resistant isolates of *Mycobacterium tuberculosis* from patients in North India. Antimicrob Agents Chemother 2002; 46: 443-50.

[35] Sekiguchi J, Miyoshi-AT, Augustynowicz-KE, *et al.* Detection of multidrug resistance in *Mycobacterium tuberculosis.* 2007; 45: 179-92.

[36] Aziz MA, Wright A, Laszlo A, *et al.* for the WHO/International Union Against Tuberculosis and Lung Disease global project on anti-tuberculosis drug resistance surveillance. Epidemiology of antituberculosis drug resistance (the Global Project on Anti-tuberculosis Drug Resistance Surveillance): an updated analysis. Lancet 2006; 368: 2142-54.

[37] Sreevatsan S, Pan X, Stockbauer KE, *et al.* Characterization of rpsL and rrs mutations in streptomycin-resistant *Mycobacterium tuberculosis* isolates from diverse geographic locations. Antimicrob Agents Chemother 1996; 40: 1024-26.

[38] Cooksey RC, Morlock GP, McQueen A, *et al.* Characterization of streptomycin resistance mechanisms among *Mycobacterium tuberculosis* isolates from patients in New York City. Antimicrob Agents Chemother 1996; 40: 1186-88.

[39] Maus CE, Pilkaytis BB, Shinnick TM. Molecular analysis of cross-resistance to capreomycin, kanamycin, amikacin and viomycin in Mycobacterium tuberculosis. Antimicrob Agents Chemother 2005; 49: 3192-97.

[40] Takayama K, Kilburn JO. Inhibition of synthesis of arabinogalactan by ethambutol in *Mycobacterium smegmatis.* Antimicrob Agents Chemother 1989; 33: 1493-99.

[41] Sreevatsan S, Stockbauer KE, Pan X, *et al.* Ethambutol resistance in *Mycobacterium tuberculosis*: critical role of embB mutations. Antimicrob Agents Chemother 1997; 41: 1677-81.

[42] Safi H, Sayers B, Hazbon MH, *et al.* Transfer of embB codon 306 mutations into clinical *Mycobacterium tuberculosis* strains alters susceptibility to ethambutol, isoniazid and rifampin. Antimicrob Agents Chemother 2008; 52: 2027-34.

[43] Starks AM, Gumusboga A, Plikaytis BB, *et al.* Mutations at embB codon 306 are an important molecular indicator of ethambutol resistance in *Mycobacterium tuberculosis.* Antimicrob Agents Chemother 2009; 53: 1061-66.

[44] Telenti A, Honore N, Bernasconi C, *et al.* Genotypic assessment of isoniazid and rifampin resistance in Mycobacterium tuberculosis: a blind study at reference laboratory level. J Clin Microbiol 1997; 35: 719-23.

[45] Ramaswamy SV, Amin AG, Göksel S, *et al.* Molecular genetic analysis of nucleotide polymorphisms associated with ethambutol resistance in human isolates of *Mycobacterium tuberculosis.* Antimicrob Agents Chemother 2000; 44: 326-36.

[46] Barco P, Cardoso RF, Hirata RD, *et al.* pncA mutations in pyrazinamide-resistant Mycobacterium tuberculosis clinical isolates from the southeast region of Brazil. J Antimicrob Chemother 2006; 58: 930-35.

[47] Scorpio A, Zhang Y. Mutations in pncA, a gene encoding pyrazinamidase/nicotinamidase, cause resistance to the antituberculous drug pyrazinamide in tubercle bacillus. Nat Med 1996; 2: 662-67.

[48] Takiff HE, Salazar L, Guerrero C, *et al.* Cloning and nucleotide sequence of *Mycobacterium tuberculosis* gyrA and gyrB genes and detection of quinolone resistance mutations. Antimicrob Agents Chemother 1994; 38: 773-80.

[49] Kocagöz T, Hackbarth CJ, Unsal I, *et al.* Gyrase mutations in laboratory-selected, fluoroquinolone-resistant mutants of Mycobacterium tuberculosis H37Ra. Antimicrob Agents Chemother 1996; 40: 1768-74.

[50] Takiff HE, Cimino M, Musso MC, *et al.* Efflux pump of the proton antiporter family confers low-level fluoroquinolone resistance in *Mycobacterium smegmatis.* Proc Natl Acad Sci USA 1996; 93: 362-66.

[51] Liu J, Takiff HE, Nikaido H. Active efflux of fluoroquinolones in *Mycobacterium smegmatis* mediated by LfrA, a multidrug efflux pump. J Bacteriol 1996; 178: 3791-95.

[52] Wilson M, DeRisi J, Kristensen HH, *et al.* Exploring drug-induced alterations in gene expression in *Myocbacterium tuberculosis* by microarray hybridization. Proc Acad Natl Sci USA 1999; 96: 123833-38.

[53] Fu LM, Shinnick TM. Understanding the action of INH on a highly INH-resistant *Mycobacterium tuberculosis* strain using GeneChips. Tuberculosis 2007a; 87: 63-70.

[54] Fu LM. Exploring drug action on *Mycobacxterium tuberculosis* using Affimatrix oligonucleotide genechips. Tuberculosis 2006; 86: 134-43.

[55]   Fu LM, Shinnick TM. Genome-wide exploration of the drug action of capreomycin on *Mycobacterium tuberculosis* using Affymetrix oligonucleotide GeneChips. J Infect 2007b; 54: 277-84.

[56]   Manjunatha UH, Boshoff H, Dowd CS, *et al.* Identification of a nitroimidazo-oxazine-specific protein involved in PA-824 resistance in *Mycobacterium tuberculosis.* PNAS 2006; 103: 431-36.

[57]   Gryadunov D, Mikhailovich V, Lapa S, *et al.* Evaluation of hybridization on oligonucleotide microarrays for analysis of drug-resistant *Mycobacterium tuberculosis.* Clin Microbiol Infect 2005; 11: 531-39.

[58]   Gupta AK, Katoch VM, Chauhan DS, *et al.* Microarray analysis of efflux pump genes in multidrug-resistant *Mycobacterium tuberculosis* during stress induced by common anti-tuberculous drugs. Microb Drug Resist 2010; 16: 21-28.

[59]   Canetti G, Fox W, Khomenko A, *et al.* Advances in techniques of testing mycobacterial drug sensitivity, and the use of sensitivity tests in tuberculosis control programmes. Bull World Health Organ 1969; 41: 21-43.

[60]   Siddiqi SH, Hwangbo CC, Silcox V, *et al.* Rapid radiometric methods to detect and differentiate *Mycobacterium tuberculosis/M. bovis* from other mycobacterial species. Am Rev Respir Dis 1984; 130: 6346-40.

[61]   Rodrigues CS, Shenai SV, Almeida DVG, *et al.* Use of bactec 460 TB system in the diagnosis of tuberculosis. *Indian J Med Microbiol* 2007; 25: 32-36.

[62]   Bemer P, Bodmer T, Munzinger J, *et al.* Multicenter evaluation of the MB/BACT system for susceptibility testing of *Mycobacterium tuberculosis.* J Clin Microbiol 2004; 42: 1030-34.

[63]   Singh P, Wesley C, Jadaun GP, *et al.* Comparative evaluation of Löwenstein-Jensen proportion method, BacT/ALERT 3D system, and enzymatic pyrazinamidase assay for pyrazinamide susceptibility testing of *Mycobacterium tuberculosis.* J Clin Microbiol 2007; 45: 76-80.

[64]   Heifets LB, Iseman MD. Radiometric method for testing susceptibility of mycobacteria to pyrazinamide in 7H12 broth. J Clin Microbiol 1985; 21: 200-04.

[65]   Pfyffer GE, Palicova F, Rüsch-Gerdes S. Testing of susceptibility to pyrazinamide with the nonradiometric BACTEC MGIT 960 system. J Clin Microbiol 2002; 40: 1670-74.

[66]   Palaci M, Ueki SYM, Sato DN, *et al.* Evaluation of Mycobacteria Growth Indicator Tube for recovery and drug susceptibility testing of *Mycobacterium tuberculosis* isolates from respiratory specimens. J Clin Microbiol 1996; 34: 762-64.

[67]   Fegou E, Jelastopulu E, Nicolaou S, *et al.* Comparison of the manual Mycobacteria Growth Indicator tube and the Etest with the method of proportion for susceptibility testing of *Mycobacterium tuberculosis.* Chemother 2006; 52: 174-77.

[68]   Dubaniewicz A, Hoppe A. The spontaneous and stimulated nitroblue tetrazolium (NBT) tests in mononuclear cells of patients with tuberculosis. Rocz Akad Med Bialymst 2004; 49: 252-55.

[69]   Bardarov S Jr, Dou H, Eisenach K, *et al.* Detection and drug-susceptibility testing of *M. tuberculosis* from sputum samples using luciferase reporter phage: comparison with the Mycobacteria Growth Indicator Tube (MGIT) system. Diagn Microbiol Infect Dis 2003; 45: 53-61.

[70]   Moore DA, Mendoza D, Gilman RH, *et al.* Tuberculosis Working Group in Peru. Microscopic observation drug susceptibility assay, a rapid, reliable diagnostic test for multidrug-resistant tuberculosis suitable for use in resource-poor settings. J Clin Microbio 2004; 42: 4432-37.

[71]   Das R, Srivastava K, Gupta P, *et al.* Comparison of Etest with MIC method of Lowenstein-Jensen medium for susceptibility testing of *Mycobacterium tuberculosis.* Curr Sci 2003; 85: 191-193.

[72]   Muralidhar S, Srivastava L. Evaluation of three methods to determine the antimicrobial susceptibility of *Mycobacterium tuberculosis.* Indian J Med Res 2004; 120: 463-67.

[73]   Pina-Vaz C, Costa-de-Oliveira S, Rodrigues AG. Safe susceptibility testing of *Mycobacterium tuberculosis* by flow cytometry with the fluorescent nucleic acid stain SYTO 16. J Med Microbiol 2005; 54: 77-81.

[74]   Palomino JC, Martin A, Camacho M, *et al.* Resazurin microtiter assay plate: simple and inexpensive method for detection of drug resistance in *Mycobacterium tuberculosis.* Antimicrob Agents Chemother 2002; 44: 2720-22.

[75]   Martin A, Camacho M, Portaels F, *et al.* Resazurin microtitre assay plate testing of *Mycobacterium tuberculosis* susceptibilities to second-line drugs: rapid, simple and inexpensive method. Antimicrob Agents Chemother 2003; 47; 3616-19.

[76]   Nateche F, Martin A, Baraka S, *et al.* Application of Resazurin microtitre assay for detection of multidrug resistance in *Mycobacterium tuberculosis* in Algiers. J Med Microbiol 2006; 55: 857-60.

[77]   Jadaun GP, Agarwal C, Sharma H, *et al.* Determination of ethambutol MICs for *Mycobacterium tuberculosis* and *Mycobacterium avium* isolates by resazurin microtitre assay. J Antimicrob Chemother 2007; 60: 152-55.

[78]   Mokrousov I, Narvskaya O, Otten T, *et al.* High prevalence of Ser315Thr substitution among isoniazid-resistant *Mycobacterium tuberculosis* clinical isolates of from Northwestern Russia, 1996e2001. Antimicrob Agents Chemother 2002; 46: 1417-24.

[79]   Ahmad S, Mokaddas E. Contribution of AGC to ACC and other mutations at codon 315 of the katG gene in isoniazid-resistant *Mycobacterium tuberculosis* isolates from the Middle East. Int J Antimicrob Agents 2004; 23: 473-79.

[80]   Ahmad S, Jaber AA, Mokaddas E. Frequency of embB codon 306 mutations in ethambutol-susceptible and -resistant clinical *Mycobacterium tuberculosis* isolates in Kuwait. Tuberculosis 2007; 87: 123-29.

[81]   Ruiz M, Torres MJ, Llanos AC, *et al.* Direct detection of rifampin- and isoniazid-resistant *Mycobacterium tuberculosis* in auramine-rhodamine-positive sputum specimens by real-time PCR. J Clin Microbiol 2004; 42: 1585-89.

[82]   Espasa M, Gonzales-Martin J, Alcaide F, *et al.* Direct detection in clinical samples of multiple gene mutations causing resistance of *Mycobacterium tuberculosis* to isoniazid and rifampicin using fluorogenic probes. J Antimicrob Chemother 2005; 55: 860-65.

[83]   Beenhouwer H, Lhiang Z, Jannes G, *et al.* Rapid detection of rifampicin resistance in sputum and biopsy specimens from tuberculosis patients by PCR and line probe assay. Tuber Lung Dis 1995; 76: 425-30.

[84]   Sharma M, Sethi S, Mishra B, *et al.* Rapid detection of mutations in rpoB gene of rifampicin resistant *Mycobacterium tuberculosis* strains by line probe assay. Indian J Med Res 2003; 117: 76-80.

[85]   Srivastava K, Das R, Jakhmola P, *et al.* Detection of mutations in *rpo*B gene region of rifampicin resistant isolates of *Mycobacterium tuberculosis* by INNO-LiPA assay. Indian J Med Res 2004; 120: 100-05.

[86]   Fortun J, Martin-Davila P, Navas E, *et al.* Linezolid for the treatment of multidrug-resistant tuberculosis. J Antimicrob Chemother 2005; 56: 180-85.

[87]   Dietze R, Hadad DJ, McGee B, *et al.* Early and extended early bactericidal activity of linezolid in pulmonary tuberculosis. Am J Respir Crit Care Med 2008; 178: 1180-85.

[88]   Dye C. Doomsday postponed? Preventing and reversing epidemics of drug-resistant tuberculosis. Nat Rev Microbiol 2009; 7: 81-87.

[89]   Iseman MD. MDR-TB and the developing world--a problem no longer to be ignored: the WHO announces 'DOTS Plus' strategy". The International Journal of Tuberculosis and Lung Disease 1998; 2: 867.

CHAPTER 7

Extended Spectrum Beta Lactamases: A Critical Update

Shazi Shakil[1], Hafiz Muhammad Ali[2], Raffaele Zarrilli[3] and Asad Ullah Khan[1]*

[1]Interdisciplinary Biotechnolology Unit, Aligarh Muslim University, Aligarh, India-202002 and [2]Signalisations et Réseaux Intégratifs en Biologie BIO-SigNE, Faculté de Médecine, Université Paris-Sud 11, Paris France, [3]Department of Preventive Medical Sciences, Hygiene Section, University of Naples 'Federico II', Naples, Italy

Abstract: Antibiotic resistance in bacteria is an increasing problem worldwide. Bacteria are challenging the scientists with a hard-hitting weapon called as 'Extended Spectrum Beta Lactamases' (ESBLs). Now, CTX-M enzymes have become the most prevalent beta-lactamases found in clinical isolates, leaving behind the TEM and SHV types. Organisms that produce both an ESBL and a carbapenemase may become resistant to virtually all β-lactams, leading to therapeutic dead-ends. Structural studies of ESBLs indicate that active site expansion and remodeling are responsible for this extended hydrolytic activity. Continuing questions still exist regarding the optimal detection method for ESBLs. Presently, the therapy relies on β-lactam/ β-lactamases inhibitor combinations, carbapenems and piperacillin - tazobactam plus aminoglycoside combination. In light of the emergence of carbapenemases, the presumed status of carbapenems as the therapy of choice against ESBL-producing pathogens is in question. Moreover, this review explores CTX-M, the most prevalent ESBL at molecular level so that the reader may appreciate "structure-function relationships" in these enzymes.

Keywords: ESBL, CTX-M, carbapenems resistance, MDR, enterobactericea, TEM, SHV, MBL.

INTRODUCTION

Bacterial cell wall had been a traditional target of attack by antibiotics. We have come a long way using β-lactams as antibiotics. Bacteria have also got them selected with hardier resistance mechanisms [1]. The Extended Spectrum Beta Lactamase (ESBL)-phenomenon was first detected in Germany [2] probably because extended-spectrum β-lactam antibiotics were used there first. There is a widespread occurrence of ESBLs, particularly in the hospital environment [3, 4]. ESBLs demonstrate resistance to 3rd-generation cephalosporins and are now a threat to hospitalized patients globally. Multidrug resistant bacteria causing therapeutic problems have become a matter of serious concern [5, 6]. ESBLs are dangerous because they are often plasmid-associated and the plasmids can exchange with a variety of bacterial species. Moreover, these plasmids can carry genes for co-resistance to other antibiotics such as aminoglycosides, fluoroquinolones, tetracyclines, chloramphenicol and sulfamethoxazole-trimethoprim. The presence of such multidrug-resistant strains limits the use of β- lactam and other antibiotics and can lead to the prescription of more broad spectrum and expensive drugs such as carbapenems. Antibiotic selection for such isolates thus becomes a therapeutic challenge.

Henceforth, we decided the present review covers recent literature dwelling upon the threat imposed by these enzymes with an aim to minimize the spread of resistance. Structure-function relationships have also been summarized so that the reader may appreciate the implications for development of potential inhibitors against these enzymes.

PRIMARY INFORMATION AND SIGNIFICANCE

ESBLs are globular proteins composed of alpha-helices and beta-pleated sheets [7]. These are β-lactamases that hydrolyze extended-spectrum cephalosporins with an oxyimino side chain. ESBLs are usually capable

---

Address correspondence to Asad Ullah Khan: Interdisciplinary Biotechnolology Unit, Aligarh Muslim University, Aligarh, India-202002; Tel: 0091-9837021912; Fax: 0091571-2721776; Email: asad.k@rediffmail.com

of hydrolyzing penicillins (*e.g.,* ampicillin and piperacillin), cephalosporins of the first-, second-, third- and fourth-generations, and the monobactam aztreonam (but not the cephamycins or carbapenems) [8]. The distinctive property of ESBLs (*e.g.* members of TEM and SHV families) of being inhibited by beta lactamase inhibitors such as clavulanic acid, tazobactam, or sulbactam, is duly exploited in the double-disk synergy test meant for ESBL-detection.

The Ambler scheme and the Bush-Medeiros-Jacoby system [8, 9] are the two systems commonly used for the classification of these enzymes (Table **1**). Typically, the ESBLs derive from genes for TEM-1, TEM-2, or SHV-1 by mutations that result in a change in the amino acid configuration around the active site of these enzymes. ESBLs are classified in group 2be in the Bush-Medeiros-Jacoby system and class A in the Ambler system. Authors have long back observed that point mutations in the SHV and TEM ß-lactamases which cause single amino acid substitutions (Asp104→Lys, Arg164→Ser, Arg164→His, Asp179→Asn, Gly238→Ser, and Glu240→Lys) are responsible for this resistance [10, 11]. Hence these enzymes are a potent weapon of bacteria and a significant research problem for scientists.

Table 1: Classification of the Extended-Spectrum Beta Lactamases.

Bush-Jacoby-Medeiros System	Major Subgroups	Ambler System	Main Attributes
Group 1 cephalosporinases	-	C (cephalosporinases)	Usually chromosomal; Resistance to all β-lactams except carbapenems; Not inhibited
Group 2 penicillinases (clavulanic acid susceptible)	2a	A(serine β-lactamases)	Staphylococcal penicillinases
	2b	A	Broad-spectrum-TEM-1, TEM-2, SHV-1
	2be	A	Extended-spectrum-TEM-3-160,SHV-2-101
	2br	A	Inhibitor resistant TEM (IRT)
	2c	A	Carbenicillin-hydrolyzing
	2e	A	Cephalosporinases inhibited by clavulanate
	2f	A	Carbapenemases inhibited by clavulanate
	2d	D (oxacillin-hydrolyzing)	Cloxacillin-hydrolyzing (OXA)
Group 3 metallo-b- 3a B (metalloenzymes)	3a	B (metalloenzymes)	Zinc-dependent carbapenemases
	3b	B	
	3c	B	
Group 4		Not classified	Miscellaneous enzymes, most not yet sequenced

EPIDEMIOLOGY

Although these enzymes were first detected in Germany in 1983 among *Klebsiella* spp [2], it was not long before that ESBLs were detected in the United States and Asia. The SENTRY surveillance program reported the frequency of ESBL-producing *K. pneumoniae* to be approximately 37% in Latin America *vs* 7% in the United States [12]. ESBLs are quite commonly encountered in the Asian Pacific region also, with prevalences of ESBL-producing *Klebsiella* spp reported to be 5%, 21.7%, 31% and 38% in Japan, Taiwan, the Philippines and Malaysia/Singapore, respectively. In addition, the prevalence of ESBL-producing *E. coli* varies from 6% to 23% within one region [13]. Several studies from India have also reported a high prevalence of ESBL producing pathogens [14-17]. Currently, the CTX-M type enzymes have started dominating the globe [18-20]. PER- and OXA type enzymes are more common in *P. aeruginosa* and *Acinetobacter* spp., but there have been sporadic reports of PER type ESBLs in *Enterobacteriacea* as well [21-23]. Plasmid-borne KPC enzymes have been reported among *K. pneumoniae* and other enterobacteria from the United States and other countries [24, 25]. These are of due concern because of their ability to inactivate carbapenems.

ESBL-DIVERSITY

TEM

TEM-1 was first reported in 1965 from an *Escherichia coli* strain isolated from a patient in Athens, Greece, named Temoneira (hence the designation TEM) [26]. TEM-1 is able to hydrolyze ampicillin at a greater rate than carbenicillin, oxacillin, or cephalothin, and has negligible activity against extended-spectrum cephalosporins. It is inhibited by clavulanic acid. TEM-1 and TEM-2 are not ESBLs. *Klebsiella pneumoniae* isolates from France were found to harbor a novel plasmid-mediated β-lactamase (CTX-1) in 1987 [27, 28]. The enzyme, now termed TEM-3, differed from TEM-2 by two amino acid substitutions [29]. But TEM-3 may not have been the first TEM-type ESBL. *Klebsiella oxytoca*, harboring a plasmid carrying a gene encoding ceftazidime resistance, was first isolated in Liverpool, England, in 1982 [30]. The gene is now designated as TEM-12. The amino acid substitutions responsible for the ESBL phenotype cluster around the active site of the enzyme and change its configuration, in such a manner that allows access to oxyimino-beta-lactams. This change also enhances the susceptibility of the enzyme to ß-lactamase inhibitors, such as clavulanic acid. Single amino acid substitutions at positions 104, 164, 238, and 240 produce the ESBL phenotype, but ESBLs with the broadest spectrum usually have more than a single amino acid substitution. Based upon different combinations of changes, currently 140 TEM-type enzymes have been described. TEM-10, TEM-12, and TEM-26 are among the most common in the United States [31-33].

SHV

Authors from Germany in 1983, reported a *Klebsiella ozaenae* isolate that harbored a β-lactamase which efficiently hydrolyzed cefotaxime, and to a lesser extent ceftazidime [2]. The enzyme, now called SHV-2 differed from SHV-1 by G238S mutation. To date, bacteria harboring SHV-2 have been reported throughout the globe [31]. SHV-type ESBLs have been detected in a wide range of Gram negative organisms including *Pseudomonas aeruginosa* and *Acinetobacter* spp as well [34, 35].

PER

PER-1 efficiently hydrolyzes penicillins and cephalosporins and is susceptible to clavulanic acid inhibition. PER-1 was first detected in *Pseudomonas aeruginosa* [36], and later in *Salmonella enterica* serovar Typhimurium and *Acinetobacter* isolates as well [37-40].The PER-type enzymes share only 25 to 27% homology with known TEM- and SHV-type ESBLs [41, 42]. PER-1 producing isolates of *Pseudomonas aeruginosa* and *Acinetobacter* spp. have been reported worldwide [43-45]. PER-2, which shares 86% homology to PER-1, has been detected in *S. enterica* serovar Typhimurium, *Escherichia coli*, *Klebsiella pneumoniae*, *Proteus mirabilis*, and *Vibrio cholerae* [41, 46]. *Pseudomonas aeruginosa* strain producing both PER-1 and the carbapenemase VIM-2 has been already reported [47]. A situation in which an ESBL and a carbapenemase is simultaneously produced in a pathogen poses a serious therapeutic challenge to clinicians. Such an organism may become resistant to virtually all β-lactams.

OXA

These β-lactamases (group 2d) are characterized by hydrolysis rates for cloxacillin and oxacillin greater than 50% that for benzylpenicillin [9]. They predominantly occur in *Pseudomonas aeruginosa* [48] but have been detected in many other gram-negative bacteria. Most OXA-type β-lactamases do not hydrolyze the extended-spectrum cephalosporins to a significant degree and are not regarded as ESBLs. However, OXA-10 hydrolyzes (weakly) cefotaxime, ceftriaxone, and aztreonam, giving most organisms reduced susceptibility to these antibiotics. Other OXA ESBLS include: OXA-11, -14, -16, -17, -19, -15, -18, -28, -31, -32, -35, and -45. These confer resistance to cefotaxime and sometimes ceftazidime and aztreonam [49].

VEB-1, BES-1 and Other ESBLs

VEB-1 has greatest homology with PER-1 and PER-2 (38%) [50]. It confers high-level resistance to ceftazidime, cefotaxime, and aztreonam, which is reversed by clavulanic acid. The gene encoding VEB-1 was found to be plasmid mediated; such plasmids also confer resistance to non-β-lactam antibiotics [50]. A variety of other β-lactamases which are plasmid-mediated or integron-associated class A enzymes have been already discovered [51-54]. Several chromosomally encoded ESBLs have also been described [55]. Other VEB enzymes have also been detected in Kuwait and China [56, 57]. GES [58-61], BES [51], TLA [54, 62], SFO [63], and IBC [64-66] are other examples of non-TEM, non-SHV ESBLs and have been reported from various countries.

CTX-M

The name CTX reflects the potent hydrolytic activity of these β-lactamases against cefotaxime. Organisms producing CTX-M-type β-lactamases typically have cefotaxime Minimum Inhibitory Concentrations (MICs) in the resistant range (>64 μg/ml), while ceftazidime MICs are usually in the apparently susceptible range (2 to 8 μg/ml). However, some CTX-M-type ESBLs may actually hydrolyze ceftazidime and confer resistance to this cephalosporin (MICs as high as 256 μg/ml) [67-69]. Aztreonam MICs are variable. CTX-M-type β-lactamases hydrolyze cefepime with high efficiency [70], and cefepime MICs are higher than observed in bacteria producing other ESBL types [71]. Another unique feature of these enzymes is that they are better inhibited by the β-lactamase inhibitor tazobactam than by sulbactam and clavulanate [72, 73]. CTX-M-type β-lactamases have 40% or less identity with TEM and SHV-type ESBLs. CTX-M beta-lactamases are commonly found in *K. pneumoniae, E. coli*, typhoid and non typhoidal *Salmonella, Shigella, Citrobacter freundii, Enterobacter*, spp., and *Serratia marcescens* [18]. Different genetic elements may be involved in the mobilization of CTX-M genes. Plasmids and Insertion Sequences (*e.g.*, IS*Ecp1* or IS*Ecp1*-like insertion sequences) have been repeatedly observed upstream of ORFs encoding the CTX-M-1, CTXM-2, CTX-M-3, CTX-M-9, CTX-M-13, CTX-M-14, CTX-M-15, CTX-M-17, CTX-M-19, CTX-M-20, and CTX-M-21 β-lactamases [74-76].

CTX-M BETA LACTAMASES - THE LEADING THERAPEUTIC CHALLENGE

These are now considered the most prevalent ESBLs worldwide [18-20] and hence will be the focus of our discussions throughout this review. Pitout *et al* have described the clonal spread of two closely related Canadian isolates harboring CTX-M-14, isolated mainly from urine samples [77, 78]. In a national survey several types of ESBLs were reported from the community in United Kingdom, among which clonally-spread *E. coli* carrying CTX-M-15 predominated, although CTX-M 9 was also represented [20].

In Hong-Kong, 42/600 (7%) of community isolates of urinary *E. coli* were ESBL producers [79]. A low prevalence (1.8%) and great diversity of enzymes and bacterial species were found among community isolates in Brazil, in contrast with Bolivian and Peruvian isolates among which *E. coli* harboring CTX-M-15 and CTX-M-9 were predominant [80, 81]. Recently we have observed a high prevalence of CTX-M-15 type ESBLs in a premier hospital of North India [Shakil S, Akram M, Danishuddin M, Khan AU- Unpublished results; Genbank Accession Nos.- FJ997864, FJ997865, FJ997866, GQ145219, GQ145220, GQ145221, GQ174503, GQ174504, GQ174506].

DIRECTION OF TRANSMISSION OF CTX-Ms

It is interesting to argue that whether the CTX-Ms arose in the nosocomial setting and spread to the community or vice-versa. A hospital is the area where the selective pressure of broad-spectrum antibiotics coupled with suboptimal infection control practices best conspires to promote the emergence and transmission of multidrug-resistant organisms. Nursing homes, in turn, may serve as reservoirs from which colonized and infected patients transfer to the community or back to the hospitals [82]. Prior to the rise of CTX-M, such a model seemed to have corresponded with the available data [83]. Even after the noted spread of bacteria producing CTX-M into the community, recent hospitalization, along with age and exposure to cephalosporins and/or quinolones, have consistently been identified as risk factors for infection with these organisms [84, 85]. Nevertheless, there are reports suggesting an opposite trend too. A report from Israel described high rates of patients with bacteremia and colonization with ESBL-producing *Enterobacteriaceae* on admission to the hospital [86]. An additional potential reservoir of resistant bacteria and genetic determinants of resistance which intersects with the community is the food supply, as illustrated by the finding of diverse ESBL-producing bacteria, including CTX-M-15, in poultry and other farm animals [87-89]. Finally, the origin of CTX-M enzymes probably lies in beta-lactamases found in environmental species, like *Kluyvera* spp. [18], further supporting the notion of a community reservoir for these enzymes. "Antibiotic resistome" is the concept that best describes the existence of resistant microorganisms that predate over the clinical use of antibiotics [90, 91]. We have also found CTX-M-15 marker located on the genomic DNA of two clinical isolates from North India [Akram M, Shakil S, Danishuddin M, Khan AU- Unpublished results; Genbank Accession Numbers- FJ997868 and FJ997869].

STRUCTURE-FUNCTION RELATIONSHIPS

The study of the atomic structures of class A ESBLs has revealed that the active site is selectively "remodeled and expanded" to accommodate the bulky R1 side chain of extended spectrum cephalosporins [92].

THE KEY PLAYERS BEHIND THE SUBSTRATE SPECIFICITY OF CTX-Ms

Amino acid residues Asn104, Asn132, Ser237, and Asp240 have been identified as the key players behind the substrate specificity of the CTX-M beta-lactamases by several studies that used comparative sequence analyses, modeling, and mutagenesis techniques [93]. Ser23, has been observed to be involved in the extension of the substrate specificities of TEM and SHV ESBLs to cefotaxime [7]. The Ser237Ala substitution in the CTX-M-4 enzyme induces a decrease both in relative hydrolytic activity against cefotaxime and in susceptibility to inhibition by clavulanate [94]. The acyl intermediate structure of Toho-1 in complex with cefotaxime shows a rotation of the Ser237 side chain, which prevents steric clashes with the methoxyimino group of cefotaxime and which allows the formation of a hydrogen bond with the carboxylate group of cefotaxime [95]. It has been suggested that this interaction assists in bringing the carbonyl group of the β-lactam ring of cephalosporins to the optimal position in the oxyanion hole for acylation [95]. The relatively low penicillinase activities of CTX-M enzymes may be caused by Van der Waals contact between residue Ser237 and the methyl group of the thiazolidine ring. Asn104, Asn132, Ser237, and Asp240 residues establish hydrogen bonds with the amide and aminothiazole groups of the acyl-amide-cefotaxime chain. This unusual acyl intermediate of CTX-M enzymes in complex with cefotaxime may therefore be involved in the activities of the oxyimino-cephalosporinases by fixing cefotaxime tightly in the binding site [95, 96].

THE OMEGA LOOP

The structure of Toho-1 revealed that the omega loop has fewer hydrogen bond interactions with the β3 strand in the vicinities of Asn170 and Asp240 than the restricted-spectrum β-lactamase of *Bacillus licheniformis*, the enzyme most closely related to Toho-1 at the structural level. No hydrogen bond has been observed between the Phe160 residue and Thr181 and Asp157 residues, which both connect the N and C termini of the omega loop in restricted-spectrum β-lactamases [96]. These structural features may increase the flexibility of the omega loop. The structures of acyl intermediates of the Toho-1 enzyme show a shift of the omega loop to helix H5 [95] as a result of a complex structural rearrangement in the hydrophobic core in the vicinity of the omega loop (the residues involved in the rearrangement are Cys69, Ser72, Met135, Phe160, and Thr165). This shift narrows the binding site, but the steric contacts of the Pro167 and Asn170 residues with the aminothiazole ring of cefotaxime are avoided.

THE STEPS OF CTX-M EVOLUTIONARY LADDER: RESIDUES SER167 AND GLY240

Mutants with point mutations in common CTX-M enzymes exhibiting improved catalytic efficiencies against ceftazidime have been observed [7]. The change in activities of CTX-Ms leading to the evolution of more variants may be due to point mutations present either inside or outside of the active site omega loop. For example the P167T mutation differentiates CTX-M-23 from CTX-M-1, CTX-M-3 and CTX-M-15 (Fig. **1**). However the CTX-Ms, having identical residues present in the omega loop may still have some difference in their enzymatic activities due to mutations present outside the omega loop. The CTX-M-15, CTX-M-16, and CTX-M-27 enzymes harbor the Asp240Gly substitution. The presence of Lys and Arg residues at position 240 are known to increase the enzymatic activities of the TEM and SHV ESBLs against ceftazidime [7]. The Lys and Arg residues are positively charged and can form an electrostatic bond with the carboxylic acid group on oxyimino substituents of Ceftazidime [97, 98]. Neutral residue Gly240 is not able to form electrostatic interactions with β-lactams but could favor the accommodation of the oxyimino-ceftazidime side chain [99, 100].

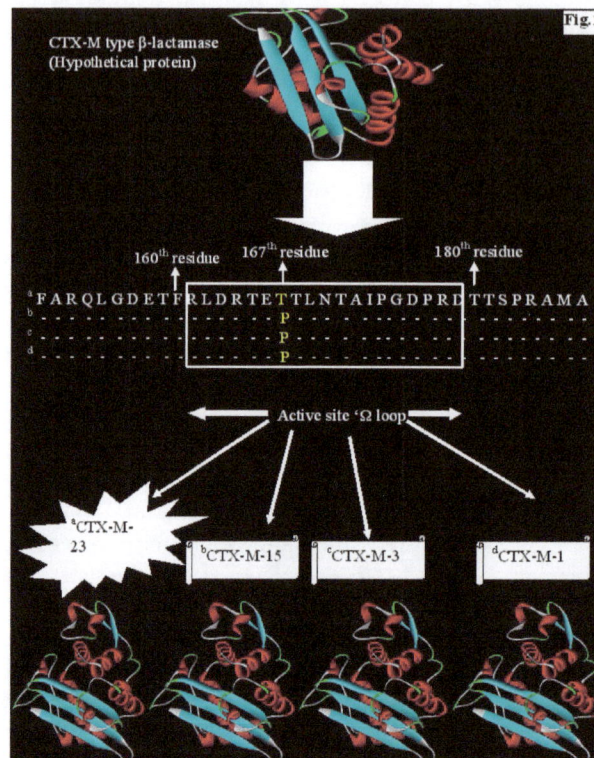

Figure 1: Amino acids profile of active site omega loop of different CTX-M variants.

DETECTION OF ESBLs

As per the Clinical Laboratory Standard Institute (CLSI) criteria, enterobacterial resistance to ceftriaxone, cefotaxime, ceftazidime, cefepime, and aztreonam is defined by MICs ≥ 16 μg/ml [101]. However, since several ESBL producers have MIC values for extended spectrum cephalosporins and aztreonam below the standard breakpoints for resistance (*e.g.*, between 2 and 8 μg/ml), the real prevalence of these organisms may go unchecked. A study in Connecticut, USA found that only 5.4% (2/130) of clinical microbiology laboratories could detect an ESBL producing challenge strain [102]. Thus, these resistant strains can be missed by routine susceptibility testing, leading to adverse therapeutic outcomes. Since the inaccurate identification of ESBL producers bears important clinical implications for antibiotic therapy and infection control measures, specific reporting guidelines are issued [101]. For all confirmed ESBL producers, the general consensus states that ESBL producers should be reported as resistant to all penicillins, cephalosporins (except for the cephamycins cefoxitin and cefotetan), and aztreonam irrespective of routine antimicrobial susceptibility results [101]. However, beta-lactam/betalactamase inhibitor combinations (*e.g.*, piperacillin-tazobactam, amoxicillin-clavulanate, and ampicillin-sulbactam) are not affected by this rule and should be reported as obtained during routine susceptibility tests.

SCREENING FOR ESBL PRODUCTION

Both broth dilution and disk diffusion methods for screening for ESBL producers are advised by CLSI. It is recommended that *E. coli*, *K. pneumoniae* and *K. oxytoca* strains with MIC ≥ 8 μg/ml for cefpodoxime or MICs ≥ 2 μg/ml against ceftazidime, cefotaxime, ceftriaxone, or aztreonam should be investigated using specific phenotypic confirmatory tests for ESBL production. For *P. mirabilis* isolates, confirmatory tests should be performed if strains demonstrate MICs ≥ 2 µg/ml for ceftazidime, cefotaxime or cefpodoxime. The use of more than one of the above agents for screening improves the sensitivity of ESBL detection. The British Society for Antimicrobial Chemotherapy (BSAC) maintains that all *Enterobacteriaceae* resistant to ceftazidime (MIC ≥ 4 µg/ml or zone inhibition ≤ 21 mm for *E. coli* and *Klebsiella* spp and ≤ 27 mm for the remaining species), cefotaxime (MIC ≥ 2 µg/ml or zone inhibition ≤ 29 mm), or cefpodoxime (MIC ≥ 2 µg/ml or zone inhibition ≤ 19 mm) should be evaluated by the ESBL confirmatory tests (Health Protection Agency, 2005). Similarly, the Société Française de Microbiologie (SFM) suggests the evaluation of all enterobacteria with the confirmatory test. Moreover, the ESBL confirmatory test should be performed when an isolate shows resistance to aminoglycosides (Comite de L'Antibiogramme de la Société Française de Microbiologie, SFM, 2007), since *bla* genes encoding ESBLs are frequently found in the same plasmid that encode resistance determinants to other classes of antibiotics such as aminoglycosides, tetracycline and sulfonamides [32].

PHENOTYPIC CONFIRMATORY TESTS FOR ESBL PRODUCTION

ESBL confirmatory testing based upon phenotype requires the use of both ceftazidime and cefotaxime alone and in combination with clavulanate according to the CLSI [101]. Several companies produce disks for use in this application. Usually, these discs contain 30 µg /disk of ceftazidime, cefotaxime with or without clavulanate (10 µg/disk). These discs have been reported to have sensitivity and specificity of greater than 95% [103, 104]. It is speculated that the use of cefepime and cefpirome with clavulanate might improve the ability to detect ESBLs [105, 106]. Accordingly, BSAC advises the use of cefpirome/clavulanate combination disks (in addition to cefpodoxime/clavulanate) for *Enterobacter* spp. and *C. freundii* as a confirmatory test (Health Protection Agency, 2005), whereas the SFM recommends to use cefepime or cefpirome with the double-disk diffusion test for all enterobacteria producing AmpC enzymes (CASFM, 2007). ESBLs are more difficult to detect in these organisms because AmpC enzymes may be induced by clavulanate (which inhibits them poorly) and may increase resistance to cephalosporins, overcoming the synergy arising from inhibition of the ESBL [107].

COMMERCIAL METHODS FOR ESBL DETECTION

The Etest strips produced by Bio-Stat (Stockport, UK) and AB Biodisk (Solna, Sweden)constitute a plastic drug-impregnated strip, one end of which generates a stable concentration gradient of cephalosporin (*i.e.*, ceftazidime 0.5-32 µg/ml, cefotaxime and cefepime 0.25-16 µg/ml) and the remaining end of which generates a gradient of cephalosporin (*i.e.*, ceftazidime and cefepime 0.064-4 µg/ml, cefotaxime 0.016-1 µg/ml) plus a constant concentration of clavulanate (4 µg/ml). ESBL production is inferred if the MIC ratio for cephalosporin alone/ cephalosporin plus clavulanate MIC is ≥ 8 µg/ml (Health Protection Agency, 2005). Accurate and precise (but more expensive than combination disks) these tests are suggested by the BSAC as a confirmatory test for ESBL production. Significantly, BSAC recommends the cefepime/ clavulanate Etest for *Enterobacter* spp (Health Protection Agency, 2005). In fact, neither ceftazidime/clavulanate nor cefotaxime/clavulanate Etest strips are able to detect the ESBLs in *Enterobacter* spp. In contrast, the cefepime/clavulanate strip is the only commercially available and highly reliable test that permits accurate detection of ESBLs within this group of organisms [105]. The BD Phoenix System (Becton-Dickinson Biosciences, Sparks, MD) uses its "expert software" to interpret the growth response to ceftazidime, cefotaxime, ceftriaxone and cefpodoxime, with or without clavulanate. Similarly, the Vitek 2 System (bioMérieux, Marcy L'Etoile, France) uses a "card" containing ceftazidime and cefotaxime alone and in combination with clavulanate. Ceftazidime or cefotaxime plus beta lactamase inhibitors are also used in the MicroScan Walkaway-96 System (Dade Behring, Inc., West Sacramento, CA). The above three semi-automated systems were compared to the conventional phenotypic confirmatory tests with regard to their ability to detect ESBL production in well characterized *Enterobacteriaceae* including *Enterobacter* spp, *C. freundii* and *S. marcescens*. The system with the highest sensitivity was Phoenix (99%), followed by Vitek 2 (86%) and MicroScan (84%) [104].

CLINICAL IMPACT AND IMPLICATIONS FOR THERAPY

Several authors have concluded that patients with infection due to ESBL-producing enterobacteria have less satisfactory outcomes than those infected by Non ESBL-producers [108-113]. In a large multicenter study analyzing bloodstream infections due to ESBL-producing *K. pneumoniae* isolates, cephalosporin monotherapy was associated with a 40% 14-day mortality rate [114]. A comparable mortality rate among patients treated empirically with cephalosporin monotherapy was observed in another related study due to CTX-M-positive *E. coli* isolates [115]. It might be concluded that extended-spectrum cephalosporin treatment is associated with high rate of treatment failure (>80%) and mortality (>35%) when the susceptibility of infecting strains is close to the CLSI breakpoints (*i.e.*, MIC ≥ 16 μg/ml). Choice of appropriate empiric therapy within the first 24-48 hours of presentation is a key factor in the outcome of infected patients. The choice becomes difficult as many ESBL-producers harbour co-resistance markers for aminoglycosides (e.g, gentamicin and tobramycin), quinolones (*e.g.*, ciprofloxacin), and sulfamethoxazole [32].

BETA-LACTAM/BETA-LACTAMASES INHIBITOR COMBINATIONS

ESBLs are usually susceptible to β-lactam / β-lactamase inhibitor combinations, but these drugs can usually be overwhelmed by particularly large amounts of enzyme and thus may show *in vivo* resistance. Treatment with this combination was shown to be inferior to treatment with imipenem or piperacillin/tazobactam plus aminoglycoside combination in an animal model [116]. Furthermore, a possible presence of chromosomal AmpC enzymes that are normally resistant to inactivation by a β-lactamase inhibitor can never be ruled out [107].

CEFEPIME

ESBL-producing bacteria may be susceptible to cefepime (MIC ≤ 8 μg/ml). Studies have analyzed the outcomes of patients treated with cefepime therapy for infection with ESBL-producing, cefepime-susceptible *E. coli* and *K. pneumoniae* [117-119]. A randomized, multicenter, evaluator-blind trial found imipenem/cilistatin (0.5g q6h by IV route) to be substantially better than cefepime (2g q8h by IV route) for treatment of nosocomial pneumonia among intensive care unit-patients [120]. From these studies it can be suggested that cefepime may not be the optimal therapy in the treatment of ESBL-producing bacteria, particularly in serious infections (*e.g.*, bacteremia and pneumonia). However, the administration of higher doses of cefepime (*i.e.*, 4-6g administered as a continuous infusion or 2g q6-8h with prolonged infusion) may result in improved outcomes [121].

QUINOLONES

Scientists have repeatedly observed co-transfer of quinolone resistance markers (*e.g.* ciprofloxacin) with ESBL markers (*e.g.* CTX-M) in ESBL-positive bacteria [122]. A multicenter prospective study of *K. pneumonia* bacteremia conducted during 1996-1997, detected ESBL production in 60% of ciprofloxacin resistant isolates, compared with 16% of ciprofloxacin-susceptible strains [123]. Hence quinolones can be drugs of choice against ESBL-producers, provided that the strains give a positive susceptibility test for the same *in vitro*.

AMINOGLYCOSIDES

Aminoglycosides may be effective therapy against ESBL producing pathogens only when the organism is susceptible to these drugs *i.e.* the aminoglycoside and ESBL resistance markers should not be associated with each other as is frequently observed. Susceptibility to amikacin seems to be preserved, in contrast to gentamicin and tobramycin, thus justifying its use as empiric therapy [122]. For other aminoglycosides [1], our views are same as for the quinolones.

TIGECYCLINE

Tigecycline is the first Food and Drug Administration approved glycylcycline antibiotic. It has shown remarkable *in vitro* activity against a wide variety of gram-positive, gram-negative and anaerobic bacteria including many multidrug resistant strains. For complicated intra-abdominal infections, tigecycline was found to be as effective as imipenem/cilastatin [124]. Adverse events related to tigecycline therapy, *i.e.*

nausea and vomiting, were tolerable [125]. Currently available data suggest that tigecycline may play an important role in the future as a monotherapy alternative to older broad-spectrum antibiotics, such as advanced generation cephalosporins and carbapenems [5, 126].

CARBAPENEMS

Studies have observed over 98% ESBL-producing *E. coli, Klebsiella* spp, and *P. mirabilis* isolates to be carbapenems-susceptible [122, 127]. As per the findings of many authors, carbapenems may be considered as the preferred treatment for infections due to ESBL-producing enterobacteria [128, 129]. In a study that included ESBL-producing *K. pneumoniae* bloodstream isolates, patients who were treated with imipenem/cilistatin during the 5-day period after onset of infections had a 14-day mortality of 4.8%, compared with 27.6% when another *in vitro* active beta-lactam was used [114]. However, in light of the emergence of carbapenemases, the presumed status of carbapenems as the therapy of choice against ESBL-producing pathogens is in question.

DORIPENEM

This latest carbapenem has been suggested to be maximally stable against carbapenem hydrolyzing beta lactamases. In a study, the authors performed docking of the enzyme Sme1 with imipenem, meropenem, ertapenem and doripenem separately to compare their effectiveness against Sme1 producing bacteria [6]. The authors suggested a relationship between total free energy of docking and MICs observed in wet lab studies. A higher negative value of free energy of docking for the enzyme-antibiotic complex was taken as an indicator of more stability. A more stable and better fitting of the carbapenem antibiotic into the active site of the carbapenem hydrolyzing enzyme would ensure an easy hydrolysis of the drug. The authors observed that the imipenem-Sme1 complex was far more stable than the complex involving doripenem. This suggested an easier hydrolysis of imipenem by Sme-1 and a poor hydrolysis of doripenem. This was in coherence with the wet studies that suggested a better activity of doripenem over other carbapenems against carbapenemase producing bacteria [6].

CONCLUSIONS

ESBLs constitute a serious threat to currently available antibiotics. Outbreaks of infections by organisms resistant to β-lactam agents due to the production of these enzymes are being increasingly reported from across the globe. Detection of ESBL-production is of paramount importance both in hospital and community isolates. CTX-M enzymes confer higher levels of resistance to cefotaxime than to ceftazidime. The MICs of ceftazidime are sometimes found to be in the susceptible range, whereas ESBL detection is frequently based on ceftazidime utilization. This argues in favor of further studies on how to adapt ESBL detection procedures to survey and contain the spread of CTX-M enzymes. Development of newer β-lactams and discovery of 'next-generation' inhibitors against these versatile enzymes are eagerly awaited. Commercial methods should be made more economic to extend their benefits to underdeveloped and developing countries like India.

REFERENCES

[1]   Shakil S, Khan R, Zarrilli R, *et al.* Aminoglycosides *vs* bacteria- a description of the action, resistance mechanism, and nosocomial battleground. J Biomed Sci 2008; 15: 5-14.

[2]   Knothe H, Shah P, Krcmery V, *et al.* Transferable resistance to cefotaxime, cefoxitin, cefamandole and cefuroxime in clinical isolates of *Klebsiella pneumoniae* and *Serratia marcescens.* Infection 1983; 11: 315-17.

[3]   Minarini LA, Clímaco EC, Guimarães DB, *et al.* Clonal transmission of ESBL-producing *Klebsiella* spp. at a university hospital in Brazil. Curr. Microbiol 2008; 56: 587-91.

[4]   Pfaller MA, Segreti J. Overview of the epidemiological profile and laboratory detection of extended-spectrum β-lactamases. Clin Infect Dis 2006; 42: S153-S163.

[5]   Shakil S, Akram M, Khan AU. Tigecycline: a critical update. J Chemother 2008; 20: 411-19.

[6]   Shakil S, Danishuddin M, Khan AU. Doripenem *vs* bacteria- an emerging battleground. J Chemother 2009; in press.

[7]   Knox JR. Extended-spectrum and inhibitor-resistant TEM-type beta-lactamases: mutations, specificity, and three-dimensional structure. Antimicrob Agents Chemother 1995; 39: 2593-601.

[8]   Ambler RP, Coulson AF, Frere JM, *et al.* A standard numbering scheme for the class A beta-lactamases. Biochem J 1991; 276: 269-70.

[9]   Bush K, Jacoby GA, Medeiros AA. A functional classification scheme for beta-lactamases and its correlation with molecular structure. Antimicrob Agents Chemother 1995; 39, 1211-33.

[10]   Philippon ALR, Jacoby G. Extended-spectrum beta-lactamases. Antimicrob Agents Chemother 1989; 33: 1131-36.

[11]   Jacoby GA, Medeiros AA. More extended-spectrum beta-lactamases. Antimicrob Agents Chemother 1991; 35: 1697-704.

[12]   Sader HS, Jones RN, Gales AC, *et al.* Antimicrobial susceptibility patterns for pathogens isolated from patients in Latin American medical centers with a diagnosis of pneumonia: analysis of results from SENTRY surveillance program (1997). SENTRY Latin America Study Group. Diagn. Microbiol Infect Dis 1998; 32: 289-301.

[13]   Parasakthi N, Ariffin H, (eds.) Consensus Guidelines for the Management of Infections by ESBL-Producing Bacteria. Ministry of Health Malaysia, Academy of Medicine of Malaysia, Malaysian Society of Infectious Diseases and Chemotherapy 2001.

[14]   Babypadmini S, Appalaraju B. Extended spectrum beta-lactamases in urinary isolates of *Escherichia coli* and *Klebsiella pneumoniae* - Prevalence and susceptibility pattern in a tertiary care hospital. Indian J Med Microbiol 2004; 22: 172-74.

[15]   Akram M, Shahid M, Khan AU. Etiology and antibiotic resistance patterns of community-acquired urinary tract infections in JNMC Hospital Aligarh, India. Ann Clin Microbiol Antimicrob 2007; 23: 6-4.

[16]   Shobha KL, Rao SG. Prevalence of Extended Spectrum Beta-Lactamases in Urinary Isolates of *Escherichia coli*, *Klebsiella* and *Citrobacter* Species and their Antimicrobial Susceptibility Pattern in a Tertiary Care Hospital. Ind J Pract Doc 2007; 3(6) (2007-01 - 2007-02).

[17]   Shakil S, Ali SZ, Akram M, *et al.* Risk factors for extended-spectrum β-lactamase producing *Escherichia coli* and *Klebsiella pneumoniae* acquisition in a neonatal intensive care unit. J Trop Pediatr 2009; in press.

[18]   Walther-Rasmussen J, Høiby N. Cefotaximases (CTX-M-ases), an expanding family of extended-spectrum β-lactamases. Can J Microbiol 2004; 50: 137-65.

[19]   Canton R, Coque TM. The CTX-M beta-lactamase pandemic. Curr Opin Microbiol 2006; 9: 466-75.

[20]   Livermore DM, Canton R, Gniadkowski M, *et al.* CTX-M: changing the face of ESBLs in Europe. J Antimicrob Chemother 2007; 59: 165-174.

[21]   Quinteros M, Radice M, Gardella N, *et al.* Extended-spectrum beta-lactamases in enterobacteriaceae in Buenos Aires, Argentina, public hospitals. Antimicrob Agents Chemother 2003; 47: 2864-67.

[22]   Lartigue M, Fortineau N, Nordmann P. Spread of novel expanded-spectrum beta-lactamases in enterobacteriaceae in a university hospital in the Paris area, France. Clin Microbiol Infect 2005; 11: 588-91.

[23]   Luzzaro F, Mezzatesta M, Mugnaioli C, *et al.* Trends in production of extended-spectrum beta-lactamases among enterobacteria of medical interest: report of the second Italian nationwide survey. J Clin Microbiol 2006; 44: 1659-64.

[24]   Goldfarb D, Harvey SB, Jessamine K, *et al.* Detection of plasmid-mediated KPC-producing *Klebsiella pneumoniae* in Ottawa, Canada: evidence of intrahospital transmission. J Clin Microbiol 2009; 47: 1920-22.

[25]   Gootz TD, Lescoe MK, Dib-Hajj F, *et al.* Genetic organization of transposase regions surrounding blaKPC carbapenemase genes on plasmids from *Klebsiella* strains isolated in a New York City hospital. Antimicrob Agents Chemother 2009; 53: 1998-2004.

[26]   Datta N, Kontomichalou P. Penicillinase synthesis controlled by infectious R factors in *Enterobacteriaceae*. Nature 1965; 208: 239-41.

[27]   Brun-Buisson C, Legrand P, Philippon A, *et al.* Transferable enzymatic resistance to third-generation cephalosporins during nosocomial outbreak of multi resistant *Klebsiella pneumoniae*. Lancet 1987; ii: 302-06.

[28]   Sirot D, Sirot J, Labia R, *et al.* Transferable resistance to third generation cephalosporins in clinical isolates of *Klebsiella pneumoniae*: identification of CTX-1, a novel beta-lactamase. J Antimicrob Chemother 1987; 20: 323-34.

[29]   Sougakoff W, Goussard S, Gerbaud G, *et al.* Plasmid mediated resistance to third-generation cephalosporins caused by point mutations in TEM-type penicillinase genes. Rev Infect Dis 1988; 10: 879-84.

[30] Du Bois SK, Marriott MS, Amyes SG. TEM- and SHV-derived extended-spectrum beta-lactamases: relationship between selection, structure and function. J Antimicrob Chemother 1995; 35: 7-22.

[31] Paterson DL, Hujer KM, Hujer AM, *et al.* Extended-spectrum beta-lactamases in *Klebsiella pneumoniae* bloodstream isolates from seven countries: dominance and widespread prevalence of SHV- and CTX-M-type beta-lactamases. Antimicrob Agents Chemother 2003; 47: 3554-60.

[32] Bradford PA. Extended-spectrum β-lactamases in the 21st century: characterization, epidemiology, and detection of this important resistance threat. Clin Microbiol Rev 2001; 48: 933-51.

[33] Jacoby GA, Munoz-Price LS. Mechanisms of disease: The New beta-Lactamases. N Engl J Med 2005; 352: 380-91.

[34] Kalai Blagui S, Achour W, Abdeladhim A, *et al.* Identification of SHV-type extended spectrum beta-lactamase genes in *Pseudomonas aeruginosa* by PCR-restriction fragment length polymorphism and insertion site restriction-PCR. Pathol Biol (Paris) 2009; 57(5): 420-24.

[35] Gür D, Gülay Z, Akan OA, *et al.* Resistance to newer beta-lactams and related ESBL types in gram-negative nosocomial isolates in Turkish hospitals: results of the multicentre HITIT study. Mikrobiyol Bul 2008; 42: 537-44.

[36] Neuhauser MM, Weinstein RA, Rydman R, *et al.* Antibiotic resistance among gram-negative bacilli in US intensive care units: implications for fluoroquinolone use. JAMA 2003; 289: 885-88.

[37] Vahaboglu H, Coskunkan F, Tansel O, *et al.* Clinical importance of extended-spectrum beta-lactamase (PER-1-type)-producing *Acinetobacter* spp. and *Pseudomonas aeruginosa* strains. J Med Microbiol 2001; 50: 642-45.

[38] Vahaboglu H, Hall LM, Mulazimoglu L, *et al.* Resistance to extended-spectrum cephalosporins, caused by PER-1 beta-lactamase, in *Salmonella typhimurium* from Istanbul, Turkey. J Med Microbiol 1995; 43: 294-99.

[39] Vahaboglu H, Ozturk R, Aygun G, *et al.* Widespread detection of PER-1-type extended-spectrum beta-lactamases among nosocomial *Acinetobacter* and *Pseudomonas aeruginosa* isolates in Turkey: a nationwide multicenter study. Antimicrob Agents Chemother 1997; 41: 2265-69.

[40] Vahaboglu H, Saribas S, Akbal H, *et al.* Activities of cefepime and five other antibiotics against nosocomial PER-1-type and/or OXA-10-type beta-lactamase-producing *Pseudomonas aeruginosa* and *Acinetobacter* spp. J Antimicrob Chemother 1998; 42: 269-70.

[41] Bauernfeind A, Stemplinger I, Jungwirth R, *et al.* Characterization of beta-lactamase gene blaPER-2, which encodes an extended-spectrum class A beta-lactamase. Antimicrob Agents Chemother 1996; 40: 616-20.

[42] Nordmann P, Naas T. Sequence analysis of PER-1 extended spectrum beta-lactamase from *Pseudomonas aeruginosa* and comparison with class A beta-lactamases. Antimicrob Agents Chemother 1994; 38: 104-14.

[43] Libisch B, Poirel L, Lepsanovic Z, *et al.* Identification of PER-1 extended-spectrum beta-lactamase producing *Pseudomonas aeruginosa* clinical isolates of the international clonal complex CC11 from Hungary and Serbia. FEMS Immunol. Med Microbiol 2008; 54: 330-38.

[44] Strateva T, Todorova A, Ouzounova-Raykova V, *et al.* Emergence of a PER-1 extended-spectrum beta-lactamase-producing *Acinetobacter baumannii* clinical isolate in Bulgaria. J Chemother 2008; 20: 391-92.

[45] Szabó D, Szentandrássy J, Juhász Z, *et al.* Imported PER-1 producing *Pseudomonas aeruginosa*, PER-1 producing *Acinetobacter baumanii* and VIM-2-producing *Pseudomonas aeruginosa* strains in Hungary. Ann. Clin Microbiol Antimicrob 2008; 30: 7-12.

[46] Petroni A, Corso A, Melano R, *et al.* Plasmidic extended-spectrum beta-lactamases in *Vibrio cholera* O1 El Tor isolates in Argentina. Antimicrob Agents Chemother 2002; 46: 1462-68.

[47] Docquier JD, Luzzaro F, Amicosante G, *et al.* Multidrug-resistant *Pseudomonas aeruginosa* producing PER-1 extended-spectrum serine-beta-lactamase and VIM-2 metallo-beta-lactamase. Emerg Infect Dis 2001; 7: 910-11.

[48] Weldhagen GF, Poirel L, Nordmann P. Ambler class A extended-spectrum beta-lactamases in *Pseudomonas aeruginosa*: novel developments and clinical impact. Antimicrob Agents Chemother 2003; 47: 2385-92.

[49] Toleman MA, Rolston K, Jones RN, *et al.* Molecular and biochemical characterization of OXA-45, an extended-spectrum class 2d beta-lactamase in *Pseudomonas aeruginosa*. Antimicrob Agents Chemother 2003; 47: 2859-63.

[50] Poirel L, Naas T, Guibert M, *et al.* Molecular and biochemical characterization of VEB-1, a novel class A extended-spectrum beta-lactamase encoded by an *Escherichia coli* integron gene. Antimicrob Agents Chemother 1999; 43: 573-81.

[51] Bonnet R, Sampaio JL, Chanal C, *et al.* A novel class A extended-spectrum beta-lactamase (BES-1) in *Serratia marcescens* isolated in Brazil. Antimicrob Agents Chemother 2000; 44: 3061-68.

[52] Mavroidi A, Tzelepi E, Tsakris A, *et al.* An integron-associated beta-lactamase (IBC-2) from *Pseudomonas aeruginosa* is a variant of the extended-spectrum beta-lactamase IBC-1. J Antimicrob Chemother 2001; 48: 627-30.

[53] Poirel L, Weldhagen GF, Naas T, *et al.* GES-2, a class A beta-lactamase from *Pseudomonas aeruginosa* with increased hydrolysis of imipenem. Antimicrob Agents Chemother 2001; 45: 2598-603.

[54] Silva J, Aguilar C, Ayala G, *et al.* TLA-1: a new plasmid-mediated extended spectrum beta-lactamase from *Escherichia coli.* Antimicrob Agents Chemother 2000; 44: 997-1003.

[55] Bellais S, Poirel L, Fortineau N, *et al.* Biochemical-genetic characterization of the chromosomally encoded extended-spectrum class A beta-lactamase from *Rahnella aquatilis.* Antimicrob Agents Chemother 2001; 45: 2965-68.

[56] Jiang X, Ni Y, Jiang Y, *et al.* Outbreak of infection caused by *Enterobacter cloacae* producing the novel VEB-3 beta-lactamase in China. J Clin Microbiol 2005; 43: 826-31.

[57] Poirel L, Rotimi VO, Mokaddas EM, *et al.* VEB-1-like extended-spectrum beta-lactamases in *Pseudomonas aeruginosa,* Kuwait. Emerg Infect Dis 2001; 7: 468-70.

[58] Castanheira M, Mendes RE, Walsh TR, *et al.* Emergence of the extended-spectrum beta-lactamase GES-1 in a *Pseudomonas aeruginosa* strain from Brazil: report from the SENTRY antimicrobial surveillance program. Antimicrob Agents Chemother 2004; 48: 2344-45.

[59] Vourli S, Giakkoupi P, Miriagou V, *et al.* Novel GES/IBC extended-spectrum beta-lactamase variants with carbapenemase activity in clinical enterobacteria. FEMS Microbiol Lett 2004; 234 : 209-13.

[60] Wachino J, Doi Y, Yamane K, *et al.* Nosocomial spread of ceftazidime-resistant *Klebsiella pneumoniae* strains producing a novel class a beta-lactamase, GES-3, in a neonatal intensive care unit in Japan. Antimicrob Agents Chemother 2004; 48: 1960-67.

[61] Weldhagen GF, Prinsloo A. Molecular detection of GES-2 extended spectrum beta-lactamase producing *Pseudomonas aeruginosa* in Pretoria, South Africa. Int. J Antimicrob Agents 2004; 24: 35-38.

[62] Alcantar-Curiel D, Tinoco JC, Gayosso C, *et al.* Nosocomial bacteremia and urinary tract infections caused by extended-spectrum beta-lactamase-producing *Klebsiella pneumoniae* with plasmids carrying both SHV-5 and TLA-1 genes. Clin Infect Dis 2004; 38: 1067-74.

[63] Matsumoto Y, Inoue M. Characterization of SFO-1, a plasmid-mediated inducible class A beta-lactamase from *Enterobacter cloacae.* Antimicrob Agents Chemother 1999; 43: 307-13.

[64] Lebessi E, Stamos G, Foustoukou M, *et al.* Performance of methods for detection of extended spectrum beta-lactamases applied to clinical enterobacterial strains producing IBC-type beta-lactamases. J Clin Microbiol 2003; 41: 912.

[65] Vourli S, Tzouvelekis LS, Tzelepi E, *et al.* Characterization of In111, a class 1 integron that carries the extended-spectrum beta-lactamase gene blaIBC-1. FEMS Microbiol Lett 2003; 225: 149-53.

[66] Galani I, Souli M, Chryssouli Z, *et al.* First identification of an *Escherichia coli* clinical isolate producing both metallo-beta-lactamase VIM-2 and extended-spectrum beta-lactamase IBC-1. Clin Microbiol Infect 2004; 10: 757-60.

[67] Baraniak A, Sadowy E, Hryniewicz W, *et al.* Two different extended-spectrum beta-lactamases (ESBLs) in one of the first ESBL-producing *Salmonella* isolates in Poland. J Clin Microbiol 2002; 40: 1095-97.

[68] Poirel L, Gniadkowski M, Nordmann P. Biochemical analysis of the ceftazidime-hydrolysing extended-spectrum beta-lactamase CTXM-15 and of its structurally related beta-lactamase CTX-M-3. J Antimicrob Chemother 2002; 50: 1031-34.

[69] Sturenburg E, Kuhn A, Mack D, *et al.* A novel extended spectrum beta-lactamase CTX-M-23 with a P167T substitution in the active-site omega loop associated with ceftazidime resistance. J Antimicrob Chemother 2004; 54: 406-09.

[70] Tzouvelekis LS, Tzelepi E, Tassios PT, *et al.* CTX-M-type beta-lactamases: an emerging group of extended-spectrum enzymes. Int. J Antimicrob Agents 2000; 14: 137-42.

[71] Yu WL, Pfaller MA, Winokur PL, *et al.* Cefepime MIC as a predictor of the extended-spectrum beta-lactamase type in *Klebsiella pneumoniae,* Taiwan. Emerg. Infect Dis 2002; 8 : 522-24.

[72] Bradford PA, Yang Y, Sahm D, *et al.* CTX-M-5, a novel cefotaxime-hydrolyzing b-lactamase from an outbreak of *Salmonella typhimurium* in Latvia. Antimicrob Agents Chemother 1998; 42: 1890-94.

[73] Ma L, Ishii Y, Ishiguro M, *et al.* Cloning and sequencing of the gene encoding Toho-2, a class A b-lactamase preferentially inhibited by tazobactam. Antimicrob Agents Chemother 1998; 42: 1181-86.

[74] Khalaf NG, Eletreby MM, Hanson ND. Characterization of CTX-M ESBLs in *Enterobacter cloacae, Escherichia coli and Klebsiella pneumoniae* clinical isolates from Cairo, Egypt. BMC Infect Dis 2009; 9: 84.

[75] Park YJ, Kim SY, Yu JK, *et al.* Spread of *Serratia marcescens* coharboring aac(6')-Ib-cr, bla CTX-M, armA, and bla OXA-1 carried by conjugative IncL/M type plasmid in Korean hospitals. Microb Drug Resist 2009; 15: 97-102.

[76] Rodríguez I, Barownick W, Helmuth R, *et al.* Extended-spectrum {beta}-lactamases and AmpC {beta}-lactamases in ceftiofur-resistant *Salmonella enterica* isolates from food and livestock obtained in Germany during 2003-07. J Antimicrob Chemother 2009; 64(2): 301-09.

[77]   Pitout JD, Church DL, Gregson DB, *et al.* Molecular epidemiology of CTX-M-producing *Escherichia coli* in the Calgary Health Region:emergence of CTX-M-15-producing isolates. Antimicrob Agents Chemother 2007; 51, 1281-1286.

[78]   Pitout JD, Nordmann P, Laupland KB, *et al.* Emergence of Enterobacteriaceae producing extended-spectrum beta-lactamases (ESBLs) in the community. J Antimicrob Chemother 2005; 56: 52-59.

[79]   Ho PL, Poon WW, Loke SL, *et al.* Community emergence of CTX-M type extended-spectrum {beta}-lactamases among urinary *Escherichia coli* from women. J Antimicrob Chemother 2007; 60: 140-44.

[80]   Minarini LA, Gales AC, Palazzo IC, *et al.* Prevalence of Community-Occurring Extended Spectrum beta-Lactamase-Producing Enterobacteriaceae in Brazil. Curr Microbiol 2007; 54: 335-41.

[81]   Pallecchi L, Bartoloni A, Fiorelli C, *et al.* Rapid Dissemination and Diversity of CTX-M Extended-Spectrum {beta}-Lactamase Genes in Commensal Escherichia coli from Healthy Children from Low-Resource Settings of Latin America. Antimicrob Agents Chemother 2007; 51(8): 2720-25.

[82]   Wiener J, Quinn JP, Bradfordm PA, *et al.* Multiple antibiotic resistant *Klebsiella* and *Escherichia coli* in nursing homes. JAMA 1999; 281: 517-23.

[83]   Arpin C, Dubois V, Maugein J, *et al.* Clinical and molecular analysis of extended-spectrum {beta}-lactamase-producing enterobacteria in the community setting. J Clin Microbiol 2005; 43: 5048-5054.

[84]   Calbo E, Romani V, Xercavins M, *et al.* Risk factors for community-onset urinary tract infections due to *Escherichia coli* harbouring extended-spectrum beta lactamases. J Antimicrob Chemother 2006; 57: 780-83.

[85]   Colodner R, Rock W, Chazan B, *et al.* Risk factors for the development of extended-spectrum beta-lactamase-producing bacteria in non hospitalized patients. Eur J Clin Microbiol Infect Dis 2004; 23: 163-67.

[86]   Ben-Ami R, Schwaber MJ, Navon-Venezia S, *et al.* Influx of extended-spectrum beta-lactamase-producing enterobacteriaceae into the hospital. Clin Infect Dis 2006; 42: 925-34.

[87]   Duan R S, Sit TH, Wong SS, *et al. Escherichia coli* producing CTX-M beta-lactamases in food animals in Hong Kong. Microb Drug Resist 2006; 12: 145-48.

[88]   Mesa RJ, Blanc V, Blanch AR, *et al.* Extended-spectrum beta-lactamase-producing Enterobacteriaceae in different environments (humans, food, animal farms and sewage). J Antimicrob Chemother 2006; 58: 211-15.

[89]   Meunier D, Jouy E, Lazizzera C, *et al.* CTX-M-1- and CTX-M-15-type betalactamases in clinical *Escherichia coli* isolates recovered from food-producing animals in France. Int. J Antimicrob Agents 2006; 28(5): 402-07.

[90]   D'Costa VM, McGrann KM, Hughes DW, *et al.* Sampling the antibiotic resistome. Science 2006; 311: 374-377.

[91]   Wright GD. The antibiotic resistome: the nexus of chemical and genetic diversity. Nat. Rev. Microbiol 2007; 5: 175-186.

[92]   Baraniak A, Fiett J, Hryniewicz W, *et al.* Ceftazidime-hydrolysing CTX-M-15 extended-spectrum beta-lactamase (ESBL) in Poland. J Antimicrob Chemother 2002; 50: 393-96.

[93]   Bauernfeind A, Stemplinger I, Jungwirth R, *et al.* Characterization of beta-lactamase gene *bla*PER-2, which encodes an extended-spectrum class A beta-lactamase. Antimicrob Agents Chemother 1996; 40: 616-20.

[94]   Gazouli M, Tzelepi E, Sidorenko SV, *et al.* Sequence of the gene encoding a plasmid-mediated cefotaxime-hydrolyzing class A β-lactamase (CTX-M-4): involvement of serine 237 in cephalosporin hydrolysis. Antimicrob Agents Chemother 1998; 42: 1259-62.

[95]   Shimamura T, Ibuka A, Fushinobu S, *et al.* Acyl-intermediate structures of the extended spectrum class A beta-lactamase, Toho-1, in complex with cefotaxime, cephalothin and benzylpenicillin J Biol Chem 2002; 277, 46601-08.

[96]   Ibuka A, Taguchi A, Ishiguro M, *et al.* Crystal structure of the E166A mutant of extended-spectrum β-lactamase Toho-1 at 1.8 A° resolution. J Mol Biol 1999; 285: 2079-87.

[97]   Cantu C, Huang W, Palzkill T. Selection and characterization of amino acid substitutions at residues 237-240 of TEM-1 β-lactamase with altered substrate specificity for aztreonam and ceftazidime. J Biol Chem 1996; 271: 22538-45.

[98]   Huletsky A, Knox JR, Levesque RC. Role of Ser-238 and Lys-240 in the hydrolysis of third-generation cephalosporins by SHV-type β-lactamases probed by site-directed mutagenesis and three-dimensional modeling. J Biol Chem 1993; 268: 3690-97.

[99]   Bonnet R, Dutour C, Sampaio JLM, *et al.* Novel cefotaximase (CTX-M-16) with increased catalytic efficiency due to substitution Asp240Gly. Antimicrob Agents Chemother 2001; 45: 2269-75.

[100]   Bonnet R, Recule C, Baraduc R, *et al.* Effect of D240G substitution in a novel ESBL CTX-M-27. J Antimicrob Chemother 2003; 52: 29-35.

[101] Clinical and Laboratory Standard Institute, Wayne, PA. CLSI document. Clinical and Laboratory Standard Methods. Performance standards for antimicrobial susceptibility testing: seventeenth informational supplement 2007; p. M100-S17.

102] Tenover FC, Mohammed MJ, Gorton TS, *et al.* Detection and reporting of organisms producing extended-spectrum β -lactamases: survey of laboratories in Connecticut. J Clin Microbiol 1999; 37, 4065-70.

[103] Carter MW, Oakton KJ, Warner M, *et al.* Detection of extended-spectrum beta-lactamases in klebsiellae with the Oxoid combination disk method. J Clin, Microbiol 2000; 38: 4228-32.

[104] Wiegand I, Geiss HK, Mack D, *et al.* Detection of extended-spectrum beta lactamases among Enterobacteriaceae by use of semiautomated microbiology systems and manual detection procedures. J Clin Microbiol 2007; 45: 1167-74.

[105] Tzelepi E, Giakkoup IP, Sofianou D, *et al.* Detection of extended spectrum beta-lactamases in clinical isolates of *Enterobacter cloacae* and *Enterobacter aerogenes.* J Clin Microbiol 2000; 38(2): 542-546.

[106] Sturenburg E, Sobottk AI, Noor D, *et al.* Evaluation of a new cefepimeclavulanate ESBL Etest to detect extended-spectrum beta-lactamases in an Enterobacteriaceae strain collection. J Antimicrob Chemother 2004; 54(1): 134-138.

[107] Hanson ND. AmpC beta-lactamases: what do we need to know for the future? J Antimicrob Chemother 2003; 52: 2-4

[108] Wong-Beringer A, Hindler J, Loeloff M, *et al.* Molecular correlation for the treatment outcomes in bloodstream infections caused by *Escherichia coli* and *Klebsiella pneumoniae* with reduced susceptibility to ceftazidime. Clin Infect Dis 15; 34(2): 135-46.

[109] Endimiani A, Luzzaro F, Brigante G, *et al. Proteus mirabilis* bloodstream infections: risk factors and treatment outcome related to the expression of extended-spectrum beta-lactamases. Antimicrob Agents Chemother 2005; 49, 2598-605.

[110] Tumbarello M, Spanu T, Sanguinetti M, *et al.* Bloodstream infections caused by extended-spectrum-beta-lactamase-producing *Klebsiella pneumoniae*: risk factors, molecular epidemiology, and clinical outcome. Antimicrob Agents Chemother 2006; 50: 498-504.

[111] Ho PL, Chan WM, Tsang KW, *et al.* Bacteremia caused by *Escherichia coli* producing extended-spectrum beta-lactamase: a case-control study of risk factors and outcomes. Scand. J Infect Dis 2002; 34: 567-573.

[112] Kim YK, Pai H, Lee HJ, *et al.* Bloodstream infections by extended-spectrum beta-lactamase-producing *Escherichia coli* and *Klebsiella pneumoniae* in children: epidemiology and clinical outcome. Antimicrob Agents Chemother 2002; 46: 1481-91.

[113] Marra AR, Wey SB, Castelo, A, *et al.* Nosocomial bloodstream infections caused by *Klebsiella pneumoniae*: impact of extended-spectrum beta-lactamase (ESBL) production on clinical outcome in a hospital with hight ESBL prevalence. BMC Infect Dis 2006; 6: 24.

[114] Paterson DL, Ko WC, Von Gottberg A, *et al.* Antibiotic therapy for *Klebsiella pneumonia* bacteremia: implications of production of extended-spectrum beta-lactamases. Clin Infect Dis 2004; 39: 31-37.

[115] Rodriguez-Bano J, Navarro MD, Romero L, *et al.* Bacteremia due to extended-spectrum beta -lactamase-producing *Escherichia coli* in the CTX-M era: a new clinical challenge. Clin Infect Dis 2006; 43: 1407-14.

[116] Karadenizli A, Mutlu B, Okay E, *et al.* Piperacillin with and without tazobactam against extended spectrum beta lactamase-producing *Pseudomonas aeruginosa* in a rat thigh abscess model. Chemotherapy 2001; 47: 292-96.

[117] Paterson D, Ko WC, Von Gottbert A, *et al.* Outcome of cephalosporin treatment for serious infections due to apparently susceptible organisms producing extended-spectrum beta-lactamases: implications for the clinical microbiology laboratory. J Clin Microbiol 2001; 39: 2206-12.

[118] Kotapati S, Kutty, JL, Nightingale CH, *et al.* Clinical implications of extended-spectrum beta lactamase (ESBL) producing *Klebsiella* species and *Escherichia coli* on cefepime effectiveness. J Infect 2005; 51: 211-17.

[119] LaBombardi VJ, Rojtman A, Tran K. Use of cefepime for the treatment of infections caused by extended spectrum beta-lactamases-producing *Klebsiella pneumoniae* and *Escherichia coli.* Diagn. Microbiol Infect Dis 2006; 56: 313-15.

[120] Zanetti G, Bally F, Greub G, *et al.* Cefepime *vs* imipenem-cilastatin for treatment of nosocomial pneumonia in intensive care unit patients: a multicenter, evaluatorblind, prospective, randomized study. Antimicrob Agents Chemother 2003; 47: 3442-47.

[121] Ambrose PG, Bhavnani SM, Jones RN. Pharmacokinetics-pharmacodynamics of cefepime and piperacillin-tazobactam against *Escherichia coli* and *Klebsiella pneumoniae* strains producing extended-spectrum beta-lactamases: report from the ARREST program. Antimicrob Agents Chemother 2003; 47, 1643-46.

[122] Hirakata Y, MatsudaJ, Miyazaki Y, *et al.* Regional variation in the prevalence of extended-spectrum beta-lactamaseproducing clinical isolates in the Asia-Pacific region (SENTRY 1998-2002). Diagn. Microbiol Infect Dis 2005. 52: 323-29.

[123] Paterson DL, Mulazimoglu L, Casellas JM, *et al.* Epidemiology of ciprofloxacin resistance and its relationship to extended-spectrum beta-lactamase production in *Klebsiella pneumoniae* isolates causing bacteremia. Clin Infect Dis 2000; 30: 473-78.

[124] Dartois N, Gioud-Paquet M, Ellis-Grosse EJ, *et al.* Tigecycline *vs* imipenem/cilastatin for treatment of complicated intra-abdominal infections. In: Programs and Abstracts of the Forty-fourth Interscience Conference on Antimicrobial Agents and Chemotherapy, Washington, DC 2004. Abstract LB-992c, pp. 12. American Society for Microbiology, Washington, DC, USA.

[125] Oliva ME, Rekha, A, Yellin A, *et al.* A multicenter trial of the efficacy and safety of tigecycline *vs* imipenem/cilastatin in patients with complicated intra-abdominal infections. BMC Infect Dis 2005; 5: 88.

[126] Hope R, Warner M, Potz NA, *et al.* Activity of tigecycline against ESBL-producing and AmpC-hyperproducing Enterobacteriaceae from south-east England. J Antimicrob Chemother 2006; 58: 1312-14.

[127] Sader HS, HsiungA, Fritsche TR *et al.* Comparative activities of cefepime and piperacillin/tazobactam tested against a global collection of *Escherichia coli* and *Klebsiella* spp. with an ESBL phenotype. Diagn Microbiol Infect Dis 2007; 57: 341-44.

[128] Wong-Beringer, A. Therapeutic challenges associated with extended-spectrum, beta-lactamase producing *Escherichia coli* and *Klebsiella pneumoniae*. Pharmacotherapy 2001; 21: 583-92.

[129] Bhavnani SM, Ambrose PG, Craig WA, *et al.* Outcomes evaluation of patients with ESBL- and non-ESBL-producing *Escherichia coli* and *Klebsiella* species as defined by CLSI reference methods: report from the SENTRY Antimicrobial Surveillance Program. Diagn Microbiol Infect Dis 2006; 54: 231-36.

CHAPTER 8

Methicillin Resistant *Staphylococcus aureus* (MRSA)

Esperanza C. Cabrera[*]

De La Salle University-Manila Philippines

Abstract: *Staphylococcus aureus* has been recognized as an extremely successful hospital pathogen that has established itself firmly in the community as well. In addition to its compendium of virulence factors, it has the immense propensity to develop resistance to antimicrobials belonging to different classes. The emergence of methicillin resistant *S. aureus* (MRSA) that carries transferable multiple antibiotic resistance to the class of β-lactams alone or to other antimicrobials as well, is a serious public health concern. The development of community-associated MRSA (CA-MRSA) from a genetic lineage different from that of hospital-associated MRSA (HA-MRSA) was unexpected, as was the observation that different strains of CA-MRSA from different parts of the world co-evolved simultaneously. Considering these observations with the virulence of the organism, and the transferable nature of the methicillin resistance genetic element, it is not surprising that MRSA is regarded as a pathogen that warrants utmost attention of the medical and scientific community. The need for urgent measures for its control cannot be overemphasized.

Keywords: MRSA, CA-MRSA, MDR, S. *aureus*, community acquired infection, hospital settings, nosocomil, β-lactams.

INTRODUCTION

Staphylococcus aureus is a facultatively anaerobic, heterotrophic, mesophilic gram-positive coccus that occurs in clusters. It is found as a normal flora in the nasal cavity of 30% of healthy individuals, and colonization is associated with a greater risk of infection with the same strain [1]. Most *S. aureus* strains are opportunistic pathogens that can cause diseases when the immune system becomes compromised. It is said to be one of the most successful and adaptable human pathogens [2], being responsible for a wide array of diseases that range from minor skin and soft tissue infections to systemic diseases such as pneumonia, sepsis, urinary tract infections, osteomyelitis, endocarditis, septic arthritis among others. The antimicrobials of choice for the treatment of staphylococcal infections include the β-lactam antibiotics, called such because of the presence of the β-lactam ring. These include the penicillins, cephalosporins, cephamycins, monobactams, cephems and carbapenems. However, resistance to this group developed significantly through the years.

Benzylpenicillin was the first introduced for clinical use in the 1940s. Clinical strains resistant to the antibiotic rose from less than 1 % in the pre-antibiotic era to approximately 80% [3], such that penicillin has ceased to be a useful therapeutic agent against staphylococcal infections. Strains resistant to penicillin G were found in 68% of the *S. aureus* isolated from outpatients who sought consult for various reasons, including but not restricted to infections [4]. In another study, as much as 97% of *S. aureus* recovered as normal flora of healthy volunteers were found to be resistant to penicillin [5]. The most common resistance mechanism to penicillin is inactivation by penicillinases [3]. These are coded by plasmid-borne *blaZ* gene that is transferred horizontally by bacteriophages, contributing to the rapid dissemination of resistance.

Methicillin, originally called celbenin [6], is a penicillinase-resistant semisynthetic penicillin that was first introduced for clinical use in Europe from 1959-1960. The first European isolate of Methicillin Resistant *S. aureus* (MRSA) was reported in 1961 [7]. It became a serious threat in the 1980s when the epidemic clones of MRSA acquired multidrug resistant traits [8] and spread worldwide to become one of the most important causative agents of hospital acquired infections [3, 8].

---

*Address correspondence to Esperanza C. Cabrera: De La Salle University-Manila Philippines; Tel & Fax: 632 536-0228; Email: esperanza.cabrera@dlsu.edu.ph

Asad U. Khan and Raffaele Zarrilli (Eds)

Surveillance studies show an increase in the incidence of MRSA infections in hospitals and community through the years in various parts of the world. A rapid emergence of nosocomial MRSA infection from 26.3% in 1986 to 77% in 2001 was established in a national university hospital in Taiwan [9]. Data from The Surveillance Network (TSN), composed of antimicrobial susceptibility test results gathered from 300 USA hospitals distributed across laboratories in North America, showed a steady increase in the overall MRSA rates from 38% in 1998 to 53.3% in March, 2005 [10]. Most of the countries in the Mediterranean region are also reported to be experiencing a surge in MRSA infections [11]. Susceptibility test results of more than 5000 invasive blood culture *S. aureus* isolates from 62 hospitals situated in Algeria, Cyprus, Egypt, Jordan, Lebanon, Malta, Morocco, Tunisia and Turkey collected from 2003 to 2005 by the ARMed project showed the median MRSA proportion was 39% (interquartile range: 27.1% to 51.1%). The highest proportions of MRSA were reported by Jordan, Egypt and Cyprus, where more than 50% of the invasive isolates were methicillin-resistant. It was noted that there was considerable variation in the proportion of MRSA in hospitals within the same country.

MECHANISM OF METHICILLIN RESISTANCE

Staphylococcus aureus has four penicillin binding proteins (PBP1, 2, 3, 4), which are involved in the synthesis of the cross-linked peptidoglycan of the bacterial cell wall. Methicillin resistance is due to the production of an altered 78kDa penicillin binding protein [12] called PBP2a or PBP2'. The altered PBP2a has decreased affinity for all beta-lactam antibiotics, resulting to multiple resistances that are not confined to methicillin alone. This low affinity of PBP2A for beta-lactams allows it to act as a transpeptidase, that together with the transglycosidase domain of the native PBP2, takes over the function of cell wall synthesis even in the presence of beta-lactam antibiotics in the environment [6].

GENETIC BASIS OF METHICILLIN RESISTANCE

The Staphylococcal Cassette Chromosome Mec

The Staphylococcal Cassette Chromosome Mec (SCC*mec*) is a 21 to 66 kb mobile genetic element comprised of the *mecA* gene, site-specific recombinase genes, regulatory genes, insertion sequence elements, terminal inverted and direct repeats, and the J regions (junkyard or joining regions). The 2.1 kb *mecA* gene encodes for the PBP2a, which is responsible for resistance to methicillin. MRSA is produced when Methicillin-Susceptible *S. aureus* (MSSA) acquires the SCC*mec*. SCC*mec* elements are the only vectors that have been identified for the *mecA* gene [13]. These mobile elements may serve to move the *mecA* gene across staphylococcal species, since *mecA* genes in other staphylococcal species have never been found in the absence of SCC*mec*-like structure [14]. However, the mechanism of transfer of SCC elements between different staphylococcal species has not been identified [13].

The *mecA* gene is considered to have originated from an evolutionary relative of the *mecA* homologue identified in *Staphylococcus sciuri*, which may perform a normal physiological function in this bacterium unrelated to β-lactam resistance [15]. Similar to the *mecA* of MRSA, the *mecA* homologue of *S. sciuri* is composed of a putative transglycosylase and a transpeptidase domain, with the latter showing all the conserved motifs typical of the active sites of the penicillin binding domain of transpeptidases. The site-specific recombinase genes of SCC*mec* belong to the invertase/resolvase family. These are designated *ccrA*, *ccr B* [16] and *ccrC* [17]. These catalyze the precise excision of the SCC*mec* from the MRSA chromosome, and site-specific as well as orientation-specific integration of the SCC*mec* into the *S. aureus* chromosome. SCC*mec* is integrated into the chromosome at a site-specific location (*attBscc*), located near the origin of replication [18]. The *attBSCC* is found downstream of an open reading frame of unknown function (*orfX*), that is well conserved among clinical strains of *S. aureus* [14]. The terminal inverted and direct repeats of SCC*mec* may be recognized by SCC*mec* specific recombinases during the integration and excision of SCC*mec* to and from the chromosome [19].

SCC*mec* also contains the regulatory genes *mecI-mecR1* and an insertion sequence element IS*431mec* or IS*1272*. [2, 20]. *mecR1* encodes the signal transducer protein MecR1, while *mecI* encodes the repressor protein MecI. The insertion sequence element IS431*mec* allows the acquisition of genes coding for resistance to non beta-lactam antibiotics, *e.g.* erythromycin, gentamicin, tetracycline and ciprofloxacin, converting MRSA to resistance to different classes of antimicrobials, in addition to its resistance to all beta-lactams. The J regions J1, J2, and J3 are located upstream, downstream and between the *mec* and *ccr* gene complexes. These may contain various genes or pseudogenes, which may include plasmid-mediated or transposon-mediated resistance genes for non-beta-lactam antibiotics or heavy metals.

SCC*mec* Types

The identification of the structural types of the SCC*mec* is an important component of molecular typing techniques to study the epidemiology of MRSA and evolutionary relationships among MRSA clones [21, 22]. For example, the composition of the SCC*mec* types has provided strong evidence for the independent derivation of hospital-acquired MRSA (HA-MRSA) and community-acquired MRSA (C-MRSA) clone [23]. In addition, the new nomenclature scheme for MRSA set by the International Union of Microbiology Societies includes the SCC*mec* type and multilocus sequence type [24]. A combination of Multilocus Sequence Type (MLST) and SCC*mec* type is frequently used as an identifier for MRSA.

SCC*mec* types are classified according to the combination of their *mecA* gene complex and the nature of the *ccr* allele. Each SCC*mec* type is further classified into subtypes on the basis of the J-region sequence [19]. The *mecA* gene complex is comprised of the *mecA* gene with the upstream *mecI-mecR1* regulatory region, IS*431* and/or IS*1272*. Four classes of the *mec* gene complex have been identified and are structured as follows: Class A, *mecI-mecR1-mecA*-IS*431*; Class B, Δ*mecR1-mecA*-IS*431*; Class C, IS*431*-Δ*mecR1-mecA*-IS*431*; and class D, IS*431-mecA*-Δ*mecR1* [25].

Based on the composition of the *mecA* gene complex and the *ccr* allele, six types of SCC*mec* have been established, with two additional types that were recently proposed [20]. The SCC*mec* type is usually designated with roman numeral designations, *e.g.* Type I, Type II. An SCC*mec* element can also be described by *ccr* type (indicated by a number and *mec* class indicated by an uppercase letter, *e.g.* Type 1B, Type 2A [26]. SCC*mec* Types I to III were classified by Ito *et al.* [14] and were numbered in the order of the year of isolation of the strains analyzed in their study. SCC*mec* Type I or Type 1B (34 kb), identified in the first MRSA strain isolated in 1961 in the United Kingdom, is composed of Class B *mec* gene complex and *ccrAB1*. SCC*mec* Type II or Type 2A (52 kb) was identified in an MRSA strain isolated in 1982 in Japan. It is comprised of Class A *mec* gene complex and Type *ccrAB2*. SCC*mec* Type III or type 3A (66 kb) was identified in an MRSA strain isolated in 1985 in New Zealand. It carries Class A *mec* gene complex and *ccrAB3*.

Type IV or Type 2B (20 to 24 kb) was first described in two community-acquired MRSA (CA-MRSA), and is comprised of Class B *mec* gene complex and *ccrAB2* [27]. SCC*mec* Type V or Type 5C2 (28kb) was characterized by Ito *et al.* [17] in a CA-MRSA isolated in Australia. This type has Class C2 *mec* gene complex and *ccrC* (or Type 5) recombinase. Similar to Type IV, it does not carry any antibiotic resistance genes besides *mecA*. Type VI or Type 4B carries Class B *mec* complex and *ccrAB4* [28]. This is a reclassification of strains formerly identified to have Type IV SCC*mec* based on the difference in the *ccr* allele. The proposed Type VII or Type 5C1 SCC*mec* (27 bp) identified in a Swedish MRSA strain, carries class C1 *mec* gene complex and *ccr* C gene complex [29]. *mecA* is the only resistance gene it carries. Type VIII or Type 4A SCC*mec* (32 kb) is composed of Class A *mec* and *ccrAB4*. It was identified in a Canadian epidemic, hospital-acquired strain of MRSA [20]. This newly described type was shown to be derived from the homologous recombination of two SCC*mec* elements from two different strains of *Staphylococcus epidermidis*, supporting the ability of SCC elements to transfer horizontally or undergo recombination to generate new SCC*mec* types.

SCC*mec* types I, II and III have commonly been identified in Hospital-Acquired MRSA (HA-MRSA), whereas types IV and V are associated with CA-MRSA. Types II and III carry both integrated plasmid sequences and transposons containing drug resistance genes that confer multiple resistances [30]. These multiple resistance genes may be suited for the survival of HA-MRSA in the presence of the selective pressure provided by the extensive use of antimicrobials in the hospital environment. On the other hand, the cost on fitness imposed by the burden of these additional antibiotic resistance genes on the micoorganisms may have restricted their spread in the community where there is less use of antibiotics for positive selection [31].

Types IV and V usually exclusively encode resistance to B-lactam antibiotics. SCC*mec* types IV and V function mainly for the transfer of the element (through the *ccr* genes) and methicillin resistance (through the *mecA* gene). The lack of nonessential functions and their small sizes (20-24 kb and 28 kb respectively) provide a lower cost for fitness that allows their acquisition and retention as mobile genetic elements for *S. aureus* in the community than any other type of SCC*mec* [17, 27, 31]. The extreme heterogeneity of the chromosome genotypes in CA-MRSA strains with Type IV suggests that this type is highly transmissible [17].

SCC*mec* Typing

Different assays have been developed for SCC*mec* typing. These include full sequence analysis of the SCC*mec* element [14, 17, 32], and PCR-restriction fragment length polymorphism assay for the *ccrB* gene [33]. Oliveira and de Lencastre [21] developed a multiplex PCR assay that classifies SCC*mec* into types I to IV based on eight loci (A to H) in the J-region located upstream and downstream of the *mecA* gene. It does not take into account the specific *ccr* gene complex. This method has been updated to better characterize SCC*mec* type IV and to include the detection of SCC*mec* type V [34]. Another multiplex PCR classifies the SCC*mec* by identifying the *ccr* gene complex, the *mec* gene complex and specific structures in the junkyard (J) regions [22]. However, there is currently no standardized SCC*mec* typing method that systematically and efficiently utilizes all known variations [35].

COMMUNITY-ASSOCIATED MRSA (CA-MRSA) AND HOSPITAL-ACQUIRED OR HEALTHCARE-ASSOCIATED MRSA (HA-MRSA)

MRSA is predominantly a nosocomial pathogen [36]. However, community-acquired or community-associated MRSA (CA-MRSA) strains have been reported in increasing frequency in the past decades [37, 38]. CA-MRSA was first described in the 1990s in persons without previous healthcare exposure. Patients infected with CA-MRSA are usually young individuals with no underlying health problems, and who lack the traditional risk factors such as recent admittance, surgery or long-term confinement in healthcare facilities [39]. Outbreaks of diseases caused by CA-MRSA have been reported among jail inmates [40-43], injection drug users [44], military personnel [45], men who have sex with men [43] and those in contact sports [46] among others.

Although the spread of MRSA from the hospital to the community was not surprising, the emergence of novel strains of CA-MRSA that are distinct from those associated with healthcare facilities was not expected [38]. The genetic background of CA-MRSA strains were shown not to correspond to those of the HA-MRSA strains from within the same continent, suggesting that CA-MRSA strains have a different genetic lineage, and thus did not emerge from local HA-MRSA [47-49]. In addition, evidences show that different CA-MRSA strains from different parts of the world co-evolved simultaneously, and were not the results of dissemination of a single clone [23, 47, 48].

A database of Pulsed-Field Gel Electrophoresis (PFGE)-generated patterns of *Sma*I-digested genomic DNA of MRSA has been established and used for genotyping MRSA strains into USA types. The USA types have been validated using multilocus sequence typing (MLST or ST) and *spa* typing [50]. Presently, five CA-MRSA lineages have been reported worldwide. These are ST1-IV (USA400); ST8-IV (USA300); ST30-IV (Pacific/Oceania); ST59-IV and V (USA1000, Taiwan) and ST80-IV (European) [48].

USA300 is the most commonly isolated CA-MRSA strain in the United States, Canada and in nine European countries [as reviewed in 51]. It has been implicated in unusually severe human diseases such as endocarditis, necrotizing fasciitis, sepsis and pneumonia. The introduction of USA300 into a new geographic area has often been associated with the displacement of locally endemic CA-MRSA strains belonging to ST1, ST30, ST59 and ST80 clonal lineages.

CA-MRSA strains generally belong to SCC*mec* type IV, and to a lesser extent, to type V [17, 47], and carry the *lukf-luks* Panton Valentine Leukocidin (PVL) genes, in contrast to HA-MRSA. In addition, they are generally susceptible to most antimicrobials that do not belong to the beta-lactam group, and are reported to grow much faster than HA-MRSA [39]. The diseases they cause range from skin and soft tissue infections to serious and even fatal infectious such as necrotizing pneumonia, necrotizing fasciitis, bloodstream infection, septic arthritis, and septic shock.

Despite the clinical and genotypic differences seen between CA-MRSA and HA-MRSA, there is still no clear definition of CA-MRSA [48, 49]. The characteristics described above can also be found in some HA-MRSA, or may be absent in CA-MRSA strains. A large proportion (80%) of HA-MRSA isolates studied in Ireland did not have the multiple resistant genotype and belonged to ST22-MRSA-IV, while PVL was found only in a small proportion of CA-MRSA studied [52]. EMRSA-15 (ST22), which is one of the five large traditional HA-MRSA lineages, carries SCC*mec* IV [48]. MRSA carriage can be acquired in the community and carried as a normal flora for a prolonged period of time before causing infection in the hospital, and is thus classified as nosocomial. On the other hand, colonization with HA-MRSA of the patient may go undetected, and eventually cause infection months after discharge into the community, and thus be classified as CA-MRSA infection [2].

Recently, CA-MRSA strains have been reported to be the cause of nosocomial infections [48-55]. This presents significant nosocomial risks that infection control personnel should address. CA-MRSA may acquire multiple antibiotic resistances in a hospital setting and become phenotypically similar to HA-MRSA. Compounding this are the higher mobility of SCC*mec* type IV that most CA-MRSA strains carry, which allows its horizontal transfer to other susceptible strains thereby converting them to resistance; and their high propensity to cause diseases even in otherwise healthy individuals such as hospital personnel, and in hospitalized patients as well.

VIRULENCE FACTORS OF CA-MRSA

Certain strains of CA-MRSA are reported to be more virulent than HA-MRSA [36]. The whole genome sequence of MW2, a typical community-acquired strain of MRSA isolated in 1998 in North Dakota, shows 19 additional virulence genes when compared to the genomes of five HA-MRSA strains [39]. These include the *lukSPV-lukF PV* (PVL or Panton-Valentine leukocidin), *bsa* (bacteriocin of *S. aureus*), *seh* (staphylococcal enterotoxin H, an extremely potent superantigen, which is involved in acute toxic-shock-like syndrome), several other enterotoxin genes *sec4, seg2, sek2, sel2* among others. However, it was not identified which among these was the most important in the pathogenesis of the organism. Conflicting results of studies involving PVL as a virulence factor (see below) demonstrates this complexity. The total pathogenic potential may be a result of the combined effect of the different factors.

The cytolytic toxins α hemolysin (or α toxin), and phenol soluble modulins have also been implicated in the virulence of CA-MRSA [reviewed in 36]. α hemolysin, similar to PVL is a pore-forming toxin, and has been shown to lyse host cells, excluding neutrophils of the leuokocytes. Phenol soluble modulins are α helical peptides that lyse host cells including neutrophils. The genes for these toxins are in the chromosome of both CA-MRSA and HA-MRSA. Thus, the difference in the virulence of these two strains that is attributed to these toxins may be caused by a difference in the gene expression. The gene regulatory network for these virulence genes is not well elucidated.

The Arginine Catabolic Mobile Element (ACME) was likewise found to be involved in the virulence, enhanced growth, survival, and dissemination of the widely-distributed CA-MRSA USA300 strain [31]. It enhances the hematogenous dissemination of the organism to target organs, and is found in most pathogenic strains of *S. aureus* studied. ACME contains two gene clusters that are homologues of genetic elements that have been implicated in pathogenesis. These are the *arc,* which encodes the arginine deiminase pathway, and *opp3,* which encodes an oligopeptide permease system. The proximity of ACME to SCC*mec* Type IV and its mobilization by the same *ccrAB* allows the co-acquisition and integration of these two elements into the chromosome. Thus, ACME enhances virulence, while SCC*mec* protects the

MRSA from the action of β-lactams, enhancing further dissemination of USA300 in the presence of antibiotic use.

The Panton Valentine Leukocidin (PVL) toxin has been found to be a stable genetic marker of CA-MRSA [47], although it was not detected in most of the CA-MRSA strains in some studies [52, 56]. The PVL gene is comprised of two co-transcribed open reading frames, *lukS-PV* and *lukF-PV*, coding for the class S and the class F components, respectively [57] and is carried by a mobile bacteriophage. PVL belongs to the pore forming toxin family. It causes lysis of human neutrophils, monocytes and macrophages. PVL has been shown to induce polymorphonuclear cell death by necrosis or apoptosis *in vitro*, depending on its concentration [58]. It creates pores in the outer mitochondrial membrane, resulting in the release of apoptogenic proteins cytochrome c and Smac/DIABLO that leads to apoptosis. PVL is directly involved in the pathophysiology of necrotizing pneumonia as evidenced by the presence of the LukS-PVL component in lung secretions of patients with this disease together with DNA fragmentation [58]. The presence of the PVL gene was shown to increase the risk of death 1.56-fold in patients with hospital-acquired pneumonia caused by MRSA [59], although hemorrhagic and necrotizing peneumonia were not shown in this group of patients.

Results of other studies however, do not show a significant role of the PVL in the pathogenicity of CA-MRSA. PVL-negative strains (*lukS/F-PV* knockout) of USA 300 and USA400 were as virulent as the wild-type strains in mouse sepsis and abscess models, and caused comparable skin diseases [60]. Lysis of human neutrophils and pathogen survival after phagocytosis were likewise similar in both strains. Another study showed that USA400 with and without PVL genes produced similar clinical characteristics [61]. More studies need to be conducted to define the role of PVL in disease causation, and to determine the discrepancy in the results of the different studies.

LABORATORY DIAGNOSIS OF METHICILLIN RESISTANCE

Methicillin-Resistant *S. aureus* (MRSA) has been defined as *S. aureus* having the *mecA* gene or showing a minimum inhibitory concentration (MIC) of oxacillin ≥4 mg/L [62]. Standard methods for the phenotypic determination of resistance to methicillin (or oxacillin in actual practice) include the screening procedure using solid culture medium supplemented with 4% NaCl and 6mg/L oxacillin, disc diffusion assay using oxacillin and cefoxitin discs, Minimum Inhibitory Concentration (MIC) determination using broth dilution, agar dilution methods or E test. PBP2A can be detected using latex agglutination test. Assays for *mecA* gene and PBP2A detection are the most accurate methods for the prediction of resistance to oxacillin [62]. It is recommended that clinical cases due to MRSA strains should not be treated with β-lactams, including β-lactam/ β-lactamase inhibitor combinations and cephems (with the exception of the newer "cephalosporins and anti-MRSA activity") due to possible treatment failure [62].

HETEROGENOUSLY RESISTANT MRSA

MRSA may be homogenously resistant or heterogeneously resistant. While both groups are positive for the *mecA* gene and express the 78-kDa PBP 2A, the latter exhibits the presence of the resistance at low frequency of 10^{-2} to 10^{-8} [63] or 10^{-4} to 10^{-7} [12] within a single population. The majority of cells within the strain show low level of resistance, while a minor subpopulation demonstrates resistance to higher concentrations of methicillin. However, heteroresistant MRSA should be considered as fully resistant when prescribing treatment, since it may evolve into fully resistant strains, and be positively selected in patients receiving β-lactam antibiotics. The level of resistance does not correlate with the amount of the PBP2a in the cell wall and the proportion of cells that express higher resistance levels is strain dependent.

The low-level methicillin resistance in MRSA can be due to the repression of the *mecA* gene by the *mecA*-associated negative regulatory element *mecI-mecR1* [3]. Deletions or mutations in *mecI* or the promoter region of *mecA* result in constitutive expression rather than variable expression of *mec*. However, the mechanisms and genes that are responsible for the change in expression from low level resistance to the different higher resistance levels are as yet unknown [64]. The conversion might be due to chromosomal mutation(s) that are not related to *mecA* [65].

Incubation at a lower temperature of 30°C, or an increase in osmolarity, such as the addition of NaCl or sucrose, or passage in beta-lactam antibiotic-containing medium has been found to increase the proportion of resistant cells [66]. These changes are phenotypic, *i.e.* heterogeneous strains that appear homogeneous and highly resistant at 30°C resume a heterogeneous pattern when the culture conditions are changed to 37°C [67].

OXACILLIN SUSCEPTIBLE MRSA (OS-MRSA)

Strains of *S. aureus* with *mecA* gene but are oxacillin susceptible (oxacillin MIC ≤2 mg/L) are increasingly reported [68]. These strains are called OS-MRSA. Petinaki *et al.* [69] gave the first report of the emergence of OS-MRSA clones in the clinical setting in Greece during 2001. The strains were *mecA* gene and PBP2a positive, but were susceptible to oxacillin. Most (80%) of the isolates were also resistant to tetracycline, fusidic acid and kanamycin The study of Hososaka *et al.* [70] found six strains of OS-MRSA out of 480 strains of *S. aureus* collected from 11 hospitals in different locations in Japan isolated from 2003 through 2005. The six strains were SCC*mec*-positive, but were susceptible to oxacillin and to seven other beta-lactam antibiotics tested.

In a study on the mechanism of OS-MRSA responsiveness to oxacillin, several mutations were detected in all *fem* genes of the OS-MRSA isolates studied that led to amino acid substitutions in the FemXAB protein [68]. The Fem (factors essential for the expression of methicillin resistance) proteins are chromosomally encoded factors involved in pentaglycine side chain formation of the peptidoglycan, and are essential for the expression of methicillin resistance [71]. Accumulation of amino acid changes in Fem proteins might affect intact cell wall synthesis without affecting the viability of the organism, but contributing to the atypical oxacillin susceptibility [68]. Insertional inactivation of *femA* or *femB* by TnS51 has been shown to increase the susceptibility of methicillin susceptible and methicillin resistant *S. aureus* strains to beta-lactams [64].

OS-MRSA may become a highly-resistant MRSA upon treatment of patients with beta-lactam antibiotics [70]. Hence, its correct identification is important for the management and control of diseases caused by this strain. It is imperative that OS-MRSA be differentiated from the fully **susceptible** MSSA.

BORDERLINE OXACILLIN-RESISTANT *STAPHYLOCOCCUS AUREUS* (BORSA)

Borderline oxacillin resistant *Staphylococcus aureus* exhibits low level resistance to oxacillin and methicillin due to the hyperproduction of beta-lactamase [72], and may mimic MRSA. The resistance is *mecA* independent, *i.e.*, BORSA does not have the *mecA* gene [73]. Differentiation between BORSA and MRSA is important for treatment of patients. Antimicrobials for infections caused by MRSA are restricted to the glycopeptides in general, while those caused by BORSA may be treated with the non-glycopeptide combination of beta-lactam and a beta-lactamase inhibitor. Another less commonly encountered mechanism that has been reported to result in borderline methicillin resistance in *S. aureus* is the overproduction of PBP4 [74]. Alterations of penicillin binding by PBPs 1, 2, and 4 in beta-lactamase-negatives, *mecA*-negative were also found in borderline clinical isolates. The changes in binding kinetics and PBP overexpression results in more enzymes that are free for cell wall synthesis in resistant than in susceptible cells when beta-lactam antibiotic is present.

ANTIMICROBIALS FOR TREATMENT OF MRSA

Incision and drainage remain the treatment of choice for cutaneous abscesses caused by *S. aureus*, irrespective of antibiotic susceptibility [36]. With respect to antimicrobials, the nontoxic and inexpensive β-lactam antibiotics are the usual empirical treatment for common skin and soft tissue infections. However, their use for both CA-MRSA and HA-MRSA infections is not recommended as this may result in treatment failure [62]. CA-MRSA strains are commonly, but not always susceptible to antimicrobials belonging to other classes such as sulfamethoxazole trimethoprim (cotrimoxazole), clindamycin, doxycycline, minocycline compared to HA-MRSA strains, which often carry genes for resistance to other classes of antimicrobials. Linezolid, the first oxazolidinone used for treatment of nosocomial MRSA pneumonia, has been shown to have high penetrability in the lung and to be highly effective for MRSA infections [75], although it's expensive cost and toxicity does not allow common usage when other antimicrobials can still be prescribed.

Vancomycin is the first-line parenteral antibiotic for severe CA-MRSA and HA-MRSA infections [36]. However, strains of *S. aureus* with reduced vancomycin susceptibility or SA-RVS (MIC $\geq$ 4ug/ml) have been reported [67, 76, 77]. These include the vancomycin intermediate *S. aureus* (VISA) and vancomycin resistant *S. aureus* (VRSA). In addition, vancomycin treatment failure rates have been reported that are associated with poor tissue penetration particularly in the lung, slow bacterial killing, and the potential for toxicity [78].

New treatment options for invasive infectious caused by MRSA with reduced susceptibility to vancomycin (MRSA-RSV) include linezolid, tigecycline, quinupristin/dalfopristin, and daptomycin, all of which have been approved for use by the US Food and Drug Administration (FDA). New anti-MRSA-RSV agents in development include novel glycopeptides dalbavancin, telavancin, and oritavancin, which are derivatives of vancomycin; and anti-MRSA β-lactams ceftobiprole and ceftaroline, both of which have high binding affinity for PBP2A [79]. These glycopeptide derivatives and β-lactams however, can only be administered parenterally. New treatment options that can be administered orally such as the oxazolidinone linezolid have to be explored.

CONCLUSION

Staphylococcus aureus has been associated with various hospital-associated and community-associated diseases that range from skin and soft tissue infections to life threatening, even fatal systemic diseases. The emergence of MRSA with transferable multiple drug resistance, compounded by the appearance of different clones of the more virulent CA-MRSA with a genetic lineage quite different from HA-MRSA, the establishment of CA-MRSA as nosocomial agents, and the development of additional resistance to anti-MRSA antimicrobials, have accumulated much concern and dread in the organism. However, despite the countless studies that have been done, much still have to be elucidated. These include the mechanisms of evolution of the different CA-MRSA strains, the mechanisms of transfer of the resistance genetic element to other organisms, their mechanisms of virulence, new treatment options for MRSA, especially orally-administered antimicrobials for strains that have become resistant to those that are identified for use against them, such as vancomycin, and the appropriate management of patients and non-patients who are carriers of MRSA as their normal flora. Frequent and regular monitoring of its prevalence/incidences in different settings in different parts of the world, and the concerted implementation of the proper preventive and curative measures are indispensable to control morbidity and mortality rates due to the organism especially in the light of man's current ease and frequency of global mobility. The collaborative efforts of the different scientific and health communities in the study of the diverse aspects of the organism are essential to the understanding and management of this organism.

REFERENCES

[1]   von Eiff C, Becker K, Machka K, *et al.* Nasal carriage as a source of Staphylococcus aureus bacteremia. N Engl J Med 2001; 344: 11-16.

[2]   Zetola N, Francis J, Nuernberger E, *et al.* Community-acquired methicillin resistant Staphylococcus aureus: an emerging threat. Lancet Inf Dis 2005; 5: 275-86.

[3]   Berger-Bachi B. Resistance mechanisms of gram-positive bacteria. Int J Med Microbiol 2002; 292: 27-35.

[4]   Lietzau S, Sturmer T, Erb A, *et al.* Prevalence and determinants of nasal colonization with antibiotic-resistant Staphylococcus aureus among unselected patients attending general practitioners in Germany. Epidemiol Infect 2004; 132: 655-62.

[5]   Sá-Leão R, Sanches IS, Couto I, *et al.* Low Prevalence of Methicillin-Resistant Strains among Staphylococcus aureus Colonizing Young and Healthy Members of the Community in Portugal. Microbial Drug Resistance 2001; 7: 237-45 as cited by Oliveira D, Tomasz A, de Lencastre H. Secrets of success of a human pathogen:

molecular evolution of pandemic clones of meticillin resistant Staphylococcus aureus. The Lancet Inf Dis 2002; 2: 180-89.

[6]   Oliveira DC, Tomasz A, de Lencastre H. Secrets of success of a human pathogen: molecular evolution of pandemic clones of meticillin resistant Staphylococcus aureus. The Lancet Inf Dis 2002; 2: 180-89.

[7]   Jevons MP. "Celbenin"-resistant staphylococci. British Med J 1961; 1: 124-45.

[8]   de Lencastre H, Oliveira D, Alexander TA. Antibiotic resistant Staphylococcus aureus: a paradigm of adaptive power. Current Opinion Microbiol 2007; 10: 428-35.

[9]   Hsueh PR, Teng LJ, Chen WH, *et al.* Increasing prevalence of methicillin-resistant Staphylococcus aureus causing nosocomial infections at a university hospital in Taiwan from 1986 to 2001. Antimicrob Agents and Chemother 2004; 48: 1361-64.

[10]   Styers D, Sheehan DJ, Hogan P, *et al.* Laboratory-based surveillance of current antimicrobial resistance patterns and trends among Staphylococcus aureus: 2005 status in the United States. Ann of Clin Microbiol Antimicrob 2006; 5: 2.

[11]   Borg MA, de Kraker M, Scicluna E, *et al.* Prevalence of methicillin-resistant Staphylococcus aureus (MRSA) in invasive isolates from southern and eastern Mediterranean countries. J Antimicrob Chemother 2007; Accessed online http://jac.oxfordjournals.org/cgi/reprint/dkm365v1 7687-92.

[12]   Georgopapadakou NH. Penicillin-binding proteins and bacterial resistance to beta-lactams. Antimicrob Agents Chemother 1993; 37: 2045-53.

[13]   Hanssen AM, Ericson JU. SCCmec in staphylococci: Genes on the move. FEMS Immuno. Med Microbiol 2005; 8-20.

[14]   Ito T, Katayama Y, Asada K, *et al.* Structural comparison of three types of staphylococcal cassette chromosome mec integrated in the chromosome in methicillin-resistant Staphylococcus aureus. Antimicrob Agents Chemother 2001; 45: 1323-36.

[15]   Wu S, PiscitelliI C, de Lencastre H, *et al.* Tracking the evolutionary origin of the methicillin resistance gene: Cloning and sequencing of a homologue of mecA from a methicillin susceptible strain of Staphylococcus sciuri Microb Drug Resist 1996; 2: 435-41.

[16]   Katayama Y, Ito T, Hiramatsu K. A new class of genetic element, Staphylococcus cassette chromosome mec, encodes methicillin resistance in Staphylococcus aureus. Antimicrob Agents Chemother 2000; 44: 1549-55.

[17]   Ito T, Ma XX, Takeuchi F, *et al.* Novel type staphylococcal cassette chromosome mec driven by a novel cassette chromosome recombinase, ccrC. Antimicrob Agents Chemother 2004; 48: 2637-51.

[18]   Kuroda M, Ohta T, Uchiyama I, *et al.* Whole genome sequencing of meticillin-resistant Staphylococcus aureus. Lancet 2001; 357: 1225-40.

[19]   Hiramatsu K, Katayama Y, Yuzawa H, *et al.* Molecular genetics of methicillin-resistant Staphylococcus aureus. Int J Med Microbiol 2002; 292: 67-74.

[20]   Zhang K, McClure J, Elsayed S, *et al.* Novel staphylococcal cassette chromosome mec type, tentatively designated type VIII, harboring class A mec and type 4 ccr gene complexes in a Canadian epidemic strain of methicillin-resistant Staphylococcus aureus. Antimicrob Agents Chemother 2009; 53: 531-40.

[21]   Oliveira D, de Lencastre H. Multiplex PCR strategy for rapid identification of structural types and variants of the mec element in methicillin-resistant Staphylococcus aureus. Antimicrob Agents Chemother 2002; 46: 2155-61.

[22]   Kondo Y, Ito T, Ma XX, *et al.* Combination of multiplex PCRs for staphylococcal cassette chromosome mec type assignment: Rapid identification system for mec, ccr, and major differences in junkyard regions. Antimicrob Agents Chemother 2007; 51: 264-74.

[23]   Okuma K, Iwakawa K, Turnidge J, *et al.* Dissemination of new methicillin resistant Staphylococcus aureus clones in the community. J Clin Microbiol 2002; 40: 4289-94.

[24]   Enright M, Robinson D, Randle G, *et al.* The evolutionary history of methicillin-resistant Staphylococcus aureus (MRSA). Proc Natl Acad Sci USA 2002; 99: 7687-92.

[25]   Katayama, Y, Ito T, Hiramatsu K. Genetic organization of the chromosome region surrounding mecA in clinical staphylococcal strains: role of IS431-mediated mecI deletion in expression of resistance in mecA-carrying, low-level methicillin-resistant Staphylococcus haemolyticus. Antimicrob Agents Chemother 2001; 45:1955-63. As cited by Ito T, Ma XX, Takeuchi F, Okuma K, Yuzawa H and Hiramatsu K. Novel type V staphylococcal cassette chromosome mec driven by a novel cassette chromosome recombinase, ccrC. Antimicrob Agents Chemother 2004; 48: 2637-51.

[26]   Chongtrakool P, Ito T, Ma X, *et al.* Staphylococcal cassette chromosome mec (SCCmec) typing of methicillin-resistant Staphylococcus aureus strains isolated in11 Asian countries: a proposal for a new nomenclature for SCCmec elements. Antimicrob Agents Chemother 2006; 50: 1001-12.

[27]   Ma XX, Ito T, Tiensasitorn C, *et al*. Novel type of staphylococcal cassette chromosome mec identified in community-acquired methicillin-resistant Staphylococcus aureus strains. Antimicrob Agents Chemother 2002; 46: 1147-52.

[28]   Oliveira D, Milheiric C, de Lencastre H. Redefining a structural variant ofstaphylococcal cassette chromosome mec, SCCmec Type VI. Antimicrob Agents and Chemother 2006; 50: 3457-59.

[29]   Berglund C, Ito T, Ikeda M, *et al*. Novel type of staphylococcal cassette chromosome mec in a methicillin-resistant Staphylococcus aureus strain isolated in Sweden. Antimicrob Agents Chemother 2008; 52: 3512-16.

[30]   Deurenberg R, Vink C, Oudhuis G, *et al*. Different clonal complexes of methicillin-resistant Staphylococcus aureus are disseminated in the Euregio Meuse-Rhine Region. Antimicrob Agents Chemother 2005; 49: 4263-71.

[31]   Diep B, Stone G, Basuino L, *et al*. The arginine catabolic mobile element and staphylococcal chromosomal cassette mec linkage: Convergence of virulence and resistance in the USA300 clone of methicillin-resistant Staphylococcus aureus. I Infect Dis 2008; 197: 1523-30.

[32]   Ito T, Katayama Y, Hiramatsu K. Cloning and nucleotide sequence determination of the entire mec DNA of pre-methicillin-resistant Staphylococcus aureus N315. Antimicrob Agents Chemother 1999; 43: 1449-58.

[33]   Yang JA, Park DW, Sohn JW, *et al*. Novel PCR-restriction fragment length polymorphism analysis for rapid typing of staphylococcal cassette chromosome mec elements. J Clin Microbiol 2006; 44: 236-38.

[34]   Milheiric C, Oliveira D, de Lencastre H. Update to the multiplex PCR strategy for assignment of mec element types in Staphylococcus aureus. Antimicrob Agents Chemother 2007; 51: 3374-77.

[35]   Stephens A, Huygens F, Philip M, *et al*. Systematic derivation of marker sets for staphylococcal cassette chromosome mec typing. Antimicrob Agents and Chemother 2007; 51: 2954-64.

[36]   DeLeo F, Otto M, Kreiswirth B, *et al*. Community-associated meticillin-resistant Staphylococcus aureus. The Lancet 2010; 375: 1557-68.

[37]   Fang YH, Hsueh PR, Hu JJ, *et al*. Community-acquired methicillin-resistantStaphylococcus aureus in children in northern Taiwan. J Microbiol Immunol Infect 2004; 37: 29-34.

[38]   Deresinski S. Methicillin resistant Staphylococcus aureus: an evolutionary, epidemiologic, and therapeutic odyssey. Clin Infect Dis 2005; 40: 562-73

[39]   Baba T, Takeuchi F, Kuroda M, *et al*. Genome and virulence determinants of high virulence community-acquired MRSA. The Lancet 2002; 359: 1819-27.

[40]   Cabrera EC, Ramirez-Argamosa D, Rodriguez R. Prevalence of community-acquired methicillin resistant Staphylococcus aureus from inmates of the Manila City Jail, characterization for SCCmec type and occurrence of Panton-Valentine leukocidin gene. Phil Sci Lett 2010; 3: 4-12.

[41]   David M, Mennella C, Mansour M, *et al*. Predominance of methicillin- resistant Staphylococcus aureus among pathogens causing skin and soft tissue infections in a large urban jail: Risk factors and recurrencerates. J Clin Microbiol 2008; 46: 3222-27.

[42]   Pan E, Diep B, Carleton H, *et al*. Increasing prevalence of methicillin-resistant Staphylococcus aureus infection in California jails. Clin Infect Dis 2003; 37: 1384-88.

[43]   CDC Centers for Disease Control and Prevention. Outbreaks of community-associated methicillin-resistant Staphylococcus aureus skin infections—Los Angeles County, California, 2002-2003. MMWR 2003a; 52: 88.

[44]   Huang H, Flynn N, King JH, et al. Comparisons of community-associated methicillin-resistant Staphylococcus aureus (MRSA) and hospital-associated MSRA infections in Sacramento, California. J Clin Micro 2006; 44: 2423-27.

[45]   Zinderman C, Conner B, Malakooti M, *et al*. Community-acquired methicillin resistant Staphylococcus aureus among military recruits. Emerg Infect Dis 2004; 10: 153-60.

[46]   CDC Centers for Disease Control and Prevention. Methicillin-resistant Staphylococcus aureus infections among competitive sports participants-Colorado, Indiana, Pennsylvania, and Los Angeles County, 2000-2003. MMWR 2003b; 52: 793-95.

[47]   Vandenesch F, Naimi T, Enright M, *et al*. Community-acquired methicillin-resistant Staphylococcus aureus carrying Panton-Valentine leukocidin genes: worldwide emergence. Emerg Infect Dis 2003; 9: 978-84.

[48]   Skov RL, Jensen KS. Community-associated meticillin-resistant Staphylococcus aureus as a cause of hospital-acquired infections. J of Hosp Infect 2009; 73: 364-70.

[49]   Millar BC, Loughrey A, Elborn JS, *et al*. Proposed definitions of community-associated meticillin-resistant Staphylococcus aureus (CA-MRSA). J Hosp Infect 2007; 67: 109-13.

[50]   McDougal L, Steward C, Killgore G, *et al*. Pulsed-field gel electrophoresis typing of oxacillin-resistant Staphylococcus aureus isolates from the United States: Establishing a national database. J Clin Microbiol 2003; 41: 5113-20

[51]   Diep B, Otto M. The role of virulence determinants in community-associated MRSA pathogenesis. Trends in Microbiol 2008; 16: 361-69.

[52]   Rossney A, Shore A, Morgan P, *et al*. The emergence and importation of diverse genotypes of methicillin-resistant Staphylococcus aureus (MRSA) harboring the Panton-Valentine leukocidin gene (pvl) reveal that pvl is a poor marker for community-acquired MRSA strains in Ireland. J Clin Microbiol 2007; 45: 2554-63.

[53]   Patel M, Waites KB, Hoesley CJ, *et al*. Emergence of USA300 MRSA in a tertiary medical centre: implications for epidemiological studies. J Hosp Infect 2008; 68: 208-13.

[54]   David MD, Kearns AM, Gossain S, *et al*. Community-associated methicillin-resistant Staphylococcus aureus: nosocomial transmission in a neonatal unit. J Hosp Infect 2006; 64: 244-50.

[55]   CDC Centers for Disease Control and Prevention. Community-associated methicillin resistant Staphylococcus aureus infection among healthy newborns- Chicago and Los Angeles County. MMWR Morb Mortal Wkly Rep 2006; 55: 329-23.

[56]   O'Brien FG, Lim TT, Chong FN, *et al*. Diversity among Community Isolates of Methicillin-Resistant Staphylococcus aureus in Australia. J Clin Microbiol 2004; 42: 3185-90.

[57]   Prévost G, Cribbier B, Couppie P, *et al*. Panton-Valentine leucocidin and gamma-hemolysin from Staphylococcus aureus ATCC 49775 are encoded by distinct genetic loci and have different biological activities. Infect Immun 1995; 63: 4121-29.

[58]   Genestier A, Michallet M, Prévost G, *et al*. Staphylococcus aureus Panton-Valentine leukocidin directly targets mitochondria and induces Bax-independent apoptosis of human neutrophils. J Clin Invest 2005; 115: 3117-27.

[59]   Lopez-Aguilar C, Perez-Roth E, Mendez-Alvarez S, *et al*. Association between the presence of the Panton-Valentine leukocidin-encoding gene and a lower rate of survival among hospitalized pulmonary patients with staphylococcal disease. J Clin Micro 2007; 45: 274-76.

[60]   Voyich JM, Otto M, Mathema B, *et al*. Is Panton-Valentine leukocidin the major virulence determinant in community-associated methicillin-resistant Staphylococcus aureus disease? J Infect Dis 2006; 194: 1761-70.

[61]   Zhang K, McClure J, Elsayed S, *et al*. Coexistence of Panton-Valentine leukocidin-positive and -negative community-associated methicillin-resistant Staphylococcus aureus USA400 sibling strains in a large Canadian health-care region. J Infect Dis 2008; 197: 195-204.

[62]   CLSI (Clinical Laboratory Standards Institute). Performance Standards for Antimicrobial Susceptibility Testing: Twentieth Informational Supplement, M100-S20 2010; 30: 60-61.

[63]   Tomasz A, Nachman S, Leaf H. Stable classes of phenotypic expression in methicillin-resistant clinical isolates of staphylococci. Antimicrob Agents Chemother 1991; 35: 124-29.

[64]   Berger-Bachi B, Strissle A, Gustafson JE, *et al*. Mapping and characterization of multiple chromosomal factors involved in methicillin resistance in Staphylococcus aureus. Antimicrob Agents Chemother 1992; 36: 1367-73.

[65]   Rinder H. Hetero-resistance: an under-recognized confounder in diagnosis and therapy? J Med Microbiol 2001; 50: 1018-20.

[66]   Sabath LD, Wallace SJ. Factors influencing methicillin resistance in staphylococci. Ann NY Acad Sci 1971; 182: 258-66.

[67]   Hartman BJ, Tomasz A. Expression of methicillin resistance in heterogeneous strains of Staphylococcus aureus. Antimicrob Agents Chemother 1986; 29: 85-92.

[68]   Giannouli S, Labrou M, Kyritsis A, *et al*. Detection of mutations in the FemXAB protein family in oxacillin-susceptible mecA-positive 633Staphylococcus aureus clinical isolates. J Antimicrob Chemother 2010; 65: 626.

[69]   Petinaki E, Kontos F, Maniatis AN. Emergence of two oxacillin-susceptible mecA-positive Staphylococcus aureus clones in a Greek hospital. J of Antimicrob Chemother 2002; 50: 1090-91.

[70]   Hososaka Y, Hanaki, H, Endo H, *et al*. Characterization of oxacillin-susceptible mecA-positive Staphylococcus aureus: a new type of MRSA. J Infect and Chemother 2007; 13: 79-86.

[71]   Hurlimann-Dalel RL, Ryffel C, Kayser FH, *et al*. Survey of the methicillin resistance-associated genes mecA, mecR1-mecI, and femA-femB in clinical isolates of methicillin-resistant Staphylococcus aureus. Antimicrob Agents Chemother 1992; 36: 2617-21.

[72]   McDougal L, Thornsberry C. The Role of β-lactamase in staphylococcal resistance to penicillinase-resistant penicillins and cephalosporins. J Clin Microbiol 1986; 23: 832-39

[73]   Nicola F, Bantar C, Canigia LF, *et al*. Comparison of several methods to determine methicillin-resistance in Staphylococcus aureus with focus on borderline strains. Diagn Microbiol Infect Dis 2000; 36: 91-93.

[74]   Tomasz A, Drugeon HB, de Lencastre HM, *et al*. New mechanism for methicillin resistance in Staphylococcus aureus: clinical isolates that lack the PBP 2a gene and contain normal penicillin-binding proteins with modified penicillin-binding capacity. Antimicrob Agents Chemother 1989 Nov; 33: 1869-74.

[75] Burkhardt O, Pletz MW, Mertgen CP, *et al.* Linezolid - the first oxazolidinone in the treatment of nosocomial MRSA pneumonia. Recent Pat Antiinfect Drug Discov 2007; 2(2): 123-30.

[76] Fridkin S, Hageman J, McDougal L, *et al.* Epidemiological and microbiological characterization of infections caused by Staphylococcus aureus with reduced susceptibility to vancomycin,United States, 1997-2001. Clinical Infectious Diseases 2003; 36: 429-39.

[77] CDC Centers for Disease Control and Prevention. Public Health Dispatch: Vancomycin-Resistant Staphylococcus aureus - Pennsylvania, 2002. MMWR 2002; 51: 902.

[78] Kollef MH. Limitations of vancomycin in the management of resistant staphylococcal infections. Clin Infect Dis 2007; 45: S191-95

[79] Micek ST. Alternatives to vancomycin for the treatment of methicillin-resistant Staphylococcus aureus infections. Clin Infect Dis 2007; 45 (Suppl 3): S184 -90.

CHAPTER 9

Multidrug-Resistant *Acinetobacter baumannii*: An Emerging Threat in Health Care Facilities

Raffaele Zarrilli[1*], Maria Triassi[1] and Asad U. Khan[2]

[1]Department of Preventive Medical Sciences, Hygiene Section, University of Naples 'Federico II', Naples, Italy and [2]Interdisciplinary Biotechnology Unit, AMU, Aligarh India

Abstract: *Acinetobacter baumannii* is an opportunistic gram-negative pathogen with increasing relevance in a variety of hospital-acquired infections especially among intensive-care-unit patients. Resistance to antimicrobial agents is the main advantage of *A. baumannii* in the hospital setting. *A. baumannii* epidemics described worldwide are caused by a limited number of genotypic clusters of multidrug-resistant strains that successfully spread among hospitals of different cities and countries. In this chapter, we will focus on the mechanisms responsible for antimicrobial drug resistance in *A. baumannii* and the epidemiology of multidrug-resistant *A. baumannii* in health-care facilities.

Keywords: *A. baumannii,* Gram negative pathogen, health care, epidemiology, MDR, ESBL.

INTRODUCTION

Acinetobacter spp. are glucose-non fermentative gram-negative coccobacilli that have emerged in recent years as a major cause of nosocomial infections associated with high morbidity and mortality [1, 2]. The genus *Acinetobacter* currently contains up to 32 described named and unnamed (genomic) species [1]. *Acinetobacter baumannii*, genomic species 3 and 13TU, three of the most clinically relevant species, are genetically and phenotypically very similar to an environmental species, *A. calcoaceticus*, and are therefore grouped together into the so-called *A. calcoaceticus-A. baumannii* (Acb) complex [1]. Because phenotypic identification of *Acinetobacter* isolates to the species level has proven to be insufficient, several genotypic methods have been developed for genomic species identification, that include amplified 16S rRNA gene restriction analysis (ARDRA), high-resolution fingerprint analysis by amplified fragment length polymorphism (AFLP), sequence analysis of the 16S-23S rRNA gene spacer region or amplification and sequence analysis of the *rpoB* gene [1, 3-5]. The species that is most commonly involved in hospital infections is *A. baumannii*, which causes a variety of health-care associated infections, comprising bacteremia, urinary tract infection, surgical-site infection, and nosocomial and ventilator-associated pneumonia, especially in Intensive-Care-Unit (ICU) patients [1, 2, 5-12]. The rates of recovery of *A. baumannii* from natural environments and its incidence in the community are low, while its rate of carriage by hospitalized patients is high and its occurrence in the hospital setting is frequent [1]. *A. baumannii* has simple growth requirements and can survive in dry conditions. This might contribute to the fitness of *A. baumannii* in the hospital environment, which represents the main reservoir of the bacterium [1, 2].

Mechanism Responsible For Antimicrobial Drug Resistance In *Acinetobacter baumannii*

Resistance to antimicrobial agents is the main advantage of *A. baumannii* in the nosocomial environment. Multidrug resistance in *A. baumannii* has been defined as resistance to more than two of the following five drug classes: antipseudomonal cephalosporins (ceftazidime or cefepime), antipseudomonal carbapenems (imipenem or meropenem), ampicillin-sulbactam, fluoroquinolones (ciprofloxacin or levofloxacin), and aminoglycosides (gentamicin, tobramycin, or amikacin) [2]. Pandrug resistance is often defined as resistance to all antimicrobials that undergo first-line susceptibility testing that have therapeutic potential

*Address correspondence to Raffaele Zarrilli: Department of Preventive Medical Sciences, Hygiene Section, University of Naples 'Federico II', Naples, Italy; Tel: +39-081-7463026; Fax: +39-081-7463352; Email: rafzarri@unina.it

against *A. baumannii*. This would include all β-lactams (including carbapenems and sulbactam), fluoroquinolones, and aminoglycosides [1,2]. However, with the increased use of the polymyxins and tigecycline, this definition have to include these two agents also. Multidrug-resistant isolates of *A. baumannii* have been reported increasingly during the last decade, probably as a consequence of extensive use of antimicrobial agents in western countries [2, 8, 13-15]. Also, as recently demonstrated by a retrospective, matched cohort study, patients with infection by multidrug-resistant *Acinetobacter* show higher mortality rate and length of hospitalization than patients with infection by susceptible *Acinetobacter* [5].

Mounting evidence indicates that *A. baumannii* possesses a broad range of mechanisms of resistance to all existing antibiotic classes as well as a prodigious capacity to acquire new determinants of resistance [1, 2]. Genome sequence analysis of a number of multidrug-resistant *A. baumannii* clinical strains has shown the presence of several large genomic islands containing multiple resistance genes interspersed with transposons, integrons, and other mobile genetic elements [9-12]. Also, plasmids carrying resistance genes and/or resistance determinants involved in horizontal gene transfer have been described in several *A. baumannii* strains [16-22]. The most relevant mechanisms of resistance to the different classes of antimicrobials in *A. baumannii* are shown in Table **1**.

Acinetobacter baumannii possesses an intrinsic class D oxacillinase and a non-inducible chromosomal AmpC cephalosporinase [23, 24]. *A. baumannii* oxacillinases belong to the OXA-51-like group of enzymes that constitutes over 40 sequence variants. OXA-51-like enzymes are able to hydrolyse penicillins (benzylpenicillin, ampicillin, ticarcillin and piperacillin) and carbapenems (imipenem and meropenem) but they do this only very weakly. They are not active against expanded-spectrum cephalosporins [23]. The expression of AmpC cephalosporinase has been demonstrated to be up-regulated by the insertion element IS*Aba1* upstream of the gene, able to act as a strong transcriptional promoter [25]. In addition to upregulation of AmpC, resistance to cephalosporins in A. *baumannii* is mediated by a wide range of class A extended spectrum β-lactamase, including those of the TEM, SHV, CTX-M, GES, SCO, PER and VEB families (Table **1**) [26-36].

The resistance of *A. baumannii* to carbapenems is mediated by all of the major resistance mechanisms that are known to occur in bacteria, including enzymatic inactivation, active efflux and decreased influx of drugs, and modification of target sites (Table **1**). The production of carbapenem-hydrolizing beta-lactamases is the most common mechanism responsible for carbapenem resistance in *A. baumannii*. Several carbapenem-hydrolyzing β-lactamases have been identified so far in *A. baumannii*. These include metallo-β-lactamases (VIM-, IMP- and SIM-types), which have been sporadically reported in some parts of the world and have been associated with class 1 integrons [1, 2, 7, 13]. Nevertheless, the most widespread carbapenemases in *A. baumannii* are class D β-lactamases. Four main acquired carbapenem-hydrolysing class D oxacillinase (CHDL) gene clusters have been identified in *A. baumannii*, represented by the bla_{OXA-23}-, $bla_{OXA-24/40}$-, bla_{OXA-58}-like genes, and $bla_{OXA-143}$ gene [13, 15-22, 37]. CHDL genes have been found either in the chromosome or in plasmids, thus suggesting that they might have been acquired through horizontal gene transfer. A family of Insertion Sequence (IS) elements at the 5' and/or the 3' of CHDL genes, such as IS*Aba1*, IS*Aba2*, IS*Aba3*, or IS*18*, has been demonstrated to regulate their acquisition and expression [10, 13, 16-21]. In addition to these CHDL genes, the chromosomal $bla_{OXA-51-like}$ gene, intrinsic to *A. baumannii* species, has been demonstrated to confer carbapenem resistance when flanked by IS elements [38]. Reduced susceptibility to carbapenems has also been associated with the modification of penicillin-binding proteins and porins or with upregulation of the AdeABC efflux system, and it has been suggested that the interplay of different mechanisms might result in high-level carbapenem resistance in *A. baumannii* (Table **1**) [39-42].

The production of aminoglycoside-modifying enzymes has been demonstrated as the main mechanism responsible for aminoglycoside resistance in *A. baumannii* [1, 2]. Acetyltransferases, nucleotidyl-transferases and phosphotransferases have all been found in *A. baumannii*, often occurring in combination. In a study of aminoglycoside resistance in epidemic *A. baumannii* clones isolated in Europe, 95% of isolates were found to contain at least one resistance gene and 84% carried between two and five genes [43]. A total of 12 different combinations were found, with *aacC1, aadA1* and *aacA4* located in association with class 1 integrons [43]. Expression of these genes leads to variable susceptibility to different aminoglycosides. Another type of enzyme, the 16s rRNA methyltransferases ArmA, which confer high-level resistance to all formulated aminoglycosides, has recently been described in *A. baumannii* [44], often found in combination with blaOXA-23 [31] (Table **1**).

Table 1: Antimicrobial resistance mechanisms in *A. baumannii*.

Antimicrobial Class	Mechanism	Note	References
Cephalosporins	β-lactam hydrolysis		
	Class C beta-lactamase	ADC 1-7	[24]
	Class A ESBL	VEB-1,-2; PER-1,-2; TEM-92,-116; SHV-12,-5; CTX-M-2,-3.	[26-30]
	Class D beta-lactamase	OXA-51-like	[23]
Carbapenems	β-lactam hydrolysis		
	class B MBLs	IMP-1, -2, -4, -5, -6, -11; VIM-2, SIM-1. Class 1 integron-associated genes.	[2,13]
	CHDLs	OXA-23 -24/40 -58 -143 clusters. Chromosomal or plasmid genes flanked by IS elements.	[2,13,16,37]
	OXA-51-like intrinsic chromosomal class D beta-lactamase	Confers carbapenem resistance if IS elements are inserted upstream of the gene	[13,38]
	Changes in OMPs		
	CarO	26 kDa OMP implicated in drug influx	[39]
	33 to 36-kDa OMPs OprD-like OMP	Other OMPs associated with carbapenem resistance	[40-42]
Aminoglycoside	Aminoglycoside modifying enzymes	AacC1/2, AadA, AadB Ant1 AphA1, AphA6	[43]
	16S rDNA methyltransferase	ArmA	[44]
Quinolones	Target alteration		
	Gyrase subunit	GyrA	[51,52]
	Topoisomerase IV subunit	ParC	[52]
Rifampicin	Drug modification	Rifampicin ADP-ribosylating transferase Arr-2	[54]
Trimethoprim/sulfamethoxazole	Dihydropteroate synthase	SulI/II	[55]
	Dihydrofolate reductase	FolA	[55]
Polymyxins	Outer membrane modification	PmrAB two component mutation	[56]
Broad (Aminoglycoside, quinolones, tetracyclines, glycylcyclines)	Efflux pumps		
	RND	AdeABC, AdeIJK	[46-49]
	MATE	AbeM	[50]
	MFS	TetA, TetB	[45,53]

ESBL, extended spectrum beta-lactamases; MBLs, class B metallo beta-lactamases; CHDLs, carbapenem hydrolyzing class D beta-lactamases; OMPs, outer membrane proteins; RND, resistance-nodulation-cell division; MATE, multidrug and toxic compound extrusion; MFS, major facilitator superfamily.

Drug removal by active efflux mechanisms contributes substantially to multidrug resistance in *A. baumannii*. Narrow-spectrum pumps of the Major Facilitator Superfamily (MFS) include those involved in tetracycline (TetA, TetB) and minocycline (TetB) resistance [45]. Neither TetA nor TetB affect tigecycline. Pumps of the Resistance-Nodulation-Cell Division (RND) type are three-component pumps with broad substrate specificity consisting of a common tripartite structure with periplasmic, inner and outer membrane components. Two systems have been characterised in *A. baumannii*, AdeABC and AdeIJK. Resistance to aminoglycosides, β-lactams, chloramphenicol, erythromycin, tetracycline and tigecycline occurs due to overexpression of adeABC, a phenomenon under the control of a two-component regulator system encoded by the adeRS genes [46-48]. The second RND pump, AdeIJK, has a substrate specificity favouring amphiphilic compounds and contributes synergistically with AdeABC to tigecycline resistance [49]. A pump belonging to the multidrug and toxic compoundextrusion (MATE) family, AbeM, has also been characterised. Overexpression of this results in reduced susceptibility to quinolones, gentamicin, kanamycin, erythromycin, chloramphenicol and trimethoprim [50].

Additional resistance mechanisms include mutations in DNA gyrase and topoisomerase IV (fluoroquinolone resistance) [51, 52], a tetracycline ribosomal protection protein (TetM) [53], a rifampicin ADP-ribosylating transferase Arr-2 (rifampicin resistance) [54], a putative dihydrofolate reductase (folA) involved in trimethoprim resistance [55] and mutations in a two-component regulator (pmrA/B) associated with resistance to polymyxins [56] (Table **1**).

GLOBAL EPIDEMIOLOGY OF MULTIDRUG-RESISTANT *Acinetobacter baumannii*

Multi-drug resistance in *A. baumannii* is now an emerging issue worldwide [1, 2]. Until recently, most isolates were susceptible to the carbapenems but there have been isolated reports of resistance since the early 1990s. Since then, the incidence of imipenem resistance has risen dramatically and constitutes a sentinel event for emerging antimicrobial resistance [2, 13-15]. Due to that reason, we will focus more on the epidemiology of carbapenem-resistant *A. baumannii*.

Surveillance studies indicate that the percentage of carbapenem-resistant isolates gradually increased over the last ten years in Europe, North America and Latin America [2, 14]. Carbapenem resistant isolates of *A. baumannii* are usually resistant to all classes of antimicrobials, show intermediate resistance to rifampin, while usually retain susceptibility to tigecycline and colistin [1, 2, 13, 57]. Numerous outbreaks of carbapenem-resistant *A. baumannii* were reported from hospitals in Europe [2, 6-8, 10, 13, 15-19, 58-67], North America and Latin America [2, 15, 68, 69], Africa [15, 70, 71] Asia [2, 15, 72-74], and Australia [15, 75]. In the majority of cases, one or two epidemic strains were detected in a given hospital. Transmission of such strains was observed between hospitals in the same city and also on a national scale [1, 2, 6, 13, 58-60, 62, 69, 70, 73-75] and a direct epidemiological link was established in several cases [6, 26, 59, 61, 62, 70, 75-79]. The inter-hospital transfer of colonised patients was demonstrated during multi-facility outbreaks occurred in The Netherlands [59], Italy [6], South Africa [70] and Tunisia [71]. The international transfer of patients colonised by carbapenem-resistant *A. baumannii* was also reported [61, 62, 75]. More recently, several cases of United Kingdom and U.S military and nonmilitary personnel returning from operations in Iraq and Afghanistan and harbouring infections caused by carbapenem-resistant *A. baumannii* were reported [77-79].

Molecular epidemiological studies showed that outbreaks of multidrug- and carbapenem-resistant *A. baumannii* described so far were demonstrated to be caused by a limited number of genotypic clusters of strains. Major outbreak clones initially named European clones I, II and III are now regarded as international [1,2,15, 80-82], and referred to, according to multilocus sequence typing, as clonal complexes 1, 2 and 3, respectively [82]. Epidemiological studies showed the prevalence of international clone II lineage world-wide during the last few years [15, 67, 80-84] and the occurrence of epidemics caused by multidrug-resistant strains belonging to novel genotypes not related to the three main clonal complexes in several Mediterranean hospitals [65, 67, 83, 84].

Genotypic characterization of carbapenem-resistance genes in *A. baumannii* strains showed the occurrence of *bla*$_{OXA-23}$-, *bla*$_{OXA-24/40}$-, or *bla*$_{OXA-58}$-like genes in multiple isolates from the same hospital or among different hospitals worldwide [2, 13, 15-18, 67, 83]. *bla*$_{OXA-23}$ was mostly detected in isolates from Asian countries [73, 74], but was also reported in South America [68, 69] and Europe [13, 17, 83]; bla_{OXA-58} was frequently found in Europe [10, 13, 16, 67, 83]. $bla_{OXA-24/40}$ was mostly found in the Iberian peninsula and Asia, but also detected in other countries [2, 18, 19, 63, 73, 79]. The bla_{OXA-58} gene flanked by IS elements was present in the majority of carbapenem-resistant genotypes analyzed from hospitals in Greece, Italy, Lebanon, and Turkey [7, 16, 67, 83]. Of note, each of the IS element flanking the 5' end of bla_{OXA-58} occurred in strains of distinct ST groups and PFGE profiles isolated in the same geographic region. Thus, IS*Aba2* element was detected in Greece and Italy, IS*18* in Lebanon and Turkey, IS*Aba1* in Turkey and Italy, suggesting that they might have been acquired through horizontal gene transfer [67]. In further support of this, plasmid-borne bla_{OXA-58} has been found in the majority of carbapenem-resistant *A. baumannii* strains isolated in Mediterranean countries [10, 16, 21, 67]. The spread of carbapenem-resistant *A. baumannii* carrying the bla_{OXA-58} gene might had also been contributed by international transfer of colonised patients, as recently demonstrated from Greece to Belgium [61], Greece to Australia [75], and Iraq to USA military services [77].

CONCLUSIONS

Outbreaks of multidrug-resistant *A. baumannii* are increasingly reported worldwide. They are sustained by clusters of highly similar strains that successfully spread among different cities and countries and are selected because of the acquisition of antimicrobial resistance genes. Multi-facility *A. baumannii* outbreaks can be also sustained by inter-hospital transfer of colonized patients. This emphasizes the need to adopt surveillance and infection control programmes to prevent colonisation and infection by multidrug-resistant *A. baumannii* in the hospital setting. These programmes would include the study of global epidemiology of multidrug-resistant *A. baumannii* using molecular typing of bacterial isolates and characterization of antibiotic resistance in order to control the spread of *A. baumannii* infections over a wide geographic region.

ACKNOWLEDGEMENTS

Work performed in the authors' laboratories was supported in part by grants from Agenzia Italiana del Farmaco, Italy (AIFA2007 contract no. FARM7X9F8K) and from Ministero dell'Istruzione, dell'Universita` e della Ricerca, Italy (PRIN 2008 to RZ).

REFERENCES

[1] Dijkshoorn L, Nemec A, Seifert H. An increasing threat in hospitals: multidrugresistant *Acinetobacter baumannii*. Nat Rev Microbiol 2007; 5: 939-51.

[2] Peleg AY, Seifert H, Paterson DL. *Acinetobacter baumannii*: emergence of a successful pathogen. Clin Microbiol Rev 2007; 21: 538-82.

[3] Dijkshoorn L, van Harsselaar B, Tjernberg I, *et al*. Evaluation of amplified ribosomal DNA restriction analysis for identification of *Acinetobacter* genomic species. Syst Appl Microbiol 2007; 21: 33-39.

[4] Chang HC, Wei YF, Dijkshoorn L, *et al*. Species-level identification of isolates of the *Acinetobacter calcoaceticus-Acinetobacter baumannii* complex by sequence analysis of the 16S-23S rRNA gene spacer region. J Clin Microbiol 2005; 43: 1632-39.

[5] Gundi VAKB, Dijkshoorn L, Burignat S, *et al*. Validation of partial *rpoB* gene sequence analysis for the identification of clinically important and emerging *Acinetobacter* species. Microbiology 2009; 155: 2333-41.

[6] Sunenshine RH, Wright M-O, Maragakis LL, *et al*. Multidrug-resistant *Acinetobacter* infection mortality rate and length of hospitalization. Emerg Infect Dis 2007; 13: 97-103.

[7] Zarrilli R, Casillo R, Di Popolo A, *et al*. Molecular epidemiology of a clonal outbreak of multidrug-resistant *Acinetobacter baumannii* in a university hospital in Italy. Clin Microbiol Infect 2007; 13: 481-89.

[8] Tsakris A, Ikonomidis A, Poulou A, *et al*. Clusters of imipenem-resistant *Acinetobacter baumannii* clones producing different carbapenemases in an intensive care unit. Clin Microbiol Infect 2008; 14: 588-94.

[9] Zarrilli R, Crispino M, Bagattini M, *et al*. Molecular epidemiology of sequential outbreaks of *Acinetobacter baumannii* in an intensive care unit shows the emergence of carbapenem resistance. J Clin Microbiol 2004; 42: 946-53.

[10]   Vallenet D, Nordmann P, Barbe V, *et al*. Comparative analysis of *Acinetobacters*: three genomes for three lifestyles. PLos ONE 2005; 3: e1805.

[11]   Iacono M., Villa L, Fortini D, *et al*. Whole genome pyrosequencing of an epidemic multidrug resistant *Acinetobacter baumannii* of the European clone II. Antimicrob Agents Chemother 2008; 52: 2616-25.

[12]   Adams MD, Goglin K, Molyneaux N, *et al*. Comparative genome sequence analysis of multidrug-resistant *Acinetobacter baumannii*. J Bacteriol 2009; 190: 8053-64.

[13]   Adams MD, Chan ER, Molyneaux ND, *et al*. Genomewide analysis of divergence of antibiotic resistance determinants in closely related isolates of *Acinetobacter baumannii*. Antimicrob Agents Chemother 2010; 54: 3559-67.

[14]   Poirel L, Nordmann P. Carbapenem resistance in *Acinetobacter baumannii*: mechanisms and epidemiology. Clin Microbiol Infect 2006; 12: 826-36.

[15]   Mera RM, Miller LA, Amrine-Madsen H, *et al*. *Acinetobacter baumannii* 2002-2008: increase of carbapenem-associated multiclass resistance in the United States Microb Drug Resist 2010; 16:209-15.

[16]   Higgins PG, Dammhayn C, Hackel M, *et al*. Global spread of carbapenem-resistant *Acinetobacter baumannii*. J Antimicrob Chemother 2009; 65: 233-38.

[17]   Poirel L, Nordmann P. Genetic structure at the origin of acquisition and expression of the carbapenem-hydrolyzing oxacillinase gene *bla*$_{OXA-58}$ in *Acinetobacter baumannii*.

[18]   Mugnier P, Poirel L, Naas T, *et al*. Worldwide dissemination of the *bla*$_{OXA-23}$ carbapenemase gene of *Acinetobacter baumannii*. Emerg Infect Dis 2010; 16: 35-40.

[19]   D'Andrea MM, Giani T, D'Arezzo S, *et al*. Characterization of pABVA01, a plasmid encoding the OXA-24 carbapenemase from Italian isolates of *Acinetobacter baumannii*. Antimicrob. Agents Chemother. 2009; 53: 3528-33.

[20]   Merino M, Acosta J, Poza M, *et al*. OXA-24 carbapenemase gene flanked by XerC/XerD-like recombination sites in different plasmids from different *Acinetobacter* species isolated during a nosocomial outbreak. Antimicrob. Agents Chemother 2010; 54: 2724-27.

[21]   Chen T-L, Wu RC-C, Shaio M-F, *et al*. Acquisition of a plasmid-borne *bla*OXA-58 gene with an upstream IS*1008* insertion conferring a high level of carbapenem resistance to *Acinetobacter baumannii*. Antimicrob Agents Chemother 2008; 52: 2573-80.

[22]   Zarrilli R, Vitale D, Di Popolo A, *et al*. A plasmid-borne *bla*$_{OXA-58}$ gene confers imipenem resistance to *Acinetobacter baumannii* isolates from a Lebanese hospital. Antimicrob Agents Chemother 2008; 52: 4115-4120.

[23]   Meric M, Kasap M, Gacar G, *et al*. Emergence and spread of carbapenem-resistant *Acinetobacter baumannii* in a tertiary care hospital in Turkey. FEMS Microbiol Lett 2008; 282: 214-18.

[24]   Héritier C, Poirel L, Fournier PE, *et al*. Characterization of the naturally occurring oxacillinase of *Acinetobacter baumannii*. Antimicrob Agents Chemother 2005; 49: 4174-9.

[25]   Bou G, Martínez-Beltrán J. Cloning, nucleotide sequencing, and analysis of the gene encoding an AmpC β-lactamase in *Acinetobacter baumannii*. Antimicrob Agents Chemother 2000; 44:428-32.

[26]   Héritier C, Poirel L, Nordmann P. Cephalosporinase over-expression resulting from insertion of ISAba1 in *Acinetobacter baumannii*. Clin Microbiol Infect 2006; 12:123-30.

[27]   Naas T, Coignard B, Carbonne A, *et al*. VEB-1 extended-spectrum β-lactamase-producing *Acinetobacter baumannii*, France. Emerg Infect Dis 2006; 12: 1214-22.

[28]   Pasterán F, Rapoport M, Petroni A, *et al*. Emergence of PER-2 and VEB-1a in *Acinetobacter baumannii* strains in the Americas. Antimicrob Agents Chemother 2006; 50: 3222-24.

[29]   Naas T, Bogaerts P, Bauraing C, *et al*. Emergence of PER and VEB extended-spectrum β-lactamases in *Acinetobacter baumannii* in Belgium. J Antimicrob Chemother 2006; 58: 178-82.

[30]   Vahaboglu H, Coskunkan F, Tansel O, *et al*. Clinical importance of extended-spectrum β-lactamase (PER-1-type)-producing Acinetobacter spp. and Pseudomonas aeruginosa strains. J Med Microbiol 2001; 50: 642-5.

[31]   Celenza G, Pellegrini C, CaccamoM, *et al*. Spread of blaCTX-M-type and blaPER-2 β-lactamase genes in clinical isolates from Bolivian hospitals. J Antimicrob Chemother 2006; 57: 975-78.

[32]   Kim JW, Heo ST, Jin JS, *et al*. Characterization of *Acinetobacter baumannii* carrying blaOXA-23, blaPER-1 and armA in a Korean hospital. Clin Microbiol Infect 2008; 14: 716-18.

[33]   Naiemi NA, Duim B, Savelkoul PH, *et al*. Widespread transfer of resistance genes between bacterial species in an intensive care unit: implications for hospital epidemiology. J Clin Microbiol 2005; 43: 4862-64.

[34]   Endimiani A, Luzzaro F, Migliavacca R, *et al*. Spread in an Italian hospital of a clonal *Acinetobacter baumannii* strain producing the TEM-92 extended spectrum β-lactamase. Antimicrob Agents Chemother 2007; 51: 2211-14.

[35]   Naas T, Namdari F, Réglier-Poupet H, *et al.* Panresistant extended-spectrum β-lactamase SHV-5-producing *Acinetobacter baumannii* from New York City. J Antimicrob Chemother 2007; 60: 1174-76.

[36]   Nagano N, Nagano Y, Cordevant C, *et al.* Nosocomial transmission of CTX-M-2 β-lactamase-producing *Acinetobacter baumannii* in a neurosurgery ward. J Clin Microbiol 2004; 42: 3978-84.

[37]   Poirel L, Corvec S, Rapoport M, *et al.* Identification of the novel narrow-spectrum β-lactamase SCO-1 in *Acinetobacter* spp. from Argentina. Antimicrob Agents Chemother 2007; 51:2179-84.

[38]   Higgins PG, Poirel L, Lehmann M, *et al.* OXA-143, a novel carbapenem hydrolyzing class D β-lactamase in *Acinetobacter baumannii* Antimicrob Agents Chemother 2009; 53: 5035-5038.

[39]   Turton JF, Ward ME, Woodford N, *et al.* The role of IS*Aba1* in expression of OXA carbapenemase genes in *Acinetobacter baumannii*. FEMS Microbiol Lett 2006; 258: 72-77.

[40]   Mussi MA, Limansky AS, Viale AM. Acquisition of resistance to carbapenems in multidrug-resistant clinical strains of *Acinetobacter baumannii*: natural insertional inactivation of a gene encoding a member of a novel family of β-barrel outer membrane proteins. Antimicrob Agents Chemother 2005; 49: 1432-40.

[41]   Dupont M, Page`s J-M, Lafitte D, *et al.* Identification of an OprD homologue in *Acinetobacter baumannii* J Proteome Res 2005; 4: 2386-90.

[42]   Fernandez-Cuenca F, Martínez-Martínez L, Conejo MC, *et al.* Relationship between beta-lactamase production, outer membrane protein and penicillin-binding protein profiles on the activity of carbapenems against clinical isolates of *Acinetobacter baumannii*. J. Antimicrob Chemother 2003; 51: 565-74.

[43]   Heritier C, Poirel L, Lambert T, *et al.* Contribution of acquired carbapenem-hydrolyzing oxacillinases to carbapenem resistance in *Acinetobacter baumannii*. Antimicrob Agents Chemother 2005; 49: 3198-3202.

[44]   Nemec A, Dolzani L, Brisse S, *et al.* Diversity of aminoglycoside-resistance genes and their association with class 1 integrons among strains of pan-European *Acinetobacter baumannii* clones. J Med Microbiol 2004; 53: 1233-40.

[45]   Yu YS, Zhou H, Yang Q, *et al.* Widespread occurrence of aminoglycoside resistance due to ArmA methylase in imipenem-resistant *Acinetobacter baumannii* isolates in China. J Antimicrob Chemother 2007; 60:454-55.

[46]   Huys G, Cnockaert M, Vaneechoutte M, *et al.* Distribution of tetracycline resistance genes in genotypically related and unrelated multiresistant *Acinetobacter baumannii* strains from different European hospitals. Res Microbiol 2005; 156: 348-55.

[47]   Magnet S, Courvalin P, Lambert T. Resistance-nodulation-cell division-type efflux pump involved in aminoglycoside resistance in *Acinetobacter baumannii* strain BM4454. Antimicrob Agents Chemother 2001; 45: 3375-80.

[48]   Ruzin A, Keeney D, Bradford PA. AdeABC multidrug efflux pump is associated with decreased susceptibility to tigecycline in *Acinetobacter calcoaceticus-Acinetobacter baumannii* complex. J Antimicrob Chemother 2007; 59: 1001-04.

[49]   Marchand I, Damier-Piolle L, Courvalin P, *et al.* Expression of the RND-type efflux pump AdeABC in *Acinetobacter baumannii* is regulated by the AdeRS two-component system. Antimicrob Agents Chemother 2004; 48: 3298-04.

[50]   Damier-Piolle L, Magnet S, Brémont S, *et al.* AdeIJK, a resistance nodulation-cell division pump effluxing multiple antibiotics in *Acinetobacter baumannii*. Antimicrob Agents Chemother 2008; 52: 557-62.

[51]   Su XZ, Chen J, Mizushima T, *et al.* AbeM, an H+-coupled *Acinetobacter baumannii* multidrug efflux pump belonging to the MATE family of transporters. Antimicrob Agents Chemother 2005; 49: 4362-64.

[52]   Vila J, Ruiz J, Goñi P, *et al.* Quinolone-resistance mutations in the topoisomerase IV parC gene of *Acinetobacter baumannii*. J Antimicrob Chemother 1997; 39: 757-62.

[53]   Hamouda A, Amyes SG. Novel gyrA and parC point mutations in two strains of *Acinetobacter baumannii* resistant to ciprofloxacin. J Antimicrob Chemother 2004; 54: 695-96

[54]   Ribera A, Roca I, Ruiz J, *et al.* Partial characterization of a transposon containing the tet(A) determinant in a clinical isolate of *Acinetobacter baumannii*. J Antimicrob Chemother 2003; 52: 477-80.

[55]   Houang ETS, Chu JW, Lo WS, *et al.* Epidemiology of rifampin ADP-ribosyltransferase (*arr-2*) and metallo-β-lactamase (*bla*IMP-4) gene cassettes in class 1 integrons in *Acinetobacter* strains isolated from blood cultures in 1997 to 2000. Antimicrob Agents Chemother 2003; 47: 1382-90.

[56]   Mak JK, Kim MJ, Pham J, *et al.* Antibiotic resistance determinants in nosocomial strains of multidrug-resistant *Acinetobacter baumannii*. J Antimicrob Chemother 2009; 63: 47-54.

[57]   Adams MD, Nickel GC, Bajaksouzian S, *et al.* Resistance to colistin in *Acinetobacter baumannii* associated with mutations in the PmrAB two-component system. Antimicrob Agents Chemother 2009; 53: 3628-34.

[58] Tripodi M-F, Durante-Mangoni E, Fortunato R, *et al.* Comparative activities of colistin, rifampicin, imipenem, sulbactam/ampicillin alone or in combination against epidemic multidrug-resistant *Acinetobacter baumannii* isolates producing OXA-58 carbapenemases. Int J Antimicrob Agents 2007; 30: 537-40.

[59] Coelho JM, Turton JF, Kaufmann ME, *et al.* Occurrence of carbapenem-resistant *Acinetobacter baumannii* clones at multiple hospitals in London and Southeast England. J Clin Microbiol 2006;44: 3623-27.

[60] van den Broek PJ, Arends J, Bernards AT, *et al.* Epidemiology of multiple *Acinetobacter* outbreaks in The Netherlands during the period 1999-2001. Clin Microbiol Infect 2006; 12: 837-43.

[61] Nemec A, Krizova L, Maixnerova M, *et al.* Emergence of carbapenem resistance in *Acinetobacter baumannii* in the Czech Republic is associated with the spread of multidrug resistant strains of European clone II. J Antimicrob Chemother 2008; 62: 484-89.

[62] Wybo I, Blommaert L, De Beer T, *et al.* Outbreak of multidrug-resistant *Acinetobacter baumannii* in a Belgian university hospital after transfer of patients from Greece. J Hosp Infect 2007; 67: 374-80.

[63] Schulte B, Goerke C, Weyrich P, *et al.* Clonal spread of meropenem-resistant *Acinetobacter baumannii* strains in hospitals in the Mediterranean region and transmission to south-west Germany. J Hosp Infect 2005; 61: 356-57.

[64] Da Silva GJ, Quintera S, Bertolo E, *et al.* Portugese Resistance Study Group. Long-term dissemination of an OXA-40 carbapenemase-producing *Acinetobacter baumannii* clone in the Iberian Peninsula. J Antimicrob Chemother 2004; 54: 255-58.

[65] D'Arezzo S, Capone A, Petrosillo N, *et al.* Epidemic multidrug-resistant *Acinetobacter baumannii* related to European clonal types I and II in Rome (Italy). Clin Microbiol Infect 2009; 15: 347-57.

[66] Giannouli M, Cuccurullo S, Crivaro V, *et al.* Molecular epidemiology of multi-drug resistant *Acinetobacter baumannii* in a tertiary care hospital in Naples, Italy, shows the emergence of a novel epidemic clone. J Clin Microbiol 2010; 48: 1223-30.

[67] Marchaim D, Navon-Venezia S, Leavitt A, *et al.* Molecular and epidemiologic study of polyclonal outbreaks of multidrug-resistant *Acinetobacter baumannii* infection in an Israeli hospital. Infect Control Hosp Epidemiol 2007; 28: 945-50.

[68] Giannouli M, Tomasone F, Agodi A, *et al.* Molecular epidemiology of carbapenem-resistant *Acinetobacter baumannii* strains in intensive care units of multiple Mediterranean hospitals. J Antimicrob Chemother 2009; 63: 828-30.

[69] Villegas MV, Kattan JN, Correa A, *et al.* Dissemination of *Acinetobacter baumannii* clones with OXA-23 carbapenemase in Colombian hospitals. Antimicrob Agents Chemother 2007; 51: 2001-04.

[70] Merkier AK, Catalano M, Ramirez MS, *et al.* Polyclonal spread of *bla*OXA-23 and *bla*OXA-58 in *Acinetobacter baumannii* isolates from Argentina. J Infect Developing Countries 2008; 2: 235-40.

[71] Marais E, de Jong G, Ferraz V, *et al.* Interhospital transfer of pan-resistant *Acinetobacter* strains in Johannesburg, South Africa. Am J Infect Control 2004; 32: 278-81.

[72] Poirel L, Mansour W, Bouallegue O, *et al.* Carbapenem-resistant *Acinetobacter baumannii* isolates from Tunisia producing the OXA-58-like carbapenem-hydrolyzing oxacillinase OXA-97. Antimicrob Agents Chemother 2008; 52: 1613-17.

[73] Hsueh P-R, Teng LJ, Chen CY, *et al.* Pandrug-resistant *Acinetobacter baumannii* causing nosocomial infections in a university hospital, Taiwan. Emerg Infect Dis 2002; 8: 827-32.

[74] Mendes RE, Bell JM, Turnidge JD, *et al.* Emergence and widespread dissemination of OXA-23,-24/40 and -58 carbapenemases among *Acinetobacter* spp. in Asia-Pacific nations: report from the SENTRY surveillance program. J Antimicrob Chemother 2009; 63: 55-59.

[75] Fu Y, Zhou J, Zhou H, *et al.* Wide dissemination of OXA-23-producing carbapenem-resistant *Acinetobacter baumannii* clonal complex 22 in multiple cities of China. J Antimicrob Chemother 2010; 65: 644-50.

[76] Peleg AY, Bell JM, Hofmeyr A, *et al.* Inter-country transfer of Gram-negative organisms carrying the VIM-4 and OXA-58 carbapenem-hydrolysing enzymes. J Antimicrob Chemother 2006; 57: 794-95.

[77] Hujer KM, Hujer AM, Bajaksouzian S, *et al.* Analysis of antibiotic resistance genes in multidrug-resistant *Acinetobacter* sp. isolates from military and civilian patients treated at the Walter Reed Army Medical Center. Antimicrob Agents Chemother 2006; 50: 4114-23.

[78] Hawley JS, Murray CK, Griffith ME, *et al.* Susceptibility of *Acinetobacter* strains isolated from deployed U.S. military personnel. Antimicrob Agents Chemother 2007; 51: 376-78.

[79] Scott P, Deye G, Srinivasan A, *et al.* An outbreak of multidrug-resistant *Acinetobacter baumannii-calcoaceticus* complex infection in the US military health care system associated with military operations in Iraq. Clin Infect Dis 2007; 44: 1577-84.

[80] Lolans K, Rice TW, Munoz-Price LS, *et al.* Multicity outbreak of carbapenem-resistant *Acinetobacter baumannii* isolates producing the carbapenemase OXA-40. Antimicrob Agents Chemother 2006; 50: 2941-45.

[81] Turton JF, Gabriel SN, Valderrey C, *et al.* Use of sequence-based typing and multiplex PCR to identify clonal lineages of outbreak strains of *Acinetobacter baumannii*. Clin Microbiol Infect 2007; 13: 807-15.

[82] Wisplinghoff H, Hippler C, Bartual SG, *et al.* Molecular epidemiology of clinical *Acinetobacter baumannii* and *Acinetobacter* genomic species 13TU isolates using a multilocus sequencing typing scheme. Clin Microbiol Infect 2008; 14: 708-15.

[83] Diancourt L, Passet V, Nemec A, *et al.* The population structure of *Acinetobacter baumannii*: expanding multiresistant clones from an ancestral susceptible genetic pool. PLoS One 2010; 5(4): e10034.

[84] Di Popolo A, Giannouli M, Triassi M, *et al.* Molecular epidemiology of multidrug-resistant. *Acinetobacter baumannii* strains in four Mediterranean countries using a multilocus sequence typing scheme. Clin Microbiol Infect 2011; 17: 197-201.

CHAPTER 10

Prevalence, Mechanisms and Dissemination of Antimicrobial Resistance in Enteric Foodborne Bacteria

Jing Han[†], Bashar W. Shaheen[†], Steven L. Foley and Rajesh Nayak[*]

United States Food and Drug Administration, National Center for Toxicological Research, Division of Microbiology, Jefferson, Arkansas 72079, USA

Abstract: Since the early 1990s, there has been a substantial increase in the emergence and dissemination of antimicrobial resistance in foodborne and zoonotic pathogens, such as *Campylobacter, Salmonella* and *Escherichia coli* causing human infections in several developed countries. This increase has been attributed to the potential use of antimicrobials for prophylactic treatment of food animals and humans. While these drugs were successful in the treatment of most diseases in animals and humans, they have contributed to the emergence of drug-resistant bacteria. Several studies have addressed the public health significance of antimicrobial resistance in foodborne pathogens. Attention has been particularly focused on the pros and cons of short term and long term use of antimicrobial agents in food of animals for growth promotion and disease prevention. The public health risk of emergence, spread and transmission of drug-resistant foodborne pathogens in the farm-to-the-fork continuum warrants appropriate actions by both the scientific community and the regulatory agencies in advocating restrictions on the approval and use of new and existing drugs. In this chapter, we have described the prevalence, specific mechanisms (based on the class of drugs) and dissemination of antimicrobial resistance in *Campylobacter, Salmonella* and *E. coli*. These three pathogens were selected because they constitute the bulk of bacterial illnesses worldwide. The review will highlight the importance of addressing the issue of conventional and emerging drug-resistant foodborne bacteria in foods, animals and humans so that steps can be taken to minimize their spread in the environment.

Keywords: *Salmonella, Campylobacter, E. coli,* antimicrobial resistance, foodborne pathogens.

INTRODUCTION

Since the serendipitous discovery of penicillin in 1928 by Sir Alexander Fleming, the use of antibiotics (henceforth referred to as antimicrobials) had been the "magic bullet" or "panacea" for treating most diseases in humans and animals. Antimicrobials have saved millions of lives since their use in the 1940's. However, repeated use of antimicrobials has led to a simultaneous increase in the emergence of drug resistant bacteria [1-3]. Resistant pathogens can pose a significant risk to human health because drugs used in the treatment of infected individuals have less potential to be effective, resulting in limited treatment options and increased severity of the disease. The findings of the potential risk posed by antimicrobial resistant bacteria to human health have been reported by the World Health Organization [4].

The use of antimicrobials in food producing animals, such as cattle, poultry and swine, for growth promotion, therapy and disease prevention has increased the potential of human pathogens with animal reservoirs, such as *Salmonella, Campylobacter* or *E. coli*, to develop cross resistance to drugs used for treatment of human infections [5]. The treatment of antimicrobials in food producing animals can also contribute to the emergence and dissemination of drug-resistant bacteria in the food chain and the environment. Furthermore, commensal bacteria, which form the natural microflora of animals and humans, may become resistant to drugs on exposure to antimicrobials and form a reservoir of resistance genes, which in turn could be transferred to foodborne pathogens. Conversely, most zoonotic pathogens harbor

---

*Address correspondence to Rajesh Nayak: United States Food and Drug Administration, National Center for Toxicological Research, Division of Microbiology, Jefferson, Arkansas 72079, USA; Tel: 870-543-7482; Fax: 870-543-7307; Email: Rajesh.Nayak@fda.hhs.gov
[†]Authors Han and Shaheen contributed equally to the manuscript.

mobile genetic elements, such as plasmids and integrons, which can be readily transferred to other bacteria. Hence, antimicrobial resistance in bacterial pathogens is a public health concern worldwide, and a particularly important food safety issue. Because of this concern, public health agencies throughout the world have developed antimicrobial resistance monitoring systems to monitor the development and persistence of resistance in these bacteria. In the United States (US), there is the National Antimicrobial Resistance Monitoring System (NARMS), which is a collaboration of the US Department of Agriculture (USDA), Centers for Disease Control and Prevention (CDC) and the US Food and Drug Administration (FDA) [6]. Other monitoring systems include the Danish Integrated Antimicrobial Resistance Monitoring and Research Programme (DANMAP), the Japanese Veterinary Antimicrobial Resistance Monitoring System (JVARM), Canadian Integrated Program for Antimicrobial Resistance Surveillance (CIPARS) Australian Group on Antimicrobial Resistance (AGAR) and Swedish Veterinary Antimicrobial Resistance Monitoring (SVARM) [7]. These monitoring systems provide valuable sets of data to improve the understanding of the emergence and dissemination of resistance in their respective countries.

In this chapter, we present an overview of the prevalence, mechanisms of action and dissemination of antimicrobial resistance in *Campylobacter, Salmonella* and *E. coli*. While statistical data are hard to find for developing countries, according to the CDC, non typhoidal *Salmonella*, *Campylobacter* and *E. coli* constitute ~47%, 27% and 5% respectively, of the bacterial foodborne illnesses in the US [8].

CAMPYLOBACTER

Background

Since its successful isolation from stools in the 1970s, *Campylobacter*, a Gram-negative microaerobic bacterium, has emerged as a major foodborne pathogen causing human enterocolitis [9]. *Campylobacter* spp. are responsible for ~400 to 500 million cases of diarrhea each year worldwide [10]. The most commonly identified species from human infections are *C. jejuni* and *C. coli*. These species commensally inhabit the intestinal tracts of domesticated animals, poultry, wild animals and birds [11]. Transmission of *Campylobacter* to humans occurs mainly through the consumption of *Campylobacter*-contaminated food, water, or milk. Poultry is by far the most important source of *Campylobacter* for humans [9]. The main clinical symptom of campylobacteriosis in humans is acute enteritis, which is characterized by acute diarrhea with abdominal cramps, fever, headache and nausea [9, 12]. The majority of *Campylobacter* infections are mild, self-limiting and usually resolved within a few days; no specific treatment is required for most patients with *Campylobacter* enteritis. However, in case of severe infections, prolonged illness or where the patient is pregnant, young, elderly, or has compromised immunity, antimicrobial treatment is usually warranted [9, 12]. Fluoroquinolones (FQ) and macrolides are used to treat human *Campylobacter* enteritis [9]. For systemic infections, tetracyclines and aminoglycosides are the drugs of choice [12]. However, due to widespread use of these antimicrobials in both animals and humans, a rapid increase in the proportion of *Campylobacter* strains resistant to antimicrobial agents [13, 14].

Prevalence of Antimicrobial Resistance in *Campylobacter*

The emergence of FQ-resistant (FQ^R) *Campylobacter* strains in human infections was first noticed in Europe in the late 1980s after the drug approval in animal production [14, 15]. Subsequently, a rapid increase in the proportion of FQ^R *Campylobacter* strains has been reported in humans and animals [14-16]. The use of FQs in poultry and livestock is associated with increased FQ^R strains in humans [17]. In the US, ~19 to 40% of *Campylobacter* strains isolated from humans were found to be resistant to ciprofloxacin [15]. In Canada, no FQ^R *Campylobacter* strains were isolated during 1980-1986, but ciprofloxacin resistance among *C. jejuni* has dramatically increased since 1992 and reached 47% in 2001 [18, 19]. FQ resistance in *Campylobacter* strains has rapidly increased in Europe during the last decade [13, 20, 21]. In Asia, FQ resistance rates have reached more than 80% in Thailand, Taiwan, and Hong Kong [22-24]. In contrast, FQ^R in *Campylobacter* strains is much lower in Australia and New Zealand than the rest of the world [13, 25]. The lack of FQ use in veterinary medicine probably accounts for the low frequency of FQ resistance in Australia and New Zealand.

Since the 1990s, an increase in the prevalence of macrolide resistance among *C. jejuni* and *C. coli* has been reported, but the rate of macrolide resistance among other *Campylobacter* species was found to be variable [17, 26]. In Spain, resistance to macrolides has been reported to be as high as 90%, but trends for macrolide resistance show stable and low rates in Japan, Sweden and Finland [27-29]. Resistance to macrolides is more prevalent in *C. coli* than in *C. jejuni* in both human and animal isolates [16, 30].

MECHANISMS OF ANTIBIOTIC RESISTANCE IN *CAMPYLOBACTER*

Fluoroquinolones

The FQ class of antimicrobials exhibits a bactericidal mechanism of action that interferes with DNA synthesis [31]. The dominant mechanisms involved in FQ resistance are 1) target (DNA gyrase and/or topoisomerase IV) modification, resulting in reduced affinity of these enzymes for fluoroquinolones, 2) reduced intracellular antibiotic accumulation by increasing efflux activity or decreasing outer membrane permeability, 3) reduced target enzyme expression, and 4) target protection mediated by the Qnr protein, which can protect DNA gyrase from inhibition by FQs [32, 33]. Of these mechanisms, the first three are encoded by chromosomal elements, while the Qnr is encoded by a plasmid and only confers a low level of resistance to FQs [32]. In *Campylobacter*, resistance to FQs is mediated by a point mutation in the Quinolone Resistance Determining Region (QRDR) of DNA gyrase subunit A (*gyrA*) [32, 34]. No mutations in DNA gyrase subunit B (*gyrB*) have been involved in FQ resistance in *Campylobacter* [35, 36]. Unlike the FQ resistance in other enteric organisms (*e.g. Escherichia coli* and *Salmonella*), acquisition of high-level FQ resistance in *Campylobacter* does not require stepwise accumulation of point mutations in *gyrA*. Instead, a single point mutation in the QRDR of *gyrA* is sufficient to lead to clinically relevant levels of resistance to FQ antimicrobials [34, 37]. The most commonly observed mutation in FQ^R isolates of *Campylobacter* is the C257T change in the *gyrA* gene, which leads to the Thr-86-Ile substitution in the gyrase A subunit and confers high-level resistance to ciprofloxacin [34, 38]. Other mutations include Thr-86 Lys, Ala-70-Thr, and Asp-90-Asn, which are less common and only confer intermediate-level FQ resistance [16, 34]. Mutations in *parC*, which encodes topoisomerase IV in many bacteria, confer high-level FQ resistance [39]; however, other studies failed to identify the *parC/parE* gene in *Campylobacter*, which excluded the role of *parC/parE* mutations in *Campylobacter* resistance to FQ antimicrobials [36, 40]. The multidrug efflux pump also contributes to FQ resistance in *Campylobacter*. The main efflux pump involved in FQ resistance in *Campylobacter* is CmeABC, which is encoded by a three-gene operon (*cmeA*, *cmeB* and *cmeC*) located on the *Campylobacter* chromosome. CmeABC functions as an energy-dependent efflux system and contributes to both intrinsic and acquired resistance of *C. jejuni* to FQ antimicrobials [34, 41-43]. CmeABC plays a major role in ciprofloxacin resistance in *C. jejuni* by reducing the accumulation of FQs in the cells [34, 41, 43]. Thus, CmeABC functions synergistically with the *gyrA* mutations in mediating FQ-resistance. All of the known FQ-resistance determinants in *Campylobacter* are chromosomally encoded, and plasmid-mediated quinolone resistance determinants, such as *qnr, aac(6')-Ib-cr* and *qepA*, have not been reported in *Campylobacter* [38].

Macrolides

There are three mechanisms involved in macrolide resistance in bacteria: 1) modification of the antimicrobial, 2) modification of the antimicrobial target, and 3) drug efflux [38]. Target modification and active efflux are commonly associated with macrolide resistance in *Campylobacter* [38, 44]. The most common mechanisms for macrolide resistance in *C. jejuni* and *C. coli* are point mutations in domain V of the 23S rRNA target gene at positions 2074 and 2075, which correspond to positions 2058 and 2059, respectively, in *E. coli* [32, 38, 44]. So far, A2074C, A2074G, A2074T, A2075G, A2075T, and A2075C mutations have been reported in erythromycin-resistant *Campylobacter* [38]. Among these, the A2074C, A2074G, and A2075G mutations confer high-level resistance to erythromycin (MIC >128 µg/ml) in *C. jejuni* and *C. coli* [45-48]. The A2075G mutation is a predominant mutation found among the clinical- and field- isolated *C. jejuni* and *C. coli* [32, 49]. The resistance-associated mutations are usually identified in all three copies of the 23S rRNA gene in *Campylobacter* chromosome [37, 48]. However, the wild-type and mutated alleles can coexist in some isolates and evidence suggests that at least two mutated copies are required to confer macrolide resistance [44, 50]. Mutations affecting macrolide binding have also been identified in the ribosome proteins L4 and L22 [46, 51]. The G221A change in the L4 protein, which leads to the Gly-74-Asp substitution and an insertion at position 86 or 98 of the L22 protein can result in low levels of macrolide resistance in *C. jejuni* [51]. As with FQ resistance, active efflux also contributes to macrolide resistance in *Campylobacter* [38, 45, 51]. The CmeABC efflux pump contributes to both intrinsic and acquired resistance to erythromycin in *C. jejuni* and *C. coli*. CmeABC functions synergistically with target mutations to confer resistance to macrolides in *Campylobacter* [46, 51, 52].

Tetracyclines

Tetracyclines have broad spectrum activity against most bacteria, chlamydias and mycoplasmas and protozoa [53, 54]. Tetracyclines exhibit bacteriostatic activity by preventing the binding of tRNA to the A site of the 30S ribosomal subunit, and thereby inhibits protein synthesis [53]. There are four mechanisms of tetracycline resistance: 1) efflux pumps that reduce drug accumulation, 2) protection of the ribosomal binding site of tetracycline by Ribosomal Protection Proteins (RPPs), 3) drug modification, and 4) ribosomal modifications that alter the ability of the antimicrobial to bind. In *C. jejuni* and *C. coli*, tetracycline resistance is mainly conferred through the ribosomal protection protein Tet(O) and the efflux pump CmeABC [38]. The *tet(O)* gene is widespread in *Campylobacter*, and it is mainly encoded in transferable plasmids, but the gene located on the chromosome has also been reported in tetracycline-resistant *Campylobacter* strains [55]. Tetracycline-resistant *Campylobacter* strains have acquired the *tet(O)* gene from Gram-positive bacteria through Horizontal Gene Transfer (HGT) [38, 56]. Tet(O) recognizes an open A site on tetracycline-blocked ribosomal complexes and binds to the A site. This binding induces a conformational change in the region of the decoding site and results in the release of the bound tetracycline molecule. The conformational changes induced by the binding of Tet(O) can persist after the release of Tet(O), thus allowing the aa -tRNA to bind to the ribosomal A site [57]. Tet(O) functions synergistically with CmeABC to confer high-level resistance to tetracycline [41, 52]. Since up to 60% of strains may be resistant to tetracycline, care should be taken before prescribing this antimicrobial [12].

Aminoglycosides

Aminoglycosides are active against Gram-negative bacilli and often have been used in combination with other antimicrobials to broaden their spectrum of activity [58]. Aminoglycosides inhibit protein synthesis through binding to 16S rRNA of the 30S ribosomal subunit [59]. Bacterial resistance to aminoglycosides is mediated by four mechanisms: 1) reduced accumulation of the drug in the intracellular environment, usually mediated by either increased efflux activity or by decreased outer membrane permeability, 2) 16S rRNA methylation that abolishes the intermolecular contacts between 16S rRNA and the drug, 3) ribosomal mutations that result in decreased affinity for the drug, and 4) enzymatic modification of the drug [38, 60]. Based on the type of reaction they catalyze, the intracellular aminoglycoside-modifying enzymes are classified into three different groups: aminoglycoside phosphotransferases, aminoglycoside adenyltransferases, and aminoglycoside acetyltransferases [13]. The modifications mediated by these enzymes result in the loss of antibacterial activity of the drug due to reduced affinity for the bacterial ribosomal aminoacyl-tRNA site [61]. So far, only 3' aminoglycoside phosphotransferases and aminoglycoside adenyltransferase have been described in *Campylobacter*; 3' aminoglycoside phosphotransferases account for the majority of aminoglycoside-modifying enzymes in *Campylobacter* spp. [38, 62].

β-Lactams

β-lactams target penicillin-binding proteins, which interfere with peptidoglycan (bacterial cell wall) synthesis [63]. Due to the emergence of methicillin resistance [64], fourth and fifth (http://www.merck.com/mmpe/sec14/ch170/ch170c.html) generation cephalosporins have been developed to overcome the β-lactamases produced by bacteria [65]. Bacterial resistance to β-lactams is mediated either by the production of enzymes that inactivate them (β-lactamases), or by the modification of their targets in the cell wall (penicillin-binding proteins, PBPs), sometimes in conjunction with mechanisms leading to decreasing outer membrane permeability or increasing efflux activity [66]. In *Campylobacter*, resistance is mediated by both intrinsic resistance and β-lactamase production [17, 67]. In general, *Campylobacter* spp. displays inherent resistance to a large number of β-lactams

[17, 67]. *C. jejuni* can produce more than one type of β-lactamases, and resistance to ampicillin and other β-lactams has been widely reported among *Campylobacter* spp. isolated from humans and poultry [68].

EMERGENCE OF ANTIMICROBIAL RESISTANCE IN *CAMPYLOBACTER*

Targeted mutations are the major mechanisms by which *Campylobacter* spp. develop resistance to FQs and macrolides. FQ^R mutants emerge rapidly from FQ-susceptible (FQ^S) populations, when exposed to FQs [40, 69, 70]. Since there are different types of spontaneous point mutations that may occur in the QRDR region of the *gyrA* gene and different point mutations confer different levels of resistance to FQ antimicrobials, the frequencies of emergence of FQ^R GyrA mutants range from $\sim10^{-6}$ to 10^{-8} in culture media, depending on the concentrations of ciprofloxacin used on the enumerating plates [71]. The expression levels of *cmeABC* can also influences the frequencies of emergence of spontaneous FQ^R mutants [72]. In chickens infected with FQ^S *Campylobacter*, treatment with enrofloxacin resulted in the emergence of FQ^R *Campylobacter* mutants, detected in feces within 24 to 48 hours after the initiation of treatment. The FQ^R population continued to expand during treatment and eventually occupied the intestinal tract at densities as high as 10^7 CFU/g feces [34, 73]. In addition, mfd (Mutation Frequency Decline), a transcription-repair coupling factor involved in strand-specific DNA repair, promotes the emergence of FQ^R mutants in *Campylobacter* [74]. Mutation of the *mfd* gene resulted in ~100-fold reduction in the rate of spontaneous mutation to ciprofloxacin resistance, while over expression of *mfd* elevated the mutation frequency. In addition, loss of *mfd* in *C. jejuni* significantly reduced the development of fluoroquinolone-resistant *Campylobacter* in culture media or chickens treated with fluoroquinolones. Considering that FQ use in poultry promotes the development of FQ^R *Campylobacter* species in an originally FQ^S population and FQ^R *Campylobacter* can be transmitted to humans *via* the food chain, the FDA withdrew its approval of the use of sarafloxacin and enrofloxacin in poultry production in 2005 in the US (http://www.fda.gov/NewsEvents/Newsroom/PressAnnouncements/2005/ucm108467.htm).

In contrast to FQ resistance, there are several distinct features associated with erythromycin resistance development in Campylobacter. First, the spontaneous mutation rates for macrolide resistance are low in Campylobacter (approximately 10^{-10}) [44]. Second, the development of macrolide resistance in Campylobacter is very slow. Treatment of chickens with therapeutic doses of tylosin in drinking water for a short time did not select for erythromycin-resistant mutants [44, 75]. This finding is in clear contrast with the emergence of FQR mutant Campylobacter in poultry, which occurred in enrofloxacin-treated chickens rapidly after the initiation of treatment [34]. However, erythromycin-resistant mutants emerged in chickens after prolonged exposure to tylosin, which suggested that development of these Campylobacter mutants need a prolonged exposure to macrolide [44, 45]. Third, the mutants with low to intermediate MIC levels [8 to 64 µg/ml) of resistance to erythromycin harbor mutation different from those found in high-level erythromycin-resistant mutants. Low-level erythromycin-resistant Campylobacter strains have mutations in the L4 and L22 proteins, which are not stable in the absence of macrolides or no detectable mutations [44, 45]. The high-level erythromycin resistant mutants (MIC $\geq$ 512 µg/ml) usually harbor a specific point mutation in the 23S rRNA gene, and most of these 23S rRNA mutations can be stably maintained in the absence of macrolides [44, 45]. Fourth, although macrolide resistance is generally more prevalent in C. coli isolates than in C. jejuni isolates, studies have shown there is no significant difference in the frequencies of emergence of erythromycin-resistant mutants between these two strains, suggesting that *C. coli* is not intrinsically more mutable then C. jejuni with regard to developing macrolide resistance [44].

TRANSFER OF ANTIMICROBIAL RESISTANCE DETERMINANTS IN *CAMPYLOBACTER*

Beside mutation-based antimicrobial resistance mechanisms, Horizontal Gene Transfer (HGT), which is mediated by transformation, conjugation and transduction, is another mechanism that is used by bacteria to acquire antimicrobial-resistance determinants [17]. All three HGT mechanisms occur and show strain-to-strain variation in *Campylobacter* [17]. In *Campylobacter*, conjugation plays a major role in the transfer of plasmid-mediated resistance. Multiple plasmids that can be transmitted by conjugation have been reported, and many of these conjugative plasmids carry genes mediating resistance to tetracyclines and aminoglycosides [17, 76]. Transfer of the *tetO* gene occurs rapidly between *C. jejuni* strains in the digestive tract of chickens in the absence of antimicrobial selection pressure, which indicated that conjugation may be responsible for the high prevalence of conjugative *tetO* plasmids in *Campylobacter* and contribute to the spread of tetracycline resistance [17, 77]. In *Campylobacter*, *in vitro* and *in vivo* studies have shown the transfer of genes encoding antimicrobial-modifying enzymes, and point mutations responsible for FQ and macrolide resistance occur by natural transformation [17, 78]. Transduction is the process by which DNA is transferred from one bacterium to another by a virus (bacteriophage). Several *Campylobacter*-infecting bacteriophages have been isolated from different *Campylobacter* species and various other sources [79]; however the exact role of these *Campylobacter*-infecting bacteriophages in transmitting antimicrobial resistance determinants has not yet been determined.

SALMONELLA

Background

Salmonellosis is a major problem worldwide. Nearly 1.6 million infections occur each year in the US and cost the economy ~14.6 billion dollars [80]. These costs are associated with loss of work, medical care, and loss of life. According to the CDC, for every reported case of salmonellosis in the US, there are 38 cases that are unreported [81]. In 2006, there were 40,666 reported cases, up from a total of 31,876 reported in 2002 [82, 83]. Nearly 95% of human cases of salmonellosis are associated with the ingestion of contaminated foods [81].

Salmonellosis symptoms can range from mild gastroenteritis to more severe manifestations, such as typhoid fever or bacteremia [84]. Salmonellosis is accompanied by diarrhea, abdominal cramps, vomiting, and fever. Typically, these symptoms develop 6 to 72 hours following *Salmonella* ingestion [85, 86] and are self-limiting. In a small percentage of cases more severe disease occurs, which includes septicemia and invasive infections of organs and tissues [87]. People at the age extremes, either very young or old, or who are immuno-compromised by underlying disease, are most susceptible to the more severe disease manifestations. The more severe cases of salmonellosis typically require antimicrobial therapy [88], for which, the recommended drugs of choice are fluoroquinolones or ceftriaxone. For pediatric patients, fluoroquinolones are not approved due to concerns about connective tissue damage; thus, ceftriaxone is most important for treatment in this age group [89].

Several *Salmonella* serotypes in the US are capable of causing human infections. The most common serovars are Typhimurium, Enteritidis, Newport, Heidelberg and Javiana [90]. Elsewhere other serovars are predominantly associated with human disease, for example, in the European Union, Enteritidis is the most common serovar and in parts of Asia, Choleraesuis is one of the top serovars [91-93]. A number of recent high profile *Salmonella* outbreaks have been associated with nut products, fresh produce and spices [94]; however, traditionally salmonellosis cases have most often been attributed to the consumption of contaminated meat, poultry, and eggs [88, 95]. In 2010, a multi state outbreak of *Salmonella* Enteritidis has been reported by the CDC that infected nearly half a billion eggs in the US (http://www.cdc.gov/salmonella/enteritidis/). When the most common serovars from human infections are compared to those from food animal sources, there is significant commonality [90]. For example, in 2006, serovar Typhimurium was the most commonly identified serovar isolated from ill humans and swine and the top six most common serovars from each of the other major food animal species (cattle, chickens and turkeys). One of the trends over the last half century in countries such as the US is that consumers have increased their consumption of meat and poultry products as well as fresh produce items, all of which have been implicated in *Salmonella* outbreaks. For example, the average consumer in the US has increased consumption of poultry products by >four-fold since 1950, while increase in beef and pork has been increased by approximately 25% [96]. Additionally, since 1985, there has been a five-fold increase in leaf lettuce and a 40% increase in fresh tomatoes available for consumption, according to data from the USDA (http://www.ers.usda.gov/data/foodconsumption/FoodGuideIndex.htm#fruit). An increase in consumption of these food items comes with an increased *Salmonella* exposure potential, unless improved safety standards are put in place. Additionally, a number of surveillance and outbreak response systems, such as the PulseNet program have been developed to rapidly respond to a disease outbreak when it occurs and to limit future exposure of consumers to contaminated foods [97, 98].

Prevalence of Antimicrobial Resistance in *Salmonella*

Since severe cases of salmonellosis require antimicrobial therapy for resolution, antimicrobial resistance is a major concern in *Salmonella*. In the US, the NARMS program carries out susceptibility testing on *Salmonella* isolates for 15 drugs, including amikacin, amoxicillin/clavulanic acid, ampicillin, cefoxitin, ceftiofur, ceftriaxone, chloramphenicol, ciprofloxacin, gentamicin, kanamycin, nalidixic acid, streptomycin, sulfamethoxazole, tetracycline, and trimethoprim/sulfamethoxazole [99]. The NARMS 2006 Executive Report outlines the susceptibility results for *Salmonella* isolates collected from veterinary sources, retail meats and human patients [100]. For non-Typhi *Salmonella* isolates collected from humans in 2006, 19.8% of the isolates were resistant to at least one antimicrobial agent, which is down from a high of 33.8% in 1996 [100]. The antimicrobials with the highest percentage of resistant isolates include tetracyclines (13.4%), sulfonamides (12.0%), ampicillin (10.9%) or streptomycin (10.7%). These percentages are down significantly from 1996, in which 22.4% of isolates were resistant to tetracyclines, 20.3% to sulfonamides, 20.7% to ampicillin, and 20.6% to streptomycin. In contrast, resistance to some of the drugs has increased over that time period; these include amoxicillin/clavulanic acid (1.1% in 1996 to 3.7% in 2006), ceftriaxone (0% to 0.2%), ceftiofur (0.2% to 3.6%) and nalidixic acid (0.4% to 2.7%) [100].

For *Salmonella* isolates collected as part of the food animal side of the NARMS program, 47% of the isolates were resistant to at least one antimicrobial [100]. As with *Salmonella* from humans, the highest percentage of resistance was observed for ampicillin, streptomycin, sulfonamides and tetracyclines. When the resistance phenotypes were compared among the different food animal sources, some differences were observed [100]. Overall resistance was lower in isolates from chickens and cattle. This phenomenon is likely due, at least in part, to the predominant serovars of isolates from the different animal species. For example, *S. Enteritidis* was the most commonly detected serovar from chickens and in general *S. Enteritidis* isolates display less antimicrobial resistance than other predominant serovars from turkey and swine (Hadar, Heidelberg and Anatum). For *Salmonella* isolates collected as part of the retail meats wing of NARMS, ~70% were resistant to at least one antimicrobial [100]. This higher level of resistance is likely due in part to the serovars most commonly isolated from the different meats (chicken breast, ground turkey, ground beef, and pork chops). The most commonly detected serovars were Heidelberg and Kentucky, each of which is known to carry drug resistance plasmids [101, 102]. As observed for the *Salmonella* strains from human sources, there was an increase in resistance to β-lactams: amoxicillin/clavulanic acid, ceftiofur and ceftriaxone from 1997 (first year of veterinary NARMS data) to 2006 [100]. These increases are a concern because the desired use of ceftriaxone to treat severe *Salmonella* infections in children.

Mechanisms of Antimicrobial Resistance in *Salmonella*

While a wide range of genes and their products are associated with resistance in *Salmonella* and related pathogens, most resistance is attributed to one of the following mechanisms: the production of drug-inactivating enzymes, activation of antimicrobial efflux pumps and competitive inhibition of biochemical pathways [103]. Some of the most common antimicrobial resistance gene classes found in *Salmonella* strains with resistance to streptomycin include *aadA* (encodes an aminoglycoside adenyltransferase) and *str* (aminoglycoside phosphoryltranferase), to gentamicin including *aadB* (aminoglycoside adenyltransferase) and *aacC* (aminoglycoside acetyltransferase), to kanamycin (*aphA*, aminoglycoside phosphoryltranferase), to the penicillins (*bla*$_{tem}$, β-lactamase), to the extended spectrum β-lactams by *bla*$_{cmy}$ (AmpC β-lactamase), to chloramphenicol by *cat* (chloramphenicol acetyltransferase) and *floR* (efflux pump), to trimethoprim (*dfrA*, dihydrofolate reductase competitive inhibitor), to the sulfonamides (*sul,* dihydropteroate synthase inhibitor), and to the tetracyclines by the *tet* genes (most associated with efflux pumps).

Aminoglycosides

Aminoglycosides are typically not utilized for treatment against *Salmonella* [54]. The mechanisms of resistance to aminoglycosides arise from decreased drug uptake or the modification of drug and ribosomal targets of the drug [104]. The resistance can be mediated by aminoglycoside-modifying enzymes [105, 106]. Three aminoglycoside-modifying enzymes have been identified, including acetyltransferases, phosphotransferases, and nucleotidyltransferases [104]. Aminoglycoside acetyltransferases (encoded by *aac*) cause changes in the aminoglycoside amino groups [104] and are found either in genomic islands [107] or associated with mobile genetic elements such as integrons [108] and plasmids [109]. The aminoglycoside acetyltransferases confer resistance to gentamicin, tobramycin, and kanamycin [59]. Aminoglycoside phosphotransferases cause phosphorylation of specific aminoglycoside hydroxyl groups [59, 104]. Aminoglycoside phosphotransferases encoded by *strA* and *strB*, respectively [104, 110], confer resistance to streptomycin [59]. Aminoglycoside nucleotidyltransferases, encoded by *aad*, confer resistance to streptomycin in *Salmonella* isolates [59, 104]. The *aadB* gene, which is found in serotype Typhimurium [111], confers resistance to gentamicin and tobramycin [59]. Integrons play an important role in mediating the transfer of genes encoded for aminoglycoside nucleotidyltransferases [111].

β-Lactams

This drug class is broadly represented by the penicillins, cephalosporins and carbapenems. There have been four generations of cephalosporins, developed in part to counteract resistance and increase the spectrums of activity [65]. The 1st and 2nd generations of cephalosporins were ineffective against *Salmonella* [54]. Resistance to carbapenems (imipenem), which has broad spectrum activity against both Gram-negative and Gram-positive bacteria [54], was reported in *Salmonella* isolates [112, 113]. One of the mechanisms associated with the increase in the resistance to β-lactam drugs, such as ampicillin, cefoxitin, and other cephalosporins (cephalothin, ceftriaxone, and cefazolin), is through a decrease in the expression of outer membrane proteins (*i.e.*, OmpC and OmpF) [114, 115]. However, the most common mechanism of resistance to β-lactams in *Salmonella* is due to the production of β-lactamases, which hydrolyze the β-lactam ring. Resistance in *Salmonella* is typically plasmid-mediated, unlike other bacterial species, where resistance is often encoded by the chromosomal genes [54, 106, 116]. Many β-lactamases have been characterized in *Salmonella* [117].

Plasmid mediated β-lactam resistance has been described against penicillins, early generation cephalosporins, and carbapenems, with the TEM β-lactamases being the most widespread among *Salmonella* isolates [54]. The bla_{TEM-1} and bla_{TEM-52} genes are commonly found in *Salmonella* serotypes [118, 119]. Cefotaximases (CTX-M), which confer resistance to ampicillin and cephalosporins, have also been identified in many *Salmonella* serotypes [120]. Other plasmid mediated β-lactamases, such as AmpC (bla_{CMY}), were found in *Salmonella* and confer resistance to cephalosporins, such as cefoxitin and ceftiofur [121, 122]. Furthermore, bla_{CMY-2}, which confers resistance to ceftiofur [122, 123], is another plasmid mediated extended spectrum cephalosporin. The appearance and dissemination of bla_{CMY-2} is worrisome because it encodes reduced susceptibility to ceftriaxone, which is important for the treatment of *Salmonella* infections in children [122]. The bla_{CMY-2} gene has been reported in serotypes Typhimurium, Agona and Newport [123, 124]. Metallo β-lactamases, which confer resistance to carbapenems, appear to be uncommon in *Salmonella* [54]. In addition, the gene bla_{OXA-1}, which confers resistance to cloxacillin and methicillin, was reported in Paratyphi [125] and bla_{OXA-30} was reported in Muenchen and Typhimurium [126, 127].

Quinolones

Nalidixic acid was first used to treat bacterial infections in 1962 [54]. High resistance to quinolones is uncommon in *Salmonella* [128, 129]. The most common mechanism of resistance to fluoroquinolones in *Salmonella* is attributed to mutations in the quinolone resistance determining regions of DNA gyrase and topoisomerase IV [130]. In addition, mutations in the regulatory genes (*e.g.*, *marRAB*) increase the expression of the AcrAB-TolC efflux system, and consequently increase the level of resistance to fluoroquinolones [131, 132]. The high level of resistance to fluoroquinolones in *Salmonella* is attributed to combined mechanisms or mutations [133, 134]. Plasmid mediated quinolone resistance is encoded by *qnr* genes that confer resistance through binding DNA gyrase and protecting it from quinolone inhibition [135]. These genes have been documented in other bacterial species, such as *E. coli* [136], *Klebsiella pneumoniae* [137], and *Salmonella* species [138]. Other resistance determinants have been found in the same plasmids carrying *qnr*; implicating the importance of horizontal transfer of antimicrobial resistance genes and the emergence of multidrug resistance phenotypes [135].

Tetracyclines

The major mechanism of resistance to tetracycline in *Salmonella* is due to specific energy dependent efflux pump, which decreases the concentration of the drug inside the cell [53]. Many genes confer resistance to tetracycline and oxytetracycline in *Salmonella*, including *tet(A), tet(B), tet(C), tet(D), tet(G)* and *tet(H)* [53, 139, 140]. The resistances mediated by these genes are carried in mobile genetic elements, such as *Salmonella* genomic island 1, integrons, and plasmids, therefore, *Salmonella* isolates often express multidrug resistance phenotypes [139, 141, 142]. Both *tet(A)* and *tet(B)* have been detected in several *Salmonella* serotypes [118, 142].

Sulfonamides and Trimethoprim

Both sulfonamides and trimethoprim have a bacteriostatic mechanism of action through inhibition of tetrahydrofolic acid synthesis [143]. Sulfonamides inhibit dihydropteroate synthetase (DHPS), whereas trimethoprim inhibits dihydrofolate reductase (DHFR) [143]. The resistance to sulfonamides in *Salmonella* isolates is typically caused by the presence of a *sul* gene [54, 144]. The *sul1* gene is carried on mobile genetic elements, such as class 1 integrons or plasmids [145] and *Salmonella* genomic island variants [146]. The *sul2* gene is carried on plasmids [144], and is found in serotypes Agona, Enteritidis, and Typhimurium [118]. The mechanism of resistance to trimethoprim is due to the increased expression of DHFR that does not bind trimethoprim [54]. Many variants of *dhfr* and *dfr* genes have been identified, including *dhfr1, dfrA1,* and *dhfr12* [118, 132, 147]. These genes were found in integron gene cassettes along with *sul1* and *sul3* [144], plasmids [109, 148] and on *Salmonella* genomic islands [147].

Phenicols

Phenicols, which include chloramphenicol and florfenicol, act by preventing peptide bond formation through binding to the peptidyltransferase of the 50S ribosomal unit [149]. Chloramphenicol has broad spectrum activity against Gram-positive and Gram-negative bacteria [54, 149]. However, its toxicity, related to bone marrow damage and aplastic anemia, and development of resistance limit its use [54, 150]. In *Salmonella,* chloramphenicol resistance is mediated by enzymatic inactivation through chloramphenicol *O*-acetyltransferase (*cat1* and *cat2*) and efflux pump system [54, 149]. The efflux pump system in *Salmonella* is mediated by *cmlA* [125] and *floR* genes [151]. The *floR* gene is associated with mobile genetic elements such as plasmids [124], and has been identified in *Salmonella* genomic islands [147].

Spread of Antimicrobial Resistance in *Salmonella*

An important mechanism that facilitates the spread of antimicrobial resistance is plasmid-mediated transfer of antimicrobial resistance genes among *Salmonella* and related species. In recent years, a number of studies that have examined plasmid-associated antimicrobial resistance in *Salmonella*, utilizing whole plasmid DNA sequencing and conjugation experiments to examine resistance transfer. Zhao *et al.* (2003) reported that plasmids from multi-drug resistant *S.* Newport isolates were transferred into susceptible recipient bacteria [152]. Likewise, other researchers have demonstrated that multidrug resistance plasmids from different strains of *S. Heidelberg* were transferred into other *Salmonella* isolates [102, 153]. These findings are concerning because the plasmids were transferred into Heidelberg, Typhimurium and Dublin, which are some of the most frequent serovars associated with development of invasive infections, which typically require antimicrobial therapy for resolution [154].

In addition to conjugation studies, a number of multi-drug resistance plasmids have been sequenced, such as a plasmid from an MDR strain of *S.* Newport [155]. Sequencing revealed that the plasmid had multiple genes encoding resistance to different antimicrobials, including sulfonamides, chloramphenicol, tetracyclines, aminoglycosides, quaternary ammonium compounds, β-lactams and mercury [155]. The authors utilized sets of PCR primers designed for the different regions of the plasmid to screen additional multi-drug resistant enteric pathogens and found similar incompatibility group A/C plasmids in a wide range of *Salmonella* serovars and other species of enteric pathogens [155]. Chiu *et al.* (2005) reported on the complete sequence of a resistance plasmid from *S. Choleraesuis* that contained genes encoding resistance to trimethoprim, sulfonamides, chloramphenicol, ampicillin, streptomycin, tetracycline, kanamycin, streptothricin, macrolides, mercury, ethidium bromide and quaternary ammonium compounds [156].

Many resistance genes in plasmids and on the chromosome are associated with integrons. Integrons are mobile genetic elements that can be integrated into the bacterial chromosome or larger mobile elements, such as plasmids [157]. The most common integrons associated with antimicrobial resistance are the class 1 integrons, which contain genes encoding an integrase, recombination site, and a gene cassette where the resistance determinants are incorporated [158, 159]. Adjacent to the gene cassette are *qacEΔ* and *sul1* genes that encode quaternary ammonium compound and sulfonamide resistance [158]. These mobile integrons have been shown to be widely disseminated in the bacterial population, thus raising concern for future resistance gene transfer among pathogens [157].

Escherichia coli

Background

E. coli is predominantly found in the gastrointestinal tracts of healthy animals and humans, and generally plays a beneficial role to the host [160]. However, pathogenic *E. coli* strains cause diseases in animals and humans. There are over 700 different serotypes of *E. coli* based on their serological antigenic groups, such as O somatic, F fimbrial, K capsular, and H flagellar antigens [161]. Certain serotypes have been found to be associated with diarrheal diseases in animals [162]. Currently, seven classes of pathogenic *E. coli* are identified: enterotoxigenic *E. coli* (ETEC), enteropathogenic *E. coli* (EPEC), enterohemorrhagic *E. coli* (EHEC), enteroinvasive *E. coli* (EIEC), diffuse-adhering *E. coli* (DAEC), necrotoxigenic *E. coli* (NTEC), and enteroaggregative *E. coli* (EAEC) [163].

E. coli strains cause colibacillosis, colisepticemia and colibacillary toxemia in young poultry, pigs, ruminants, dogs, cats and horses [164], and urinary tract infections, pyometra, and mastitis in adult animals [165, 166]. Antimicrobials have been prescribed to treat infections caused by *E. coli*. In veterinary medicine, antimicrobial agents were also used to prevent disease-associated economic losses or as growth promoters in food animals. As a result of extensive use of antimicrobials, drug resistance has emerged and caused high mortality in humans and economic losses due to therapeutic failure in many countries [167]. In addition, antimicrobial drug resistance is a global health concern due to the potential transfer/dissemination of resistant organisms between humans and animals [168].

Prevalence of Antimicrobial Resistance in *E. coli*

Poultry

E. coli is a major cause of colibacillosis-associated morbidity and mortality in many countries [169, 170]. The disease is caused by avian pathogenic *E. coli* (APEC) and attributed to virulence factors, such as the increased serum survival protein (Iss), K1 capsule and type 1 and P fimbriae [169, 170]. Studies have reported an increase in *E. coli* resistance to antimicrobial agents used to treat colibacillosis [118, 171-173]. APEC strains have been found to be resistant to ampicillin, nalidixic acid, enrofloxacin, streptomycin, tetracycline, sulfonamides, kanamycin and tetracycline in several countries [174, 175]. Antimicrobial resistance was also observed among *E. coli* isolates from turkeys. One study reported a high incidence of resistance to ciprofloxacin, flumequine, and enrofloxacin in turkeys and broilers compared to the laying-hen population [176]. Similarly, greater resistance to sulfanomides, trimethoprim and nalidixic acid was observed among *E. coli* isolates from turkeys than those isolated from chickens [172]. Nearly 49%, 48%, and 40% of *E. coli* O78:K89 isolates recovered from turkeys were resistant to nalidixic acid, flumequine and enrofloxacin, respectively [177]. In the US, a trend of increased resistance among APEC to fluoroquinolones was observed from 1996 to 1999 [151]. These authors reported that this increase was associated with the approval of fluoroquinolone use to treat avian *E. coli* infections between 1995 and 1996 [151]. Resistance of *E. coli* to β-lactams and extended spectrum β-lactams has also been recognized in many countries. In Belgium, researchers found ~60% of *E. coli* isolates from broiler cloacal swabs were resistant to ceftiofur [178]. *E. coli* recovered from shell eggs in the US were found to be resistant to tetracycline [179], while those isolated from laying hens exhibited resistance to tetracycline and sulfonamides (26%) and streptomycin [17%) [166].

Food Animals

In calves, *E. coli* is the major cause of calf scours, associated with high mortality and diarrhea [180, 181]. The disease is caused by ETEC harboring virulence genes F5 (K99), heat-stable (STs or STb) and/or heat-labile (LT) enterotoxins [180, 181]. Antimicrobial resistance has been reported in ruminants as a result of using drugs to treat infections caused by *E. coli* [182]. *E. coli* strains recovered from healthy fecal samples of calves in UK were resistant to tetracycline, sulfonamides, streptomycin, ampicillin, neomycin and chloramphenicol [182]. The authors attributed the emergence of resistance to the use of antimicrobials as feed additives [182]. A study of *E. coli* from Danish piglets and calves showed multi drug resistance to sulfonamides, streptomycin, tetracycline and ampicillin [183]. In the UK, *E. coli* resistance to apramycin increased from 1982 to 1994 [184]; this increase coincided with the approval of this drug for use in veterinary medicine in 1980 [184]. Similar patterns of resistance to tetracycline, streptomycin and sulfamethoxazole among bovine *E. coli* were observed in the US [185]. ETEC is one of the major causes of diarrhea in neonatal and young pigs [186]. To control morbidity and mortality associated with the disease, antimicrobials have been prescribed to treat *E. coli* infections [187]. *E. coli* isolated from fecal and diarrheal samples in pigs exhibited resistance to ampicillin, trimethoprim, neomycin, tetracycline, streptomycin, and sulfonamide [187]. An investigation by the FDA indicated that fecal *E. coli* from swine, dairy, calves and cattle displayed a higher prevalence of resistance in herds receiving antimicrobials as feed additives than in those without drug treatment [188]. *E. coli* causes bovine mastitis by colonizing the udder [189]. *E. coli* isolates from coliform mastitis were resistant to tetracycline and dihydrostreptomycin [190]. In the US, *E. coli* isolates from milk samples of suspected bovine mastitis were resistant to ampicillin and cephalothin [165]. A larger study conducted from 1994 to 2001 in Wisconsin showed that *E. coli* isolates were resistant to tetracycline (37%), cephalothin (28%), ampicillin (22%) and sulfisoxazole (16%) [191].

Companion Animals

E. coli is a common cause of urinary tract infection and pyometra in dogs and cats [192-195]. Several antimicrobials have been indicated to treat these infections in companion animals [196]. An early report indicated that *E. coli* isolates from dogs and cats with urinary tract infection exhibited resistance to streptomycin, tetracycline, ampicillin, chloramphenicol, and sulfa drugs [197]. One of the largest investigations in the UK reported an increase in the trend of resistance to streptomycin and amoxicillin-clavulanic acid among *E. coli* isolates from 1989 to 1997 [198]. A study in the US between 1990 and 1998 showed that *E. coli* isolates exhibited resistance towards amoxicillin, carbencillin, and cephalothin [199]. Multidrug resistant *E. coli* from dogs with nocosomial infections exhibited resistance to extended spectrum β-lactams [166, 193, 200]. The emergence of resistance to fluoroquinolones has increased especially after the approval of drugs to treat infections in companion animals [196, 201].

Humans

In humans, *E. coli* cause a range of infections such as diarrhea, urinary tract infection, meningitis, peritonitis, septicemia, and pneumonia [173]. Isolates of *E. coli* from meat products have been associated with intestinal pathogenic *E. coli* and extra-intestinal infections (*e.g.* urinary tract infections) [202-205]. The diseases caused by *E. coli* in humans vary from uncomplicated urinary tract infection to serious septicemic disease. Due to the extensive use of antimicrobial agents in food animal production, *E. coli* isolates from food animals frequently carry resistance genes and confer resistance to critically important drugs used to treat human diseases. Some antimicrobial agents, such as cephalosporins (third and fourth generation), quinolones, and aminoglycosides, are important in treating *E. coli* infections in humans [173]. The emergence of *E. coli* strains expressing the CTX-M-type extended-spectrum β-lactamases has been reported worldwide and in the US [206-208]. The alternative uses of antimicrobials to treat community acquired urinary tract infections have led to the emergence of resistance to other drugs [15]. For example, *E. coli* strains resistant to trimethoprim-sulfamethoxazole [209] and increased resistance to fluoroquinolones (ciprofloxacin and levofloxacin) have been described in community-acquired *E. coli* isolates [210] . Fluoroquinolone-resistant *E. coli* strains also expressed co-resistance to cephalosporins [210]. One study suggests that the emergence of fluoroquinolone-resistant *E. coli* isolates from children was derived from the use of fluoroquinolones in food animals [211].

Mechanisms of Antimicrobial Resistance in *E. coli*

β-Lactams

In *E. coli*, chromosomally encoded AmpC-type β-lactamases or cephalosporinases are constitutively expressed [212]. Other β-lactamases, such as those encoded by *ampD, ampE* and *ampG* are also present in *E. coli* [213]. Mutations in the promoter region of *ampC* have been identified to confer high resistance to penicillins, monobactams and cephalosporins (including cephamycins and oxyimino cephalosporins) among clinical *E. coli* isolates from humans and animals [214]. In addition, the plasmid-mediated genes encoding CMY β-lactamases (cephamycinases), which hydrolyze cephalosporins, are widely distributed among *E. coli* isolates [135]. These genes were found to be associated with transposons and integrons, and their dissemination is common among *E. coli* isolates from food animals [153, 215, 216]. ESBLs (TEM, SHV, OXA and CTX-M) are other plasmid mediated β-lactamases predominant in *E. coli*. The CTX-M family, hydrolyzing cefotaxime, confers high level resistance to aminopenicillins, carboxypenicillins, ureidopenicillins, and multiple generations of cephalosporins [217]. CTX-M-14 was found in *E. coli* from fecal samples of healthy chickens and conferred resistance to cefotaxime, ceftazidime, ceftriaxone and penicillins [218]. Other CTX-M enzymes, such as CTX-M-1, CTX-M-2, CTX-M-3, CTX-M-9, CTX-M-14 or CTX-M-28 have been reported in *E. coli* isolates from animal and meat products in different countries [67].

Fluoroquinolones

In *E. coli,* a substitution at codons 83 or 87 alters the binding of quinolones at the *gyrA* site [219, 220]. In addition, double mutations in *gyrA* and/or the topoisomerase IV genes (*parC* or *parE*) confer a higher level of resistance to fluoroquinolone compared to a single mutation [221-223]. The most common mutation in veterinary *E. coli* isolates occurs at Ser83, which involves a substitution of serine with leucine [177, 224]. An additional mutation at Asp87 confers a higher level of resistance to fluoroquinolones [225]. Mutations in ParC were found only in *E. coli* isolates with MIC ≥ 0.5 mg/L [226, 227], and these mutations lead to substitutions at Ser80 and Glu84 [222]. Beside mutations in gyrase/topoisomerase IV gene, studies suggested that the Resistance Nodulation Division (RND) system mediated by the AcrAB efflux pump plays an important role in resistance to fluoroquinolones [228]. Plasmid mediated quinolone resistance (PMQR) is another mechanism that confers resistance to fluoroquinolones [229]. Several genes, including *qnr, aac (6')-Ib-cr,* and a novel efflux pump gene, *qepA,* have been identified [229]. The PMQR in *E. coli* has been identified in many countries, including the US [137, 230].

Tetracyclines

Resistance to tetracycline in *E. coli* is mediated by Tet proteins belonging to the Major Facilitator Superfamily (MFS) [231]. Seven different *tet* efflux genes have been identified in *E. coli,* including *tet*(A), *tet*(B), *tet*(C), *tet*(D), *tet*(E), *tet*(I) and *tet*(Y) [53]. All the *tet* efflux genes encode for efflux proteins that decrease the intracellular concentration of tetracycline and protect the ribosomes [53]. The *tet*(B) gene confers resistance to both tetracycline and minocycline [232]. Tetracycline is a substrate of the RND efflux system in *E. coli* [233], which confers resistance to multiple drugs [228, 234]. Mutations in the chromosomal *marR* region have also been associated with increased *E. coli* resistance to tetracycline. The over-expression of transcription activator MarA decreased the accumulation of tetracycline (by increasing the expression of OmpF porin), and increased the expression of the AcrAB system in *E. coli,* thereby conferring a multi-drug resistant phenotype [235, 236].

Chloramphenicols

Chloramphenicol acetyltransferases (CATs) cause structural modification of the drug that confers resistance to chloramphenicols [237]. Two types of CATs (A and B) have been identified in a wide variety of bacteria [238]. The *cat* gene of group A-1 was first identified in *E. coli* transposon Tn9 [239], whereas the *catB2* gene was identified in transposon Tn2424 [240]. Other integron-based *catB* genes, such as *catB3-catB6 and catB8,* encode multidrug resistance in *E. coli* [136, 241, 242]. *E. coli* isolates carrying the *cmlA* gene demonstrate resistance to chloramphenicol (MIC ≥ 32 μg/ml) [181, 243]. *E. coli* isolates from cattle carrying the *floR* gene, which has been found on plasmids, and in the chromosome of *E. coli* from food animals [181, 243, 244], exhibited higher MIC values (≥616 µg/ml) to chloramphenicol [181, 243]. The multidrug efflux system also confers resistance to chloramphenicol. However, the level of resistance conferred by this mechanism is lower than those mediated by specific efflux pumps [149]. Over-expression of this system or mutations in the regulatory genes increased the chloramphenicol MIC values (16 to 32 µg/ml) in *E. coli* above the resistance breakpoint [245, 246].

Sulfonamides and Trimethoprim

Sulfonamide resistance in *E. coli* is caused by *sul*1 and *sul*2, encoding dihydropteroate synthases [247]. These genes are associated with integrons or plasmids. Resistance to trimethoprim in *E. coli* is because of the *dfr* genes, encoding for dihydrofolate reductase. The *dfr* genes are disseminated among *E. coli* due to their association with Class 1 and 2 integrons or plasmids [248].

Aminoglycosides

The efflux pump, AcrD, confers resistance to aminoglycosides [249]. One study showed that inactivation of the gene encoding the AcrD protein in *E. coli* caused an increase in susceptibility to aminoglycosides [250]. Enzymatic drug modification is another mechanism of resistance to aminoglycosides in *E. coli* [251]. The following aminoglycoside modifying enzymes have been identified in *E. coli*: N-acetyltransferases (AAC), O-adenyltransferases and O-phosphotransferases [104]. The gene encoding for AAC (3)-IV was identified in *E. coli* from human and animal sources in Belgium [252]. Nearly 83% and 75% of aminoglycoside resistance in *E.coli* strains from humans and food-producing animals, respectively, was encoded by the *aacC2* gene [253]. Resistance was also mediated by transferable plasmids of multiple incompatibility groups, such as IncI1, IncF and IncN [253].

Spread of Antimicrobial Resistance in *E. coli*

The dissemination of antimicrobial resistance genes in *E. coli* is mediated through plasmids, transposons, genomic islands or integrons and natural transformation [254]. For example, the IncP-1 β resistance plasmid R751 in *E. coli* confers resistance to trimethoprim (*dhfrIIc*) and quaternary ammonium compounds (*qacE*) [255]. A study demonstrated that gentamicin- and sulfonamide-resistant *E. coli* isolates from pigs colonized 8 of 9 humans for at least 2 weeks without consumption of antimicrobials for a month during the study [173]. The intestine can provide a favorable environment for dissemination of antimicrobial resistance genes in *E. coli* [256, 257]. The commensal human gastrointestinal microflora can act as a reservoir of antimicrobial resistance genes [258]. Using *in vivo* intestinal models, studies have demonstrated the transferability of tetracycline resistance genes in *E. coli* from animals to humans [203, 205, 257]. A study in the US found similar antimicrobial resistance profiles between resistant isolates of *E. coli* from humans and poultry [259]. The authors suggested that antimicrobial-resistant *E. coli* isolates from human feces could originate from poultry [259]. The risk of transmission of antimicrobial resistant *E. coli* between companion animals and humans is also a significant public health concern.

CONCLUDING REMARKS

The rapid increase in antimicrobial-resistant zoonotic pathogens and patients with resistant infections has become a major public health issue due to the potential treatment failure, and thus a challenge for food safety and public health professionals. Furthermore, the economic burden in terms of health care and productivity costs of treating diseases caused by drug-resistant pathogens can be difficult to surmount. While steps have been taken worldwide to address the issue of antimicrobial resistance, there is more that can be done. Since the late 1990's, the WHO and the US National Academy of Science's Institute of Medicine have recommended discontinuing the use of growth promoters that have been used in human medicine [3]. The European Union and Denmark have banned the used of growth promoters in animal agriculture [3, 260]. Some studies have shown that the ban on growth promoters had limited ill effect on the health of animals (broilers and pigs) or farmers' profits in Denmark (http://www.who.int/gfn/en/Expertsreportgrowthpromoterdenmark.pdf).

We have highlighted the following points to be considered when examining ways to confront antimicrobial resistance in enteric pathogens:

1. Developing guidelines (FDA Guidance #209) for prudent use of antimicrobials in food animals and infection control in humans could be the first step toward limiting the emergence and spread of multi drug resistant pathogens (http://www.fda.gov/downloads/Animal Veterinary/GuidanceComplianceEnforcement/GuidanceforIndustry/UCM216936.pdf).

2. Developing rapid detection technologies for drug resistance would help prevent delays by physicians in identifying the most appropriate antimicrobials for treating human diseases, thereby allowing for the most appropriate treatment to minimize resistance development.

3. Implementing surveillance programs, such as NARMS, WHO Advisory Group on Integrated Surveillance of Antimicrobial Resistance (AGISAR) and European Antimicrobial Resistance Surveillance System (EARSS) to monitor the emergence, spread and transmission of antimicrobial resistant pathogens in foods, animals and humans.

4. Improving partnerships between academia, industry, veterinary and medical communities and public health/governmental agencies will be critical to identify knowledge gaps (*i.e.* risk assessment, surveillance data in the developing countries), leverage resources and develop risk management strategies for use of existing and new drugs approved for humans and animals.

5. Developing intervention strategies at the pre- and post harvest stages of production to reduce and/or eliminate the resistant pathogens.

6. Conducting research to identify the mechanisms by which bacteria develop drug resistance and identify tools to disrupt mechanisms of resistance without negatively affecting commensal bacteria.

Antimicrobial resistance in enteric pathogens is an issue that warrants considerable attention. Humans have been in a constant battle with bacteria for survival, and pathogens have found ways to evolve and counteract the antimicrobials that have been used against them. There is a need to researching novel targets and strategies to develop newer drugs (such as fifth generation β-lactams for methicillin-resistant *Staphylococcus aureus*) for treating pathogens that develop resistance to existing antimicrobials.

ACKNOWLEDGEMENTS

We thank Drs. Carl Cerniglia, Sangeeta Khare and John Sutherland for their useful comments and suggestions in shaping this manuscript. Drs. Jing Han and Bashar Shaheen acknowledge support of their fellowships from the Oak Ridge Institute for Science and Education, administered through an interagency agreement between the US Department of Energy and the US Food and Drug Administration.

DISCLAIMER

The views presented in this manuscript do not necessarily represent the views of the US Food and Drug Administration. The authors have no conflicting financial interests.

REFERENCES

[1]   Molbak K. Human health consequences of antimicrobial drug-resistant *Salmonella* and other foodborne pathogens. Clin Infect Dis 2005; 41(11): 1613-20.
[2]   Threlfall EJ, Ward LR, Frost JA, *et al.* The emergence and spread of antibiotic resistance in food-borne bacteria. Int J Food Microbiol 2000 5; 62(1-2): 1-5.
[3]   Angulo FJ, Baker NL, Olsen SJ, *et al.* Antimicrobial use in agriculture: controlling the transfer of antimicrobial resistance to humans. Semin Pediatr Infect Dis 2004; 15(2): 78-85.

[4]   WHO. Report of the third session of the codex ad hoc intergovernmental task force on antimicrobial resistance. Jeju, Republic of Korea: World Health Organization 2009.

[5]   Mathew AG, Cissell R, Liamthong S. Antibiotic resistance in bacteria associated with food animals: a United States perspective of livestock production. Foodborne Pathog Dis 2007; 4(2): 115-33.

[6]   Tollefson L, Angulo FJ, Fedorka-Cray PJ National surveillance for antibiotic resistance in zoonotic enteric pathogens. Vet Clin North Am Food Anim Pract 1998; 14(1): 141-50.

[7]   Hammerum AM, Heuer OE, Emborg HD, *et al.* Danish integrated antimicrobial resistance monitoring and research program. Emerg Infect Dis 2007; 13(11): 1632-39.

[8]   Mead PS, Slutsker L, Dietz V, *et al.* Food-related illness and death in the United States. Emerging Inf Dis 1999; 5: 607-25.

[9]   Allos B. *Campylobacter jejuni* Infections: Update on Emerging Issues and Trends. Clinical Infectious Diseases 2001; 32(8): 1201-06.

[10]   Ruiz-Palacios GM. The health burden of *Campylobacter* infection and the impact of antimicrobial resistance: playing chicken. Clin Infect Dis 2007; 44(5): 701-03.

[11]   Humphrey T, O'Brien S, Madsen M. Campylobacters as zoonotic pathogens: A food production perspective. Interl J Food Microbiol 2007; 117(3): 237-57.

[12]   Blaser MJ, Engberg J Clinical Aspects of *Campylobacter jejuni* and *Campylobacter coli* Infections. *Campyloabcter*, American Society for Microbiology, Washington, DC. 2008; 3rd: 99-121.

[13]   Alfredson DA, Korolik V. Antibiotic resistance and resistance mechanisms in *Campylobacter jejuni* and *Campylobacter coli*. FEMS Microbiol Lett 2007; 277(2): 123-32.

[14]   Moore JE, Barton MD, Blair IS, *et al.* The epidemiology of antibiotic resistance in *Campylobacter*. Microbes Infect 2006; 8(7): 1955-66.

[15]   Gupta A, Nelson JM, Barrett TJ, *et al.* Antimicrobial resistance among *Campylobacter* strains, United States, 1997-2001. Emerging infectious diseases 2004; 10(6): 1102-09.

[16]   Engberg J, Aarestrup FM, Taylor DE, *et al.* Quinolone and macrolide resistance in *Campylobacter jejuni* and C. coli: resistance mechanisms and trends in human isolates. Emerging infectious diseases. 2001; 7(1): 24-34.

[17]   Luangtongkum T, Jeon B, Han J, *et al.* Antibiotic resistance in *Campylobacter*: emergence, transmission and persistence. Future Microbiol 2009; 4(2): 189-200.

[18]   Gaudreau C, Gilbert H. Antimicrobial resistance of clinical strains of *Campylobacter jejuni* subsp. *jejuni* isolated from 1985 to 1997 in Quebec, Canada. Antimicrobial agents and chemotherapy. 1998; 42(8): 2106-08.

[19]   Gaudreau C, Gilbert H. Antimicrobial resistance of *Campylobacter jejuni* subsp. *jejuni* strains isolated from humans in 1998 to 2001 in Montreal, Canada. Antimicrob Agents Chemotherapy 2003; 47(6): 2027-29.

[20]   Papavasileiou E, Voyatzi A, Papavasileiou K, *et al.* Antimicrobial susceptibilities of *Campylobacter jejuni* isolates from hospitalized children in Athens, Greece, collected during 2004-2005. Eur J Epidemiol 2007; 22(1): 77-78.

[21]   Gallay A, Prouzet-Mauleon V, Kempf I, *et al. Campylobacter* antimicrobial drug resistance among humans, broiler chickens, and pigs, France. Emerg Inf Dis 2007; 13(2): 259-66.

[22]   Isenbarger DW, Hoge CW, Srijan A, *et al.* Comparative antibiotic resistance of diarrheal pathogens from Vietnam and Thailand, 1996-1999. Emerging infectious diseases 2002; 8(2): 175-80.

[23]   Chu YW, Chu MY, Luey KY, *et al.* Genetic relatedness and quinolone resistance of *Campylobacter jejuni* strains isolated in 2002 in Hong Kong. J Clin Microbiol 2004; 42(7): 3321-23.

[24]   Tjaniadi P, Lesmana M, Subekti D, *et al.* Antimicrobial resistance of bacterial pathogens associated with diarrheal patients in Indonesia. Am J Trop Med Hyg 2003; 68(6): 666-70.

[25]   Sharma H, Unicomb L, Forbes W, *et al.* Antibiotic resistance in *Campylobacter jejuni* isolated from humans in the Hunter Region, New South Wales. Commun Dis Intell 2003; 27 Suppl: S80-88.

[26]   Belanger AE, Shryock TR. Macrolide-resistant *Campylobacter*: the meat of the matter. J Antimicrob Chemother 2007; 60(4): 715-23.

[27]   Niwa H, Asai Y, Yamai S, *et al.* Antimicrobial resistance of *Campylobacter jejuni* and *Campylobacter coli* isolates in Japan. Vet Rec 2004 25; 155(13): 395-96.

[28]   Hakkinen M, Heiska H, Hanninen ML. Prevalence of *Campylobacter* spp. in cattle in Finland and antimicrobial susceptibilities of bovine *Campylobacter jejuni* strains. Appl Environ Microbiol 2007; 73(10): 3232-38.

[29]   Osterlund A, Hermann M, Kahlmeter G. Antibiotic resistance among *Campylobacter jejuni*/coli strains acquired in Sweden and abroad: a longitudinal study. Scand J Infect Dis 2003; 35(8): 478-81.

[30]   Padungton P, Kaneene JB. *Campylobacter* spp in human, chickens, pigs and their antimicrobial resistance. J Vet Med Sci 2003; 65(2): 161-70.

[31] Wolfson JS, Hooper DC. Fluoroquinolone antimicrobial agents. Clin Microbiol Rev 1989; 2(4): 378-424.

[32] Payot S, Bolla JM, Corcoran D, *et al.* Mechanisms of fluoroquinolone and macrolide resistance in *Campylobacter* spp. Microbes Infect 2006; 8(7): 1967-71.

[33] Tran JH, Jacoby GA, Hooper DC. Interaction of the plasmid-encoded quinolone resistance protein Qnr with *Escherichia coli* DNA gyrase. Antimicrobial agents and chemotherapy 2005; 49(1): 118-25.

[34] Luo N, Sahin O, Lin J, *et al. In Vivo* Selection of *Campylobacter* Isolates with High Levels of Fluoroquinolone Resistance Associated with gyrA Mutations and the Function of the CmeABC Efflux Pump. Antimicrob Agents Chemother 2003; 47(1): 390-94.

[35] Payot S, Cloeckaert A, Chaslus-Dancla E. Selection and characterization of fluoroquinolone-resistant mutants of *Campylobacter jejuni* using enrofloxacin. Microb Drug Resist 2002; 8(4): 335-43.

[36] Piddock LJ, Ricci V, Pumbwe L, *et al.* Fluoroquinolone resistance in *Campylobacter* species from man and animals: detection of mutations in topoisomerase genes. J Antimicrob Chemother 2003; 51(1): 19-26.

[37] Fouts DE, Mongodin EF, Mandrell RE, *et al.* Major structural differences and novel potential virulence mechanisms from the genomes of multiple *Campylobacter* species. PLoS Biol 2005; 3(1): e15.

[38] Zhang Q, Plummer P. Mechanisms of Antibiotic Resistance in *Campylobacter* Campyloabcter, American Society for Microbiology, Washington, DC. 2008; 3rd: 263.

[39] Gibreel A, Sjogren E, Kaijser B, *et al.* Rapid emergence of high-level resistance to quinolones in *Campylobacter jejuni* associated with mutational changes in gyrA and parC. Antimicrobial agents and chemotherapy 1998; 42(12): 3276-78.

[40] Luo N, Sahin O, Lin J, *et al. In vivo* selection of *Campylobacter* isolates with high levels of fluoroquinolone resistance associated with gyrA mutations and the function of the CmeABC efflux pump. Antimicrob Agents Chemother 2003; 47(1): 390-94.

[41] Lin J, Michel LO, Zhang Q. CmeABC Functions as a Multidrug Efflux System in *Campylobacter jejuni*. Antimicrob Agents Chemother 2002; 46(7): 2124-31.

[42] Pumbwe L, Piddock LJV. Identification and molecular characterisation of CmeB, a *Campylobacter jejuni* multidrug efflux pump. FEMS Microbiology Letters 2002; 206(2): 185-89.

[43] Ge B, McDermott PF, White DG, *et al.* Role of Efflux Pumps and Topoisomerase Mutations in Fluoroquinolone Resistance in *Campylobacter jejuni* and *Campylobacter coli*. Antimicrob Agents Chemother 2005; 49(8): 3347-54.

[44] Lin J, Yan M, Sahin O, *et al.* Effect of Macrolide Usage on Emergence of Erythromycin-Resistant *Campylobacter* Isolates in Chickens. Antimicrob Agents Chemother 2007; 51(5): 1678-86.

[45] Caldwell DB, Wang Y, Lin J Development, stability, and molecular mechanisms of macrolide resistance in *Campylobacter jejuni*. Antimicrobial agents and chemotherapy 2008; 52(11): 3947-54.

[46] Corcoran D, Quinn T, Cotter L, *et al.* An investigation of the molecular mechanisms contributing to high-level erythromycin resistance in *Campylobacter*. International journal of antimicrobial agents 2006; 27(1): 40-45.

[47] Lin J, Yan M, Sahin O, *et al.* Effect of macrolide usage on emergence of erythromycin-resistant *Campylobacter* isolates in chickens. Antimicrob Agents Chemother 2007; 51(5): 1678-86.

[48] D, Plummer P. Mechanisms of antibiotic resistance in *Campylobacter*. 3rd ed. Washington DC: American Society of Microbiology; 2008.

[49] Kurincic M, Botteldoorn N, Herman L, *et al.* Mechanisms of erythromycin resistance of *Campylobacter* spp. isolated from food, animals and humans. Int J Food Microbiol 2007 30; 120(1-2): 186-90.

[50] Gibreel A, Kos VN, Keelan M, *et al.* Macrolide resistance in *Campylobacter jejuni* and *Campylobacter coli*: molecular mechanism and stability of the resistance phenotype. Antimicrobial Agents and Chemotherapy 2005; 49(7): 2753-59.

[51] Cédric C, Christian M, Axel C, *et al.* Synergy between Efflux Pump CmeABC and Modifications in Ribosomal Proteins L4 and L22 in Conferring Macrolide Resistance in *Campylobacter jejuni* and *Campylobacter coli*. Antimicrobial agents and chemotherapy 2006; 50(11): 3893-96.

[52] Gibreel A, Wetsch NM, Taylor DE. Contribution of the CmeABC efflux pump to macrolide and tetracycline resistance in *Campylobacter jejuni*. Antimicrobial agents and chemotherapy 2007; 51(9): 3212-16.

[53] Chopra I, Roberts M. Tetracycline antibiotics: mode of action, applications, molecular biology, and epidemiology of bacterial resistance. Microbiol Mol Biol Rev 2001; 65(2): 232-60.

[54] Alcaine SD, Warnick LD, Wiedmann M. Antimicrobial resistance in nontyphoidal *Salmonella*. J Food Prot 2007; 70(3): 780-90.

[55] Dasti JI, Gross U, Pohl S, *et al.* Role of the plasmid-encoded tet(O) gene in tetracycline-resistant clinical isolates of *Campylobacter jejuni* and *Campylobacter coli*. J Med Microbiol 2007; 56(Pt 6): 833-37.

[56] Batchelor RA, Pearson BM, Friis LM, *et al.* Nucleotide sequences and comparison of two large conjugative plasmids from different *Campylobacter* species. Microbiology. 2004 Oct; 150(Pt 10): 3507-17.

[57] Connell SR, Trieber CA, Dinos GP, *et al.* Mechanism of Tet(O)-mediated tetracycline resistance. EMBO J 2003 17; 22(4): 945-53.

[58] Gonzalez LS, Spencer JP. Aminoglycosides: a practical review. Am Fam Physician 1998; 58(8): 1811-20.

[59] Russell SM, Axtell SP. Monochloramine *vs* sodium hypochlorite as antimicrobial agents for reducing populations of bacteria on broiler chicken carcasses. J Food Prot. 2005 Apr; 68(4): 758-63.

[60] Jana S, Deb JK. Molecular understanding of aminoglycoside action and resistance. Appl Microbiol Biotechnol. 2006 Mar; 70(2): 140-50.

[61] Llano-Sotelo B, Azucena EF, Kotra LP, *et al.* Aminoglycosides modified by resistance enzymes display diminished binding to the bacterial ribosomal aminoacyl-tRNA site. Chem Biol 2002 Apr; 9(4): 455-463.

[62] Gibreel A, Skold O, Taylor DE. Characterization of plasmid-mediated aphA-3 kanamycin resistance in *Campylobacter jejuni*. Microb Drug Resist. 2004; 10(2): 98-105.

[63] Kong KF, Schneper L, Mathee K. Beta-lactam antibiotics: from antibiosis to resistance and bacteriology. APMIS 2010; 118(1): 1-36.

[64] Angulo FJ, Johnson KR, Tauxe RV, *et al.* Origins and consequences of antimicrobial-resistant nontyphoidal *Salmonella*: implications for the use of fluoroquinolones in food animals. Microb Drug Resist 2000; 6(1): 77-83.

[65] Hornish RE, Kotarski SF. Cephalosporins in veterinary medicine - ceftiofur use in food animals. Curr Top Med Chem 2002; 2(7): 717-31.

[66] Poole K. Resistance to beta-lactam antibiotics. Cell Mol Life Sci. 2004 Sep; 61(17): 2200-2223.

[67] Li XZ, Mehrotra M, Ghimire S, *et al.* Beta-Lactam resistance and beta-lactamases in bacteria of animal origin. Vet Microbiol 2007; 121(3-4): 197-214.

[68] Griggs DJ, Peake L, Johnson MM, *et al.* Beta-lactamase-mediated beta-lactam resistance in *Campylobacter* species: prevalence of Cj0299 (bla OXA-61) and evidence for a novel beta-Lactamase in C. *jejuni.* Antimicrob Agents Chemother 2009; 53(8): 3357-64.

[69] Griggs DJ, Johnson MM, Frost JA, *et al.* Incidence and mechanism of ciprofloxacin resistance in *Campylobacter* spp. isolated from commercial poultry flocks in the United Kingdom before, during, and after fluoroquinolone treatment. Antimicrob Agents Chemother 2005; 49(2): 699-707.

[70] van Boven M, Veldman KT, de Jong MC, *et al.* Rapid selection of quinolone resistance in *Campylobacter jejuni* but not in *Escherichia coli* in individually housed broilers. J Antimicrob Chemother 2003; 52(4): 719-23.

[71] Yan M, Sahin O, Lin J, *et al.* Role of the CmeABC efflux pump in the emergence of fluoroquinolone-resistant *Campylobacter* under selection pressure. J Antimicrob Chemother 2006, 2006; 58(6): 1154-59.

[72] Yanagawa Y, Takahashi M, Itoh T. The role of flagella of *Campylobacter jejuni* in colonization in the intestinal tract in mice and the cultured-cell infectivity. Nippon Saikingaku Zasshi. 1994; 49(2): 395-403.

[73] van Boven M, Veldman KT, de Jong MCM, *et al.* Rapid selection of quinolone resistance in *Campylobacter jejuni* but not in *Escherichia coli* in individually housed broilers. J Antimicrob Chemother 2003, 2003; 52(4): 719-23.

[74] Han J, Sahin O, Barton YW, *et al.* Key role of Mfd in the development of fluoroquinolone resistance in *Campylobacter jejuni*. PLoS Pathog 2008; 4(6): e1000083.

[75] Ladely SR, Harrison MA, Fedorka-Cray PJ, *et al.* Development of macrolide-resistant *Campylobacter* in broilers administered subtherapeutic or therapeutic concentrations of tylosin. J Food Prot 2007; 70(8): 1945-51.

[76] Pratt A, Korolik V. Tetracycline resistance of Australian *Campylobacter jejuni* and *Campylobacter coli* isolates. J Antimicrob Chemother 2005; 55(4): 452-60.

[77] Avrain L, Vernozy-Rozand C, Kempf I. Evidence for natural horizontal transfer of tetO gene between *Campylobacter jejuni* strains in chickens. J Appl Microbiol 2004; 97(1): 134-40.

[78] Jeon B, Muraoka W, Sahin O, *et al.* Role of Cj1211 in natural transformation and transfer of antibiotic resistance determinants in *Campylobacter jejuni*. Antimicrob Agents Chemother 2008; 52(8): 2699-708.

[79] Hansen VM, Rosenquist H, Baggesen DL, *et al.* Characterization of *Campylobacter* phages including analysis of host range by selected *Campylobacter* Penner serotypes. BMC Microbiol 2007; 7: 90.

[80] Scharff RL. Health-related Costs from Foodborne Illness in the United States. Washington, D.C.: Georgetown University 2010; 3/3/2010.

[81] Mead PS, Slutsker L, Dietz V, *et al.* Food-related illness and death in the United States. 1999; 5(5): 607-25.

[82] Centers for Disease Control and Prevention. *Salmonella* Surveillance: Annual Summary, 2006. Atlanta, GA: Centers for Disease Control and Prevention 2008.

[83]   McNabb SJ, Jajosky RA, Hall-Baker PA, *et al.* Summary of notifiable diseases - United States, 2005. MMWR Morb Mortal Wkly Rep 2007; 54(53): 1-92.

[84]   Darwin KH, Miller VL. Molecular basis of the interaction of *Salmonella* with the intestinal mucosa. Clin Microbiol Rev 1999; 12(3): 405-28.

[85]   Pegues DA, Ohl ME, Miller SI. *Salmonella* species, including *Salmonella* Typhi. In: Mandell GL, Bennett JE, Dolin R, editors. Principles and Practice of Infectious Diseases. 6th ed. Philadelphia, PA: Elsevier Churchill Livingstone 2005; pp. 2636-54.

[86]   Centers for Disease Control and Prevention. Diagnosis and management of foodborne illnesses: a primer for physicians. MMWR Recomm Rep. 2001; 50(RR-2): 1-69.

[87]   Cohen JI, Bartlett JA, Corey GR. Extra-intestinal manifestations of *Salmonella* infections. Medicine (Baltimore) 1987; 66(5): 349-88.

[88]   Benenson AS, Chin J, Benenson AS, Chin J Control of Communicable Diseases Manual. Washington, D.C.: American Public Health Association; 1995.

[89]   Gilbert DN, Moellering RC, Eliopoulos GM, *et al.* The Sanford guide to antimicrobial therapy. 34 ed. Hyde Park, VT: Antimicrobial Therapy, Inc; 2004.

[90]   Centers for Disease Control and Prevention. *Salmonella* Surveillance: Annual Summary, 2004. Atlanta, GA: Centers for Disease Control and Prevention; 2005.

[91]   de Jong B, Ekdahl K. The comparative burden of salmonellosis in the European Union member states, associated and candidate countries. BMC Public Health 2006; 6: 4.

[92]   Centers for Disease Control and Prevention. *Salmonella* Surveillance: Annual Summary, 2005. Atlanta, GA: Centers for Disease Control and Prevention; 2006.

[93]   Chiu CH, Su LH, Chu C. *Salmonella* enterica serotype Choleraesuis: epidemiology, pathogenesis, clinical disease, and treatment. Clin Microbiol Rev 2004; 17(2): 311-22.

[94]   Maki DG. Coming to grips with foodborne infection--peanut butter, peppers, and nationwide *Salmonella* outbreaks. N Engl J Med 2009; 360(10): 949-53.

[95]   Tauxe RV. *Salmonella*: a postmodern pathogen. J Food Protect 1991; 54(7): 563-68.

[96]   Buzby JC, Farah HA. Chicken consumption continues long run rise. Amber Waves 2006; 4(2): 5.

[97]   Swaminathan B, Barrett TJ, Hunter SB, *et al.* PulseNet: the molecular subtyping network for foodborne bacterial disease surveillance, United States. Emerg Infect Dis 2001; 7(3): 382-89.

[98]   Rose BE, Hill WE, Umholtz R, *et al.* Testing for *Salmonella* in raw meat and poultry products collected at federally inspected establishments in the United States, 1998 through 2000. J Food Prot 2002; 65(6): 937-47.

[99]   Food and Drug Administration. National Antimicrobial Resistance Monitoring System-Enteric Bacteria (NARMS): 2003 Executive Report. Rockville, MD: U.S. Department of Health and Human Services, U.S. FDA; 2006.

[100]   Food and Drug Administration. National Antimicrobial Resistance Monitoring System-Enteric Bacteria (NARMS): 2006 Executive Report. Rockville, MD: U.S. Department of Health and Human Services, U.S. FDA; 2009.

[101]   Fricke WF, McDermott PF, Mammel MK, *et al.* Antimicrobial resistance-conferring plasmids with similarity to virulence plasmids from avian pathogenic *Escherichia coli* strains in *Salmonella* enterica serovar Kentucky isolates from poultry. Appl Environ Microbiol 2009; 75(18): 5963-71.

[102]   Kaldhone P, Nayak R, Lynne AM, *et al.* Characterization of *Salmonella* enterica serovar Heidelberg from turkey-associated sources. Appl Environ Microbiol 2008; 74(16): 5038-46.

[103]   Sefton AM. Mechanisms of antimicrobial resistance: their clinical relevance in the new millennium. Journal name 2002; 62(4): 557-66.

[104]   Shaw KJ, Rather PN, Hare RS, *et al.* Molecular genetics of aminoglycoside resistance genes and familial relationships of the aminoglycoside-modifying enzymes. Microbiol Rev 1993; 57(1): 138-63.

[105]   Gebreyes WA, Altier C. Molecular characterization of multidrug-resistant *Salmonella* enterica subsp. enterica serovar Typhimurium isolates from swine. J Clin Microbiol 2002; 40(8): 2813-22.

[106]   Guerra B, Soto S, Helmuth R, *et al.* Characterization of a self-transferable plasmid from *Salmonella* enterica serotype typhimurium clinical isolates carrying two integron-borne gene cassettes together with virulence and drug resistance genes. Antimicrob Agents Chemother 2002; 46(9): 2977-81.

[107]   Doublet B, Weill FX, Fabre L, *et al.* Variant *Salmonella* genomic island 1 antibiotic resistance gene cluster containing a novel 3'-N-aminoglycoside acetyltransferase gene cassette, aac(3)-Id, in *Salmonella* enterica serovar newport. Antimicrob Agents Chemother 2004; 48(10): 3806-12.

[108] Levings RS, Partridge SR, Lightfoot D, *et al.* New integron-associated gene cassette encoding a 3-N-aminoglycoside acetyltransferase. Antimicrob Agents Chemother 2005 Mar; 49(3): 1238-1241.

[109] Guerra B, Soto SM, Arguelles JM, *et al.* Multidrug resistance is mediated by large plasmids carrying a class 1 integron in the emergent *Salmonella* enterica serotype [4,5,12:i:-]. Antimicrob Agents Chemother 2001; 45(4): 1305-08.

[110] Madsen L, Aarestrup FM, Olsen JE. Characterisation of streptomycin resistance determinants in Danish isolates of *Salmonella* Typhimurium. Vet Microbiol 2000; 75(1): 73-82.

[111] Carattoli A, Villa L, Pezzella C, *et al.* Expanding drug resistance through integron acquisition by IncFI plasmids of *Salmonella* enterica Typhimurium. Emerg Infect Dis 2001; 7(3): 444-47.

[112] Armand-Lefevre L, Leflon-Guibout V, Bredin J, *et al.* Imipenem resistance in *Salmonella* enterica serovar Wien related to porin loss and CMY-4 beta-lactamase production. Antimicrob Agents Chemother 2003; 47(3): 1165-68.

[113] Miriagou V, Tzouvelekis LS, Rossiter S, *et al.* Imipenem resistance in a *Salmonella* clinical strain due to plasmid-mediated class A carbapenemase KPC-2. Antimicrob Agents Chemother 2003; 47(4): 1297-300.

[114] Bellido F, Vladoianu IR, Auckenthaler R, *et al.* Permeability and penicillin-binding protein alterations in *Salmonella* muenchen: stepwise resistance acquired during beta-lactam therapy. Antimicrob Agents Chemother 1989; 33(7): 1113-15

[115] Medeiros AA, O'Brien TF, Rosenberg EY, *et al.* Loss of OmpC porin in a strain of *Salmonella* typhimurium causes increased resistance to cephalosporins during therapy. J Infect Dis 1987; 156(5): 751-57.

[116] Bauernfeind A, Stemplinger I, Jungwirth R, *et al.* Characterization of the plasmidic beta-lactamase CMY-2, which is responsible for cephamycin resistance. Antimicrob Agents Chemother 1996; 40(1): 221-224.

[117] Ambler RP. The structure of beta-lactamases. Philos Trans R Soc Lond B Biol Sci 1980; 289(1036): 321-31.

[118] Chen S, Zhao S, White DG, *et al.* Characterization of multiple-antimicrobial-resistant *Salmonella* serovars isolated from retail meats. Appl Environ Microbiol 2004; 70(1): 1-7.

[119] Weill FX, Demartin M, Fabre L, *et al.* Extended-spectrum-beta-lactamase (TEM-52)-producing strains of *Salmonella* enterica of various serotypes isolated in France. J Clin Microbiol 2004; 42(7): 3359-62.

[120] Batchelor M, Hopkins K, Threlfall EJ, *et al.* bla(CTX-M) genes in clinical *Salmonella* isolates recovered from humans in England and Wales from 1992 to 2003. Antimicrob Agents Chemother 2005; 49(4): 1319-22.

[121] Morosini MI, Ayala JA, Baquero F, *et al.* Biological cost of AmpC production for *Salmonella* enterica serotype Typhimurium. Antimicrob Agents Chemother 2000; 44(11): 3137-43.

[122] Winokur PL, Brueggemann A, DeSalvo DL, *et al.* Animal and human multidrug-resistant, cephalosporin-resistant *Salmonella* isolates expressing a plasmid-mediated CMY-2 AmpC beta-lactamase. Antimicrob Agents Chemother 2000; 44(10): 2777-83.

[123] Alcaine SD, Sukhnanand SS, Warnick LD, *et al.* Ceftiofur-resistant *Salmonella* strains isolated from dairy farms represent multiple widely distributed subtypes that evolved by independent horizontal gene transfer. Antimicrob Agents Chemother 2005; 49(10): 4061-67.

[124] Doublet B, Carattoli A, Whichard JM, *et al.* Plasmid-mediated florfenicol and ceftriaxone resistance encoded by the floR and bla(CMY-2) genes in *Salmonella* enterica serovars Typhimurium and Newport isolated in the United States. FEMS Microbiol Lett 2004; 233(2): 301-05.

[125] Cabrera R, Ruiz J, Marco F, *et al.* Mechanism of resistance to several antimicrobial agents in *Salmonella* Clinical isolates causing traveler's diarrhea. Antimicrob Agents Chemother 2004; 48(10): 3934-39.

[126] Gebreyes WA, Thakur S. Multidrug-resistant *Salmonella* enterica serovar Muenchen from pigs and humans and potential interserovar transfer of antimicrobial resistance. Antimicrob Agents Chemother 2005; 49(2): 503-11.

[127] Antunes P, Machado J, Sousa JC, *et al.* Dissemination amongst humans and food products of animal origin of a *Salmonella* typhimurium clone expressing an integron-borne OXA-30 beta-lactamase. J Antimicrob Chemother 2004; 54(2): 429-34.

[128] Casin I, Breuil J, Darchis JP, *et al.* Fluoroquinolone resistance linked to GyrA, GyrB and ParC mutations in *Salmonella* enterica typhimurium isolates in humans. Emerg Infect Dis 2003; 9(11): 1455-57.

[129] Olsen SJ, DeBess EE, McGivern TE, *et al.* A nosocomial outbreak of fluoroquinolone-resistant *Salmonella* infection. N Engl J Med 2001; 344(21): 1572-79.

[130] Baucheron S, Chaslus-Dancla E, Cloeckaert A. Role of TolC and parC mutation in high-level fluoroquinolone resistance in *Salmonella* enterica serotype Typhimurium DT204. J Antimicrob Chemother 2004; 53(4): 657-59.

[131] Olliver A, Valle M, Chaslus-Dancla E, *et al.* Overexpression of the multidrug efflux operon acrEF by insertional activation with IS1 or IS10 elements in *Salmonella* enterica serovar typhimurium DT204 acrB mutants selected with fluoroquinolones. Antimicrob Agents Chemother 2005; 49(1): 289-301.

[132] Levings RS, Lightfoot D, Partridge SR, *et al.* The genomic island SGI1, containing the multiple antibiotic resistance region of *Salmonella* enterica serovar Typhimurium DT104 or variants of it, is widely distributed in other S. enterica serovars. J Bacteriol 2005; 187(13): 4401-09.

[133] Giraud E, Cloeckaert A, Baucheron S, *et al.* Fitness cost of fluoroquinolone resistance in *Salmonella* enterica serovar Typhimurium. J Med Microbiol 2003; 52(Pt 8): 697-703.

[134] Heisig P. High-level fluoroquinolone resistance in a *Salmonella* typhimurium isolate due to alterations in both gyrA and gyrB genes. J Antimicrob Chemother 1993; 32(3): 367-77.

[135] Li XZ. Quinolone resistance in bacteria: emphasis on plasmid-mediated mechanisms. Int J Antimicrob Agents 2005; 25(6): 453-63.

[136] Wang M, Tran JH, Jacoby GA, *et al.* Plasmid-mediated quinolone resistance in clinical isolates of *Escherichia coli* from Shanghai, China. Antimicrob Agents Chemother 2003; 47(7): 2242-48.

[137] Wang M, Sahm DF, Jacoby GA, *et al.* Emerging plasmid-mediated quinolone resistance associated with the qnr gene in Klebsiella pneumoniae clinical isolates in the United States. Antimicrob Agents Chemother 2004; 48(4): 1295-99.

[138] Cheung TK, Chu YW, Chu MY, *et al.* Plasmid-mediated resistance to ciprofloxacin and cefotaxime in clinical isolates of *Salmonella* enterica serotype Enteritidis in Hong Kong. J Antimicrob Chemother 2005; 56(3): 586-89.

[139] Carattoli A, Filetici E, Villa L, *et al.* Antibiotic resistance genes and *Salmonella* genomic island 1 in *Salmonella* enterica serovar Typhimurium isolated in Italy. Antimicrob Agents Chemother 2002; 46(9): 2821-28.

[140] Frech G, Kehrenberg C, Schwarz S. Resistance phenotypes and genotypes of multiresistant *Salmonella* enterica subsp. enterica serovar Typhimurium var. Copenhagen isolates from animal sources. J Antimicrob Chemother 2003; 51(1): 180-82.

[141] Briggs CE, Fratamico PM. Molecular characterization of an antibiotic resistance gene cluster of *Salmonella* typhimurium DT104. Antimicrob Agents Chemother 1999; 43(4): 846-49.

[142] Pezzella C, Ricci A, DiGiannatale E, *et al.* Tetracycline and streptomycin resistance genes, transposons, and plasmids in *Salmonella* enterica isolates from animals in Italy. Antimicrob Agents Chemother 2004; 48(3): 903-08.

[143] Skold O. Resistance to trimethoprim and sulfonamides. Vet Res. 2001 May-Aug; 32(3-4): 261-273.

[144] Antunes P, Machado J, Sousa JC, *et al.* Dissemination of sulfonamide resistance genes (sul1, sul2, and sul3) in Portuguese *Salmonella* enterica strains and relation with integrons. Antimicrob Agents Chemother 2005; 49(2): 836-39.

[145] Guerra B, Soto S, Cal S, *et al.* Antimicrobial resistance and spread of class 1 integrons among *Salmonella* serotypes. Antimicrob Agents Chemother 2000; 44(8): 2166-69.

[146] Boyd D, Cloeckaert A, Chaslus-Dancla E, *et al.* Characterization of variant *Salmonella* genomic island 1 multidrug resistance regions from serovars Typhimurium DT104 and Agona. Antimicrob Agents Chemother 2002; 46(6): 1714-22.

[147] Doublet B, Lailler R, Meunier D, *et al.* Variant *Salmonella* genomic island 1 antibiotic resistance gene cluster in *Salmonella* enterica serovar Albany. Emerg Infect Dis 2003; 9(5): 585-91.

[148] Villa L, Carattoli A. Integrons and transposons on the *Salmonella* enterica serovar typhimurium virulence plasmid. Antimicrob Agents Chemother 2005; 49(3): 1194-97.

[149] Schwarz S, Kehrenberg C, Doublet B, *et al.* Molecular basis of bacterial resistance to chloramphenicol and florfenicol. FEMS Microbiol Rev. 2004; 28(5): 519-42.

[150] Yunis AA. Chloramphenicol toxicity: 25 years of research. Am J Med. 1989 Sep; 87(3N): 44N-48N.

[151] White DG, Piddock LJ, Maurer JJ, *et al.* Characterization of fluoroquinolone resistance among veterinary isolates of avian *Escherichia coli*. Antimicrob Agents Chemother 2000; 44(10): 2897-99.

[152] Zhao S, Qaiyumi S, Friedman S, *et al.* Characterization of *Salmonella* enterica serotype newport isolated from humans and food animals. J Clin Microbiol 2003; 41(12): 5366-71.

[153] Aarestrup FM, Hasman H, Olsen I, *et al.* International spread of bla(CMY-2)-mediated cephalosporin resistance in a multiresistant *Salmonella* enterica serovar Heidelberg isolate stemming from the importation of a boar by Denmark from Canada. Antimicrob Agents Chemother 2004; 48(5): 1916-17.

[154] Helms M, Vastrup P, Gerner-Smidt P, *et al.* Short and long term mortality associated with foodborne bacterial gastrointestinal infections: registry based study. BmJ 2003 15; 326(7385): 57.

[155] Welch TJ, Fricke WF, McDermott PF, *et al.* Multiple antimicrobial resistance in plague: an emerging public health risk. PLoS ONE 2007; 2: e309.

[156] Chiu CH, Tang P, Chu C, *et al.* The genome sequence of *Salmonella* enterica serovar Choleraesuis, a highly invasive and resistant zoonotic pathogen. Nucleic Acids Res 2005; 33(5): 1690-98.

[157] Bennett PM. Integrons and gene cassettes: a genetic construction kit for bacteria. J Antimicrob Chemother 1999; 43(1): 1-4.

[158] Fluit AC, Schmitz FJ Resistance integrons and super-integrons. Clin Microbiol Infect 2004; 10(4): 272-88.

[159] Mazel D. Integrons: agents of bacterial evolution. Nat Rev Microbiol 2006; 4(8): 608-20.

[160] Chang DE, Smalley DJ, Tucker DL, *et al.* Carbon nutrition of *Escherichia coli* in the mouse intestine. Proc Natl Acad Sci U S A. 2004 May 11; 101(19): 7427-7432.

[161] Robins-Browne RM, Hartland EL. *Escherichia coli* as a cause of diarrhea. J Gastroenterol Hepatol. 2002; 17(4): 467-75.

[162] Orskov F, Orskov I. The serology of capsular antigens. Curr Top Microbiol Immunol 1990; 150: 43-63.

[163] Wasteson Y. Zoonotic *Escherichia coli*. Acta Vet Scand Suppl 2001; 95: 79-84.

[164] Ramirez RM, Almanza Y, Gonzalez R, *et al.* Avian pathogenic *Escherichia coli* bind fibronectin and laminin. Vet Res Commun 2009; 33(4): 379-86.

[165] Erskine RJ, Walker RD, Bolin CA, *et al.* Trends in antibacterial susceptibility of mastitis pathogens during a seven-year period. J Dairy Sci 2002; 85(5): 1111-18.

[166] Lanz R, Kuhnert P, Boerlin P. Antimicrobial resistance and resistance gene determinants in clinical *Escherichia coli* from different animal species in Switzerland. Vet Microbiol 2003; 91(1): 73-84.

[167] Williams RJ, Heymann DL. Containment of antibiotic resistance. Science 1998; 279(5354): 1153-54.

[168] Schwartz B, Bell DM, Hughes JM. Preventing the emergence of antimicrobial resistance. A call for action by clinicians, public health officials, and patients. JAMA 1997; 278(11): 944-945.

[169] Delicato ER, de Brito BG, Gaziri LC, *et al.* Virulence-associated genes in *Escherichia coli* isolates from poultry with colibacillosis. Vet Microbiol 2003; 94(2): 97-103.

[170] Dias da Silveira W, Ferreira A, Brocchi M, *et al.* Biological characteristics and pathogenicity of avian *Escherichia coli* strains. Vet Microbiol 2002; 85(1): 47-53.

[171] Altekruse SF, Elvinger F, Lee KY, *et al.* Antimicrobial susceptibilities of *Escherichia coli* strains from a turkey operation. J Am Vet Med Assoc 2002; 221(3): 411-16.

[172] Cormican M, Buckley V, Corbett-Feeney G, *et al.* Antimicrobial resistance in *Escherichia coli* isolates from turkeys and hens in Ireland. J Antimicrob Chemother 2001; 48(4): 587-88.

[173] Trobos M, Lester CH, Olsen JE, *et al.* Natural transfer of sulphonamide and ampicillin resistance between *Escherichia coli* residing in the human intestine. J Antimicrob Chemother 2009; 63(1): 80-86.

[174] Kanai H, Hashimoto H, Mitsuhashi S. Drug resistance and R plasmids in *Escherichia coli* strains isolated from broilers. Microbiol Immunol 1983; 27(6): 471-78.

[175] Yang H, Chen S, White DG, *et al.* Characterization of multiple-antimicrobial-resistant *Escherichia coli* isolates from diseased chickens and swine in China. J Clin Microbiol 2004; 42(8): 3483-89.

[176] van den Bogaard AE, London N, Driessen C, *et al.* Antibiotic resistance of faecal *Escherichia coli* in poultry, poultry farmers and poultry slaughterers. J Antimicrob Chemother 2001; 47(6): 763-71.

[177] Giraud E, Leroy-Setrin S, Flaujac G, *et al.* Characterization of high-level fluoroquinolone resistance in *Escherichia coli* O78: K80 isolated from turkeys. J Antimicrob Chemother 2001; 47(3): 341-43.

[178] Smet A, Martel A, Persoons D, *et al.* Diversity of extended-spectrum beta-lactamases and class C beta-lactamases among cloacal *Escherichia coli* Isolates in Belgian broiler farms. Antimicrob Agents Chemother 2008; 52(4): 1238-43.

[179] Musgrove MT, Jones DR, Northcutt JK, *et al.* Antimicrobial resistance in *Salmonella* and *Escherichia coli* isolated from commercial shell eggs. Poult Sci 2006; 85(9): 1665-69.

[180] Jay CM, Bhaskaran S, Rathore KS, *et al.* Enterotoxigenic K99+ *Escherichia coli* attachment to host cell receptors inhibited by recombinant pili protein. Vet Microbiol 2004; 101(3): 153-60.

[181] White DG, Hudson C, Maurer JJ, *et al.* Characterization of chloramphenicol and florfenicol resistance in *Escherichia coli* associated with bovine diarrhea. J Clin Microbiol 2000; 38(12): 4593-98.

[182] Walton JR. Infectious drug resistance in *Escherichia coli* isolated from healthy farm animals. Lancet. 1966; 2(7476): 1300-02.

[183] Aarestrup FM. Association between the consumption of antimicrobial agents in animal husbandry and the occurrence of resistant bacteria among food animals. Int J Antimicrob Agents 1999; 12(4): 279-85.

[184] Wray C, Hedges RW, Shannon KP, *et al.* Apramycin and gentamicin resistance in *Escherichia coli* and *Salmonella* isolated from farm animals. J Hyg (Lond) 1986; 97(3): 445-56.

[185] Aden DP, Reed ND, Underdahl NR, *et al.* Transferable drug resistance among Enterobacteriaceae isolated from cases of neonatal diarrhea in calves and piglets. Appl Microbiol 1969; 18(6): 961-64.

[186] Nagy B, Fekete PZ. Enterotoxigenic *Escherichia coli* (ETEC) in farm animals. Vet Res 1999; 30(2-3): 259-84.

[187] Maynard C, Fairbrother JM, Bekal S, *et al.* Antimicrobial resistance genes in enterotoxigenic *Escherichia coli* O149: K91 isolates obtained over a 23-year period from pigs. Antimicrob Agents Chemother 2003; 47(10): 3214-21.

[188] Mercer HD, Pocurull D, Gaines S, *et al.* Characteristics of antimicrobial resistance of *Escherichia coli* from animals: relationship to veterinary and management uses of antimicrobial agents. Appl Microbiol 1971; 22(4): 700-05.

[189] Lehtolainen T, Shwimmer A, Shpigel NY, *et al. In vitro* antimicrobial susceptibility of *Escherichia coli* isolates from clinical bovine mastitis in Finland and Israel. J Dairy Sci 2003; 86(12): 3927-32.

[190] Sogaard H. In-vitro antibiotic susceptibility of *E. coli* isolated from acute and chronic bovine mastitis with reference to clinical efficacy. Nord Vet Med 1982; 34(7-9): 248-54.

[191] Makovec JA, Ruegg PL. Antimicrobial resistance of bacteria isolated from dairy cow milk samples submitted for bacterial culture: 8,905 samples (1994-2001). J Am Vet Med Assoc 2003; 222(11): 1582-89.

[192] Chen YM, Wright PJ, Lee CS, *et al.* Uropathogenic virulence factors in isolates of *Escherichia coli* from clinical cases of canine pyometra and feces of healthy bitches. Vet Microbiol 2003; 94(1): 57-69.

[193] Feria C, Ferreira E, Correia JD, *et al.* Patterns and mechanisms of resistance to beta-lactams and beta-lactamase inhibitors in uropathogenic *Escherichia coli* isolated from dogs in Portugal. J Antimicrob Chemother 2002; 49(1): 77-85.

[194] Hagman R, Kuhn I. *Escherichia coli* strains isolated from the uterus and urinary bladder of bitches suffering from pyometra: comparison by restriction enzyme digestion and pulsed-field gel electrophoresis. Vet Microbiol 2002; 84(1-2): 143-53.

[195] Wernicki A, Krzyzanowski J, Puchalski A. Characterization of *Escherichia coli* strains associated with canine pyometra. Pol J Vet Sci 2002; 5(2): 51-56.

[196] Guardabassi L, Schwarz S, Lloyd DH. Pet animals as reservoirs of antimicrobial-resistant bacteria. J Antimicrob Chemother 2004; 54(2): 321-32.

[197] Hirsh DC. Multiple antimicrobial resistances in *Escherichia coli* isolated from the urine of dogs and cats with cystitis. J Am Vet Med Assoc 1973; 162(10): 885-87.

[198] Normand EH, Gibson NR, Reid SW, *et al.* Antimicrobial-resistance trends in bacterial isolates from companion-animal community practice in the UK. Prev Vet Med 2000; 46(4): 267-78.

[199] Oluoch AO, Kim CH, Weisiger RM, *et al.* Nonenteric *Escherichia coli* isolates from dogs: 674 cases (1990-1998). J Am Vet Med Assoc 2001; 218(3): 381-84.

[200] Sanchez S, McCrackin SMA, Hudson CR, *et al.* Characterization of multidrug-resistant *Escherichia coli* isolates associated with nosocomial infections in dogs. J Clin Microbiol 2002; 40(10): 3586-95.

[201] Cohn LA, Gary AT, Fales WH, *et al.* Trends in fluoroquinolone resistance of bacteria isolated from canine urinary tracts. J Vet Diagn Invest 2003; 15(4): 338-43.

[202] Griggs DJ, Johnson MM, Frost JA, *et al.* Incidence and Mechanism of Ciprofloxacin Resistance in *Campylobacter* spp. Isolated from Commercial Poultry Flocks in the United Kingdom before, during, and after Fluoroquinolone Treatment. Antimicrob Agents Chemother 2005, 2005; 49(2): 699-707.

[203] Johnson JR, Delavari P, O'Bryan TT, *et al.* Contamination of retail foods, particularly turkey, from community markets (Minnesota, 1999-2000) with antimicrobial-resistant and extraintestinal pathogenic *Escherichia coli*. Foodborne Pathog Dis 2005; 2(1): 38-49.

[204] Nemoy LL, Kotetishvili M, Tigno J, *et al.* Multilocus sequence typing *vs* pulsed-field gel electrophoresis for characterization of extended-spectrum beta-lactamase-producing *Escherichia coli* isolates. J Clin Microbiol 2005; 43(4): 1776-81.

[205] Ramchandani M, Manges AR, DebRoy C, *et al.* Possible animal origin of human-associated, multidrug-resistant, uropathogenic *Escherichia coli*. Clin Infect Dis 2005; 40(2): 251-57.

[206] Zahar JR, Lortholary O, Martin C, *et al.* Addressing the challenge of extended-spectrum beta-lactamases. Curr Opin Investig Drugs 2009; 10(2): 172-80.

[207] Lewis JS, Herrera M, Wickes B, *et al.* First report of the emergence of CTX-M-type extended-spectrum beta-lactamases (ESBLs) as the predominant ESBL isolated in a U.S. health care system. Antimicrob Agents Chemother 2007; 51(11): 4015-21.

[208]   Castanheira M, Mendes RE, Rhomberg PR, *et al.* Rapid emergence of blaCTX-M among Enterobacteriaceae in U.S. Medical Centers: molecular evaluation from the MYSTIC Program (2007). Microb Drug Resist 2008; 14(3): 211-16.

[209]   Manges AR, Johnson JR, Foxman B, *et al.* Widespread distribution of urinary tract infections caused by a multidrug-resistant *Escherichia coli* clonal group. N Engl J Med 2001; 345(14): 1007-13.

[210]   Cagnacci S, Gualco L, Debbia E, *et al.* European emergence of ciprofloxacin-resistant *Escherichia coli* clonal groups O25: H4-ST 131 and O15: K52: H1 causing community-acquired uncomplicated cystitis. J Clin Microbiol 2008; 46(8): 2605-12.

[211]   Li Y, Odumeru JA, Griffiths M, *et al.* Effect of environmental stresses on the mean and distribution of individual cell lag times of *Escherichia coli* O157: H7. International Journal of Food Microbiology 2006; 110(3): 278-85.

[212]   Bush K, Jacoby GA, Medeiros AA. A functional classification scheme for beta-lactamases and its correlation with molecular structure. Antimicrob Agents Chemother 1995; 39(6): 1211-33.

[213]   Blattner FR, Plunkett G, 3rd, Bloch CA, Perna NT, Burland V, Riley M, *et al.* The complete genome sequence of *Escherichia coli* K-12. Science 1997; 277(5331): 1453-62.

[214]   Siu LK, Lu PL, Chen JY, *et al.* High-level expression of ampC beta-lactamase due to insertion of nucleotides between -10 and -35 promoter sequences in *Escherichia coli* clinical isolates: cases not responsive to extended-spectrum-cephalosporin treatment. Antimicrob Agents Chemother 2003; 47(7): 2138-44.

[215]   Cobbold RN, Rice DH, Davis MA, *et al.* Long-term persistence of multi-drug-resistant *Salmonella* enterica serovar Newport in two dairy herds. J Am Vet Med Assoc 2006; 228(4): 585-91.

[216]   Whichard JM, Joyce K, Fey PD, *et al.* Beta-lactam resistance and Enterobacteriaceae, United States. Emerg Infect Dis 2005; 11(9): 1464-66.

[217]   Bonnet R. Growing group of extended-spectrum beta-lactamases: the CTX-M enzymes. Antimicrob Agents Chemother 2004; 48(1): 1-14.

[218]   Brinas L, Moreno MA, Zarazaga M, *et al.* Detection of CMY-2, CTX-M-14, and SHV-12 beta-lactamases in *Escherichia coli* fecal-sample isolates from healthy chickens. Antimicrob Agents Chemother 2003; 47(6): 2056-58.

[219]   Hopkins KL, Davies RH, Threlfall EJ Mechanisms of quinolone resistance in *Escherichia coli* and *Salmonella*: recent developments. Int J Antimicrob Agents 2005; 25(5): 358-73.

[220]   Shaheen BW, Wang C, Johnson CM, *et al.* Detection of fluoroquinolone resistance level in clinical canine and feline *Escherichia coli* pathogens using rapid real-time PCR assay. Vet Microbiol 2009; 139(3-4): 379-85.

[221]   Ozeki S, Deguchi T, Yasuda M, *et al.* Development of a rapid assay for detecting gyrA mutations in *Escherichia coli* and determination of incidence of gyrA mutations in clinical strains isolated from patients with complicated urinary tract infections. J Clin Microbiol 1997; 35(9): 2315-19.

[222]   Vila J, Ruiz J, Goni P, *et al.* Detection of mutations in parC in quinolone-resistant clinical isolates of *Escherichia coli*. Antimicrob Agents Chemother 1996; 40(2): 491-93.

[223]   Weigel LM, Steward CD, Tenover FC. gyrA mutations associated with fluoroquinolone resistance in eight species of Enterobacteriaceae. Antimicrob Agents Chemother 1998; 42(10): 2661-67.

[224]   Chen JY, Siu LK, Chen YH, *et al.* Molecular epidemiology and mutations at gyrA and parC genes of ciprofloxacin-resistant *Escherichia coli* isolates from a Taiwan medical center. Microb Drug Resist 2001; 7(1): 47-53.

[225]   Saenz Y, Zarazaga M, Brinas L, *et al.* Mutations in gyrA and parC genes in nalidixic acid-resistant *Escherichia coli* strains from food products, humans and animals. J Antimicrob Chemother 2003; 51(4): 1001-05.

[226]   Everett MJ, Jin YF, Ricci V, *et al.* Contributions of individual mechanisms to fluoroquinolone resistance in 36 *Escherichia coli* strains isolated from humans and animals. Antimicrob Agents Chemother 1996; 40(10): 2380-86.

[227]   Komp LP, Karlsson A, Hughes D. Mutation rate and evolution of fluoroquinolone resistance in *Escherichia coli* isolates from patients with urinary tract infections. Antimicrob Agents Chemother 2003; 47(10): 3222-32.

[228]   Piddock LJ Clinically relevant chromosomally encoded multidrug resistance efflux pumps in bacteria. Clin Microbiol Rev 2006; 19(2): 382-402.

[229]   Strahilevitz J, Jacoby GA, Hooper DC, *et al.* Plasmid-mediated quinolone resistance: a multifaceted threat. Clin Microbiol Rev 2009; 22(4): 664-89.

[230]   Jacoby GA, Chow N, Waites KB. Prevalence of plasmid-mediated quinolone resistance. Antimicrob Agents Chemother 2003; 47(2): 559-62.

[231]   Ouellette M, Kundig C. Microbial multidrug resistance. Int J Antimicrob Agents 1997; 8(3): 179-87.

[232] Testa RT, Petersen PJ, Jacobus NV, *et al. In vitro* and *in vivo* antibacterial activities of the glycylcyclines, a new class of semisynthetic tetracyclines. Antimicrob Agents Chemother 1993; 37(11): 2270-77.

[233] Nikaido H. Multiple antibiotic resistance and efflux. Curr Opin Microbiol 1998; 1(5): 516-23.

[234] Alonso A, Martinez JL. Multiple antibiotic resistance in Stenotrophomonas maltophilia. Antimicrob Agents Chemother 1997; 41(5): 1140-42.

[235] Levy SB. Active efflux mechanisms for antimicrobial resistance. Antimicrob Agents Chemother 1992; 36(4): 695-03.

[236] Oethinger M, Kern WV, Jellen-Ritter AS, *et al.* Ineffectiveness of topoisomerase mutations in mediating clinically significant fluoroquinolone resistance in *Escherichia coli* in the absence of the AcrAB efflux pump. Antimicrob Agents Chemother 2000; 44(1): 10-13.

[237] Cannon M, Harford S, Davies J A comparative study on the inhibitory actions of chloramphenicol, thiamphenicol and some fluorinated derivatives. J Antimicrob Chemother 1990; 26(3): 307-17.

[238] Murray IA, Shaw WV. O-Acetyltransferases for chloramphenicol and other natural products. Antimicrob Agents Chemother 1997; 41(1): 1-6.

[239] Alton NK, Vapnek D. Nucleotide sequence analysis of the chloramphenicol resistance transposon Tn9. Nature 1979; 282(5741): 864-69.

[240] Parent R, Roy PH. The chloramphenicol acetyltransferase gene of Tn2424: a new breed of cat. J Bacteriol 1992; 174(9): 2891-97.

[241] Houang ET, Chu YW, Lo WS, *et al.* Epidemiology of rifampin ADP-ribosyltransferase (arr-2) and metallo-beta-lactamase (blaIMP-4) gene cassettes in class 1 integrons in Acinetobacter strains isolated from blood cultures in 1997 to 2000. Antimicrob Agents Chemother 2003; 47(4): 1382-90.

[242] Pai H, Byeon JH, Yu S, *et al. Salmonella* enterica serovar typhi strains isolated in Korea containing a multidrug resistance class 1 integron. Antimicrob Agents Chemother 2003; 47(6): 2006-08.

[243] Bischoff KM, White DG, McDermott PF, *et al.* Characterization of chloramphenicol resistance in beta-hemolytic *Escherichia coli* associated with diarrhea in neonatal swine. J Clin Microbiol 2002; 40(2): 389-94.

[244] Blickwede M, Schwarz S. Molecular analysis of florfenicol-resistant *Escherichia coli* isolates from pigs. J Antimicrob Chemother 2004; 53(1): 58-64.

[245] Baucheron S, Imberechts H, Chaslus-Dancla E, *et al.* The AcrB multidrug transporter plays a major role in high-level fluoroquinolone resistance in *Salmonella* enterica serovar typhimurium phage type DT204. Microb Drug Resist 2002; 8(4): 281-89.

[246] Lee A, Mao W, Warren MS, *et al.* Interplay between efflux pumps may provide either additive or multiplicative effects on drug resistance. J Bacteriol 2000; 182(11): 3142-50.

[247] Radstrom P, Swedberg G. RSF1010 and a conjugative plasmid contain sulII, one of two known genes for plasmid-borne sulfonamide resistance dihydropteroate synthase. Antimicrob Agents Chemother 1988; 32(11): 1684-92.

[248] Adrian PV, Thomson CJ, Klugman KP, *et al.* New gene cassettes for trimethoprim resistance, dfr13, and Streptomycin-spectinomycin resistance, aadA4, inserted on a class 1 integron. Antimicrob Agents Chemother 2000; 44(2): 355-61.

[249] Yu EW, Aires JR, Nikaido H. AcrB multidrug efflux pump of *Escherichia coli*: composite substrate-binding cavity of exceptional flexibility generates its extremely wide substrate specificity. J Bacteriol 2003; 185(19): 5657-64.

[250] Rosenberg EY, Ma D, Nikaido H. AcrD of *Escherichia coli* is an aminoglycoside efflux pump. J Bacteriol 2000; 182(6): 1754-56.

[251] Schwarz S, Chaslus-Dancla E. Use of antimicrobials in veterinary medicine and mechanisms of resistance. Vet Res 2001; 32(3-4): 201-25.

[252] Pohl P, Glupczynski Y, Marin M, *et al.* Replicon typing characterization of plasmids encoding resistance to gentamicin and apramycin in *Escherichia coli* and *Salmonella* typhimurium isolated from human and animal sources in Belgium. Epidemiol Infect 1993; 111(2): 229-38.

[253] Ho PL, Wong RC, Lo SW, *et al.* Genetic identity of aminoglycoside resistance genes in *Escherichia coli* isolates from human and animal sources. J Med Microbiol 2010 25(6): 702-07.

[254] Osborn AM, Boltner D. When phage, plasmids, and transposons collide: genomic islands, and conjugative- and mobilizable-transposons as a mosaic continuum. Plasmid 2002; 48(3): 202-12.

[255] Thorsted PB, Macartney DP, Akhtar P, *et al.* Complete sequence of the IncPbeta plasmid R751: implications for evolution and organisation of the IncP backbone. J Mol Biol 1998; 282(5): 969-90.

[256] Licht TR, Struve C, Christensen BB, *et al.* Evidence of increased spread and establishment of plasmid RP4 in the intestine under sub-inhibitory tetracycline concentrations. FEMS Microbiol Ecol. 2003; 44(2): 217-23.

[257] Hart WS, Heuzenroeder MW, Barton MD. A study of the transfer of tetracycline resistance genes between *Escherichia coli* in the intestinal tract of a mouse and a chicken model. J Vet Med B Infect Dis Vet Public Health 2006; 53(7): 333-40.

[258] Salyers AA, Gupta A, Wang Y. Human intestinal bacteria as reservoirs for antibiotic resistance genes. Trends Microbiol 2004; 12(9): 412-16.

[259] Johnson JR, Sannes MR, Croy C, *et al.* Antimicrobial drug-resistant *Escherichia coli* from humans and poultry products, Minnesota and Wisconsin, 2002-2004. Emerg Infect Dis 2007; 13(6): 838-46.

[260] Aarestrup FM, Seyfarth AM, Emborg HD, *et al.* Effect of abolishment of the use of antimicrobial agents for growth promotion on occurrence of antimicrobial resistance in fecal enterococci from food animals in Denmark. Antimicrob Agents Chemother 2001; 45(7): 2054-59.

CHAPTER 11

The Scope of Bacterial Resistance to Antibiotics in Some Countries in the Middle East and North Africa

Noha Gamal Khalaf[1*] and Nancy D. Hanson[2]

[1]Department of Microbiology and Immunology, Faculty of Pharmacy, Modern Science and Art University, Cario, Egypt and [2]Creighton University School of Medicine, Center for Research in Anti-Infectives and Biotechnology, Department of Medical Microbiology and Immunology, 2500 California Plaza, Omaha, NE 68178, USA

Abstract: Data available on bacterial resistance to antibiotics in the Middle East and some African countries mainly comprised sporadic nosocomial outbreaks. However, some surveillance studies, such as the PEARLS and ARMed have examined resistance determinants and patterns of common nosocomial pathogens in some Middle Eastern and North African countries. But no national surveillance figures have been published in any of these individual countries. In this chapter we will present reported rates of bacterial resistance to antibiotics in clinically important pathogens such as MRSA, *Escherichia coli* and other selected Enterobacteriaceae in this geographical region. In addition, we will discuss studies on nosocomial pathogens notorious for multidrug resistance such as *Acinetobacter baumannii*, *Pseudomonas aeruginosa*, as well as ESBL producers of the Enterobacteriaceae that are prevalent in some Middle Eastern and African countries. These clinically important pathogens were reported to possess various ESBL genes of the TEM-, SHV-, CTX-M-families; as well as the carbapenem hydrolyzing metallo- and OXA-type β-lactamases. Other resistance determinants were also reported and include the integron associated *qnr* gene, and the *aac (6')*-Ib-cr gene which codes for aminoglycoside resistance and reduced susceptibility to ciprofloxacin. In addition, community acquired infections caused by MRSA and ESBL producers of the Enterobacteriaceae that have been reported in this geographical region will be covered. Because of the disturbing high rates of bacterial resistance to antibiotics in this geographical region, some countries found it compelling to initiate Infection Control programs to hamper the spread of resistant pathogens.

Keywords: *Escherichia coli, Acinetobacter baumannii, Pseudomonas aeruginosa,* OXA-type β-lactamases, Enterobacteriaceae, TEM, SHV, CTX-M-families, MRSA.

INTRODUCTION

Prolonged hospital stays and higher mortality rates are more often observed in patients with infections caused by resistant bacteria than in patients infected with susceptible bacteria [1]. The spread of antibiotic resistance adds economic burden on the healthcare sector as well as on patients, particularly in low income countries where affordable first line treatments are not effective [2]. The economic burden is significant in countries where the average hospital cost of a single patient suffering from hospital acquired infection is equivalent to the national gross income per capita [3].

The evolution and spread of drug resistance have been driven by the increasing use of antibiotics, the insufficient control on dispensing antibiotics, lack of infection control, low wages for healthcare workers especially in low income countries, and more importantly the limited or lack of attention paid by the Governments with respect to increasing resistance rates [2].

Antibiotics are still available without prescription in some European countries, and are frequently prescribed to outpatients with urinary tract and respiratory tract infections in primary care practices [4, 5]. Studies from Belgium and France were carried out to raise awareness of prudent antibiotic use for outpatients and primary care prescribers [6, 7]. The uncontrolled use of antibiotics and the availability of

Address correspondence to Noha Gamal Khalaf: Department of Microbiology and Immunology, Faculty of Pharmacy, Modern Science and Art University, Cario, Egypt; Tel: +202 383 715 17; Fax: +202 383 715 43; Email: ng_khalaf@yahoo.com

antibiotics without prescriptions in the Middle East and Africa have been documented [8-11]. Self-medication of antibiotics is mainly based on previous experience of effectiveness, and antibiotics are usually available over the counter at the pharmacies besides previously prescribed antibiotics stored in households [10, 11] . Furthermore, patients more often skip physician and laboratory visits and seek antibiotic treatment directly from the pharmacist, especially those patients without health insurance [12]. Governments of limited resource countries that have high prevalence of resistance to antibiotics may need to follow the steps taken by European governments [13] to endorse events that raise the awareness of the public and health care professionals to the prudent use of antibiotics. This can be done through financial support, organizing press meetings, and encouraging members of the health ministries to actively participate in the events. Non-governmental agencies such as pharmaceutical companies, professional associations and pharmacies can also be involved [13]. There is a need to control the availability of antibiotics without prescription in the community, which may be enforced by decision makers in Health ministries in these countries, and also to encourage hospitals to strictly follow antibiotic prescribing guidelines. Finally, governments in certain countries may also need to consider paying sufficient wages and offering proper incentives so that healthcare workers adhere to guidelines.

The next section will briefly discuss current situations in antibiotic consumption for some hospitals in the region as well as limitations of antibiotic consumption in other hospitals in spite of the presence of hospital policies and prescribing guidelines in some countries in this geographical region. The prevalence of antibiotic resistance in Gram Negative rods, notably Enterobacteriaceae as well as *Pseudomonas aeruginosa* in North African countries and some countries in the Middle East will be discussed in the next section. In addition, resistance rates to methicillin in *Staphylococcus aureus* in hospital and community settings will be presented.

In section III, the molecular mechanisms of Gram negative resistance in countries of this region to different antibiotic classes will be thoroughly discussed. This will cover ESBL producers of the Enterobacteriaceae and *P. aeruginosa* as well as carbapenem resistant *Acinetobacter baumannii*. Finally, section IV will address intervention programs that have been initiated in some countries such as Egypt, Jordan and Lebanon, with highlights on the Infection Control program implemented in Egypt, and the current situation on the Infection Control practices in the region.

It is evident that we have a long way to go to address all the problems associated with healthcare infections. But these problems present an economic burden on the healthcare system in the countries of this region. This chapter points out that antibiotic resistance is a problem which is multifaceted and that is one of the reasons it is hard to control. The multifaceted aspects of antibiotic resistance including the bugs and resistance mechanisms themselves as well as use and availability of antibiotics, and how all these aspects are related will be presented in this chapter.

REPORTED RESISTANCE RATES OF GRAM-NEGATIVE AND GRAM-POSITIVE BACTERIA TO ANTIBIOTICS

Public health surveillance of bacterial infections contributes to a better understanding of the current health status of the population and rates of infectious diseases. These types of surveillance data enable health authorities and ministries of health to intervene in order to reduce rates and risks of infectious diseases caused by nosocomial and community acquired resistant bacteria [14]. Intercontinental, regional and national surveillance studies have reported resistance rates of nosocomial pathogens in the Middle East region and North Africa (Table **1**) [15-19].

Rates of Antimicrobial Resistance in Gram-Negative Bacteria in the Region

In the Pan-European Antimicrobial Resistance Using Local Surveillance (PEARLS) study during the year 2001-2002, comparisons of resistance rates among some countries in the region with some European countries was made possible. Extended Spectrum β-Lactamase (ESBL) production among Enterobacteriaceae isolates was as low as 2% in the Netherlands and as high as 38% in Egypt [16]. However, compared to Egypt, lower percentages of ESBL producers (18%) were reported for Enterobacteriaceae isolates from Lebanon and Saudi Arabia [16] although the data presented for Egypt with respect to ESBL producers may be skewed given the low number (26 isolates) of Enterobacteriaceae evaluated [16]. More representative figures were reported in the Antibiotic Resistance Surveillance & Control in the Mediterranean Region (ARMed) study, where susceptibility data from 58 laboratories serving 64 hospitals in some southern and eastern Mediterranean countries were collected from 2003-2005 [18, 19].

In the ARMed study, resistance of *E. coli* to 3rd generation cephalosporins was lowest in Malta (1%) and highest in Egypt (70%) in 2005. From 2003 to 2005, resistance to 3rd generation cephalosporins increased from 7% to 33% in Morocco, while a significant decrease was seen in Tunisia (from 20% to 11%) [19]. In a retrospective multicenter study during the year (1999-2000), microbiology laboratory records from five hospitals in Cairo, Egypt were analyzed [15]. The resistance rate to 3rd generation cephalosporins in *E. coli* and *K. pneumoniae* was 40-60%. *P. aeruginosa* resistance to 3rd generation cephalosporins in this multicenter study reached up to 38-45%, and was 50-68% in clinical *P. aeruginosa* isolates collected from three hospitals in another multicenter study carried out in Minia, Egypt [15-20]. It is worth mentioning that hospital environmental *P. aeruginosa* isolates collected from the three hospitals in the study from Minia were 90-100% resistant to 3rd generation cephalosporins. This worrisome finding calls for immediate attention of the Infection Control teams in these hospitals and the need to investigate the clonal relationships of these environmental isolates with the clinical isolates. Carbapenems can be considered the most potent β-lactam that can be used in hospitals as resistance rates to this drug remain as low as 5-9% in the Southern-Eastern Mediterranean region (Borg *et al.*, 2008) [19]. In spite of the high prevalence of resistance to 3rd generation cephalosporins among Gram-negative isolates from Egypt, 70-100% susceptibility to carbapenems among Enterobacteriaceae and *P. aeruginosa* was noted [15-20].

The ARMed surveillance study reported a significant increase in fluoroquinolone resistance among *E. coli* in Egypt and Turkey over the study period (2003-2005). A low percentage of fluoroquinolone resistance (5%) was seen in Algeria and ≥40% resistance was seen in Egypt, Lebanon and Turkey from 2003-2005 [19]. These data are in contrast with an earlier multicenter study from Cairo hospitals in Egypt, where only 20% *E. coli*, *K. pneumoniae*, and *Enterobacter* spp. strains were resistant to fluoroquinolones [15]. The rate of resistance of *P. aeruginosa* isolates to ciprofloxacin from the same multicenter study in Cairo was low (4%) [15]. A slightly higher resistance rate (29%) of clinical *P. aeruginosa* isolates to fluoroquinolones from three hospitals in Minia, Egypt was reported [20]. This rate is close to the resistance rates exhibited by Enterobacteriaceae isolates from the latter multicenter study in Cairo [15]. Interestingly, hospital environmental *P. aeruginosa* isolates collected from furniture, medical appliances, patients' beds, tables, ward sinks and surgical equipment during the multicenter study from Minia showed a much higher rate of resistance to ciprofloxacin (62%) [20]. The authors have noticed that the hospital environmental isolates possessed higher resistance rates to antibiotics than the clinical samples [20].

The highest proportion of resistance to aminoglycosides among *E. coli* isolates, collected during 2003-2005 in the ARMed study, was seen in Egypt (60%) [19]. This percentage of resistant isolates was similar to the resistance rate (50-70%) for all Gram-negative bacilli evaluated in the multicenter study from Cairo in 1999-2000 [15]. Resistance among Enterobacteriaceae to multiple drug classes including 3rd generation cephalosporins, aminoglycosides and fluoroquinolones have also been evaluated in the eastern and southern Mediterranean countries. During 2005, thirty percent of *E. coli* isolates from Egypt were resistant to 3rd generation cephalosporins, aminoglycosides and fluoroquinolones. In contrast, participating hospitals in Algeria, Cyprus and Malta showed resistance rates below 5% for these three antibiotic classes. Egypt, Jordan and Morocco saw a significant increase in multidrug resistance from 2003 to 2005 [19].

Rates of Antimicrobial Resistance in *Staphylococcus aureus* in the Region

With regard to resistance in Gram-positive organisms *S. aureus* was most notable. Methicillin resistance in *S. aureus* (MRSA) was observed in the Middle Eastern and North African countries during 2003-2005 [19]. The intercontinental surveillance study PEARLS evaluated during the year 2001-2002 showed that the incidence of MRSA was highest in Egypt, reporting 44% [16], with a very low incidence (4%) reported for

Lebanon and no MRSA isolates reported from Saudi Arabia [16]. However, the numbers of isolates evaluated for those countries were low (9 *S. aureus* isolates from Egypt and 25 isolates from each of Lebanon and Saudi Arabia) and therefore most likely an under representation of the number of resistant isolates in those patient populations.

High rates of MRSA in Middle Eastern and North African countries have been reported in some national studies from Algeria, Tunisia, Jordan, Lebanon, and Saudi Arabia [21-25]. In the ARMed surveillance study, spanning 2003-2005, a very high prevalence of MRSA was identified from Egyptian hospitals, where >50% of *S. aureus* isolates were resistant to methicillin. This study also identified that the highest proportion of MRSA was reported from Jordan and Egypt [18]. In a multicenter retrospective study covering patients from different socioeconomic strata in Cairo, Egypt during 1999-2000, methicillin resistance rates among both *S. aureus* and coagulase negative staphylococci were 70% [15]. The patient population in this study represented pediatric and adult patients, and covered a diverse socioeconomic patient population ranging from high socioeconomic class patients admitted to private hospitals to low-income patients admitted to university hospitals. However, the study did not indicate whether the methicillin resistant *S. aureus* were prevalent among a specific socioeconomic class of patients. A variation between prevalence rates of MRSA in individual hospitals in the same country was seen in the ARMed study during the years 2003-2005 [18]. Major differences in the numbers of MRSA isolates observed between hospitals were found in Egypt and Turkey, while the smallest differences were found in Morocco and Tunisia. Vancomycin resistance among the Gram positive cocci was not detected in *S. aureus* isolates from Egypt, Saudi Arabia or from Lebanon [15, 16].

Healthcare is more concentrated in urban areas, thus it is difficult to estimate the percentage of population covered from rural areas [16]. In the ARMed surveillance [2003-2005], nine hospitals from Egypt were represented but with coverage of only 17% of the population. No data was available on the geographical distribution of participating hospitals in Egypt. In contrast, 5 and 3 hospitals in Cyprus and Malta; respectively participated in the study evaluating resistance in *S. aureus*, but that number of hospitals covered a high percentage of the population (95-100%). Although 11 hospitals participated in the study from Turkey, only 6% of the population was evaluated but those hospitals were evenly distributed across the country and perhaps more representative of the whole population [18, 19].

Genetic Basis of Methicillin Resistance in *S. aureus* and Molecular Epidemiology of Community Acquired MRSA (CA-MRSA) in the Region

Methicillin resistance in *Staphylococcus aureus* is due to the PBP-2a, a penicillin binding protein that has low affinity for β-lactams and is encoded by the *mecA* gene. This gene is harbored on a mobile genetic element known as the SCC*mec* cassette [26]. The SCC*mec* cassette is classified into types I, II, III, IV, and V. SCC*mec* types IV and V are small in size and are detected in community acquired MRSA isolates [27, 28]. Type IV has been shown to transfer between different Staphylococcal species as well as within the same species [29]. Community acquired MRSA (CA-MRSA) infections are caused by MRSA isolates in healthy individuals with no prior hospital exposure. However, recent reports documented hospital acquired infections caused by CA-MRSA [30]. CA-MRSA isolates harbor genes encoding skin and soft tissue toxins such as Panton Valentine Leukocidin (PVL) genes [31].

It is noteworthy to mention that community acquired MRSA has been identified in this geographical region. A case of brain abscess due to PVL positive MRSA was reported in a patient with a history of hepatitis and diabetes from Egypt [32]. The isolated PVL positive MRSA belonged to ST30 and possessed the gene cassette SCC*mec* V [32]. The same research group further studied the molecular characteristics of PVL positive CA-MRSA isolates from Egypt and found these isolates belonged to different ST clones (ST30, 80 and 1010) [33]. Intravenous and inhalational opiate drug abusers were found to be at high risk for CA-MRSA infections [34]. A comparataive study from Cairo, Egypt was performed between patients that abused drugs and those that did not in which samples of sputum, blood, nasal and throat were evaluated for the presence of CA-MRSA. CA-MRSA colonized or was responsible for causing infections in 50% of drug abuser group compared to 10% colonization and/or infection in the non-abuser group. In order to exclude hospital acquired MRSA from the study, samples were collected from patients in each group within 48h of hospitalization, and patients who had previous exposures to healthcare facilities such as hospitalization, dialysis, surgery or working in a medical specialty were excluded from the study [34].

In Algeria, a hospital outbreak was caused by PVL positive MRSA that belonged to the ST80 clone and possessed SCC*mec* IV. The PVL positive MRSA was obtained from patients with community acquired and hospital acquired infections in the dermatology unit [21]. In Jordan, nasal carriage of *S. aureus* was detected in 40% of the healthy young adult population. Methicillin resistance was detected in 19% of the healthy group and in 57% of nosocomial isolates collected during the same period with the *mecA* gene detected in all MRSA isolates from both groups [23]. Chongtrakool and coworkers studied the molecular characteristics of MRSA clones from Asian countries, including Saudi Arabia [35]. The SCC*mec* type III predominated in isolates from Saudi Arabia, India, Sri Lanka, Singapore, Indonesia, Thailand, Vietnam, Philippines and China. Eighteen isolates of the MRSA from the Saudi hospital possessed SCC*mec* III and one isolate was positive for SCC*mec* IV [35].

Antibiotic Consumption in the Region

Antibiotic resistance has been linked to the consumption of antibiotics in hospitals [36]. The compiled data on the prevalence of multidrug resistant hospital pathogens in the Mediterranean region [37] has encouraged data collection on antibiotic consumption in southern and eastern Mediterranean countries [38]. Eight hospitals in Egypt, 3 in Jordan, and one hospital in both Lebanon and Tunisia were included in this study, as well as hospitals in Malta, Cyprus and Turkey. The consumption of penicillins with and without inhibitor combinations, together with first generation cephalosporins was high among 15 of the 25 hospitals included in the study. Third generation cephalosporins were among the top 5 classes consumed In five hospitals in Egypt, glycopeptides and carbapenems were never used. This most likely occurs because these hospitals rely on donations and both drug classes may be too expensive to be included in the hospitals' formulary. It was noticed that hospitals with a high utilization of third generation cephalosporins also consumed carbapenems at a similar rate. The use of macrolides was low and tetracyclines and chloramphenicol were rarely used in any of the hospitals analyzed [38]. The high antibiotic consumption was similar to other countries in the Mediterranean region [39]. To explain the high rates of resistance previously identified by the ARMed project [17-19], the authors hypothesized that this was due to frequent use of 3rd generation cephalosporins, quinolones, and carbapenems for empiric treatment in those hospitals; in spite of the fact that alternative first line effective therapy was available [38].

In instances where resistance to antibiotics is linked to heavy antibiotic consumption, the problem of resistance can be addressed by controlling the administration of antibiotics [36]. In hospitals, this can be achieved by paying close attention to establishing as well as enforcing adherence to antibiotic prescribing guidelines. Only 33% of participating hospitals in the Southern and Eastern Mediterranean countries follow guidelines regarding prescribing practice [40]. These guidelines are often hard to adhere to in some hospitals in the Middle East and North Africa as these hospitals rely on antibiotic donations while others receive bulk amounts of one particular drug at any given time [40]. The influence of pharmaceutical representatives on the deviation from prescribing guidelines may be a contributing factor since 69% of locations reported receiving samples and gifts from representatives. In addition, there is unregulated access of pharmaceutical representatives to physicians in 90% of the locations reported [40].

There is an immediate need for epidemiologists and staff members to initiate aggressive real time surveillance studies to track the presence and emergence of antibiotic resistant organisms in limited resource countries. These real time data are needed to implement and then oversee recommendations which will reduce the emergence and/or spread of resistant pathogens [41]. Moreover, governments of countries with a high prevalence of resistance to antibiotics, especially those limited in resources, need to take active steps to reduce the spread and emergence of resistance. These steps should begin with the implementation of national surveillance studies to identify the prevalence of the resistant organisms known to cause treatment failures and added economic burden.

Table 1: Surveillance Studies from North Africa and The Mediterranean Region[a].

Study	No. of Countries	Centers/ Hospitals	Duration of Study	Specimens	Total no. of Isolates	Microorganism (Number of Isolates)	Refs.
PEARLS	17	38	2001-2002	Blood cultures, respiratory tract, Urine, Wound swab, Fluids	9000	*S. aureus* (908) (32% MR[b]) *Enterococcus faecium* (949) (8.7% VR[c]) *K. pneumoniae* (2206) (18.2 % ESBL +ve[d]) *E. coli* (2609) (5.4% ESBL +ve) Enterobacter spp. (2328) (8% ESBL +ve)	[16][g]
ARMed	9	64	2003-2005	Blood cultures, CSF[e]	5091	*E. coli*	[17][h]
				Blood cultures	5353	*S. aureus* (5353) (39% MR)	[17][h]
Multicenter Pilot Survey in Mediterranean Area	3	9	N/A	N/A	N/A	*Enterobacteriaceae* resistant to 3rd generation cephalosporins in Tunisia and Algeria MRSA with highest incidence in France *A. baumannii* resistant to imipenem in Tunisia	[42][i]
Multicenter Retrospective Surveillance Cairo-Egypt	1	5	1999-2000	Blood cultures	1529	*S. aureus* (77) (70% MR) CoNS[f] (365) (77% MR) *K. pneumoniae* (149) *E. coli* (50) *Citrobacter* spp. (24) *Enterobacter* spp. (532) *Acinetobacter* spp. (29) *P. aeruginosa* (303)	[15][j]

[a]The number of isolates, sites of isolation and number of centers are shown, besides percentage data on some resistance determinants

[b]MR: Methicillin resistant

[c]VR: Vancomycin resistant

[d]ESBL +ve: Extended Spectrum β-lactamase positive

[e]CSF: cerebrospinal fluid

[f]CoNS: Coagulase negative staphylococci

[g] (16)   Bouchillon *et al.*, 2004   [i] (42) Amazian *et al.*, 2006

[h] (17)   Borg *et al.*, 2006   [j] (15) El Kholy *et al.*, 2003

MOLECULAR MECHANISMS OF RESISTANCE IN GRAM NEGATIVE RODS

The selective pressure exerted by extended spectrum cephalosporins and the trend of antibiotic use in the region (please refer to section II) seem to play an important role in the spread of extended spectrum β-lactamase (ESBL)-producing Enterobacteriaceae. This section will focus on the most recent findings regarding the characterization and epidemiology of ESBLs in this geographical region. These recent findings will enable healthcare professionals to monitor the increase of ESBL producing organisms in hospitals and in the community in order to intervene to prevent their global spread. In addition, other resistance mechanisms playing a role in β-lactam resistance as well as other classes of antibiotics in Gram negative bacteria will be addressed. The majority of bacteria that overcome the action of β-lactams produce β-lactamases that hydrolyze the β-lactam ring of the drug [43]. The majority of Extended Spectrum β-

Lactamases (ESBLs) are plasmid-encoded molecular class A enzymes [44], which are inhibited by clavulanic acid. They are capable of hydrolyzing penicillins, 1st, 2nd, and 3rd- generation cephalosporins, and monobactams, but not cephamycins or carbapenems [45]. These enzymes differ from their parent enzymes by one or more amino acid changes. Numerous types of ESBLs have been characterized, and more than 400 ESBLs can be found in the website hosted by Dr. Goerge Jacoby and Dr. Karen Bush (www.lahey.org/studies/webt.asp) [46]. ESBLs have been reported from more than 30 countries in the five continents, with TEM-, SHV-, and CTX-Ms being the most prevalent ESBLs. A very recent and simplified ESBL nomenclature scheme has been proposed by Giske *et al.* [47] for clinicians and health care professionals who are not involved in ESBL research. In this new nomenclature, ESBLs are not confined to class A β-lactamases that are inhibited by clavulanate, but they are expanded to include β-lactamases that hydrolyze extended spectrum cephalosporins and carbapenems [47]. Class A ESBLs are designated as $ESBL_A$; plasmid mediated AmpCs and OXA-ESBLs are designated as miscellaneous ESBLs ($ESBL_M$); and ESBLs with hydrolytic activity against carbapenems are designated as $ESBL_{CARBA}$, which is further divided into classes A, B and D carbapenemases [47].

ESBLs belonging to class D are capable of hydrolyzing oxacillin. OXA ESBLs hydrolyze ceftazidime, and/or cefotaxime, cefepime, cefpirome, aztreonam and moxalactams [48]. OXA ESBLs are encoded by genes carried on plasmids that are frequently observed in *P. aeruginosa* [48-50] and to a lesser extent in *Enterobacteriaceae*. OXA ESBLs are derived by point mutations of OXA-2 (such as OXA-15, OXA-32) [51-52]; and OXA-10 (such as OXA-11 to OXA-14, OXA-16 to OXA-19, and OXA-28) [48]. OXA ESBLs also include OXA-18 [53] and OXA-45 [50]. Only the latter two enzymes are inhibited by clavulanic acid. OXA-45 confers resistance to ceftazidime and aztreonam in *E. coli* transconjugants [50].

Many studies carried out in the Middle East and North Africa were limited to phenotypic detection of ESBLs and susceptibility testing. During a 2-months outbreak in 2001, *K. pneumoniae* accounted for 73% of isolates obtained from neonates with a positive blood culture in a NICU in a Cairo hospital in Egypt [54]. Fifty-eight percent of these *K. pneumoniae* isolates were positive for ESBLs [54]. In a more recent study performed in a pediatric hospital in Mansoura, 1600 pediatric patients were suspected of septicemia and 45% were positive for Gram negative septicemia. *K. pneumonia, E. cloacae, Serratia marcescens* and *E. coli* were identified from the blood samples collected from these patients and 45% of the isolates produced ESBLs [55].

The percentage of resistant *K. pneumonia, E. cloacae,* and *E.coli* to more than one extended spectrum β-lactam in a Jordanian hospital ICU in 1994 was 25-43% [56]. Three years later, the rate of *K. pneumoniae* and *E. coli* ESBL producers in the ICU wards in the same hospital were determined [57]. A significant difference in the susceptibility data to ceftazidime and aztreonam was noted. *Klebsiella* spp. showed an increase in resistance from 33 to 65% to aztreonam, and an increase in resistance rate to ceftazidime from 29% to 80% [57]. *Enterobacter* spp. showed an increase in resistance from 29% to 54% to aztreonam and an increase in resistance to cefotaxime from 43 % to 62%, compared to the data from 1996. Fifty four percent of ESBL *E. coli* producers were resistant to aztreonam compared to the 29% resistance in 1994 [57].

Hospital acquired *K. pneumoniae* bacteremia was investigated during a 2 year study at a 500-bed hospital and a tertiary care center in Eastern Saudi Arabia [58]. Ten out of 26 *K. pneumoniae* positive blood cultures were ESBL producers. Prior treatment with 3rd generation cephalosporins and the use of invasive devices were risk factors for the acquisition of ESBL producing *K. pneumonia*. In a 2003-2004 survey in a hospital in Saudi Arabia, 600 Enterobacteriaceae isolates were tested for ESBL production [59]. ESBL positive strains of *K. pneumonia, E. coli* and *E. cloacae* isolates were identified and constituted 15.8% of the total isolates in the study [59]. The authors of this study pointed out the diagnostic and therapeutic challenges health care professionals face to manage infections caused by ESBL positive isolates. Further evidence of this was demonstrated by a study examining the prevalence of ESBL production among 2455 *E. coli* and *K. pneumoniae* isolates collected from a hospital in Khobar, Saudi Arabia. Eleven percent of the isolates possessed ESBLs and therefore carbapenems proved to be an effective therapy [60]. Another study tested 6750 Gram negative isolates obtained from in-patients and out-patients for ESBL production in a centralized laboratory in Eastern Saudi Arabia [61]. During the period of January 2004 through December

2005, 409 isolates (6%) possessed ESBLs with ESBL producing *E. coli* frequently isolated from urine samples of inpatients.

The number of citations on ESBLs has increased sharply in the recent years as illustrated in the review of Paterson and Bonomo (2005) [62]. In the recent past, characterization of β-lactamases at the molecular level has been carried out in countries of the Middle East and North Africa. These studies highlighted how widespread genes encoding ESBLs such as CTX-M-15 and SHV types had become to this region.

CTX-M ESBLs Family

CTX-Ms are class A ESBLs that are most active against cefotaxime [63]. However, some CTX-Ms, such as CTX-M-15 and CTX-M-19, can hydrolyze ceftazidime [64]. Different types of CTX-M enzymes have been identified and classified into groups based on their nucleotide sequence. Group I comprises CTX-M-1, -3, -15, -28; and CTX-M-9, -14, -16, -27 belong to group IV [63, 65]. Paterson and Bonomo have commented on the distribution of CTX-M ESBLs. Previously, they were more frequently found in South America, the Far East, and Eastern Europe. However, in recent years, increased reports from almost all parts of the world have been cited, pointing out the global incidence of this family of ESBLs [62].

CTX-M-15 is the most prevalent ESBL in the Middle East and North African countries and for that matter, in the world. During the years 2005 and 2006, CTX-M-15-producing *E. coli*, *Enterobacter cloacae* and *K. pneumoniae* isolates were reported from Egypt, Algeria, Tunisia, United Arab Emirates (UAE) and Lebanon [66-71]. CTX-M-15 producing *Salmonella* spp. were reported in Lebanon in 2005 [72] and later in Kuwait and United Arab Emirates (UAE) [73].

Other CTX-M enzymes have also been reported in this region and include the group-1 enzymes CTX-M-1, -3; and CTX-M-9, -14, -16, -27 which belong to group IV (Table **2**). *K. pneumoniae* producing CTX-M-14 in the region was first reported in Egypt [74]. CTX-M-28 (Group I) was detected among Enterobacteriaceae from Tunisia and Algeria [75, 76]. These enzymes are widely disseminated in *K. pneumonia*, *E. coli* and to a lesser extent in *E. cloacae*. Similar findings on the widespread prevalence of CTX-M-15 in Europe have been reported. A recent review on the distribution of ESBLs in Europe showed that CTX-M-15 and CTX-M group 1 variants have spread throughout Northern and Southern Europe and the United Kingdom [77], while group 9 (CTX-M-9 and CTX-M-14) was dominant in Spain [78]. Moreover, CTX-M-3 was prevalent in Eastern Europe, in addition to the widespread distribution of *K. pneumoniae* isolates producing CTX-M-15 in Hungary and Bulgaria [77].

ESBLs of the TEM- and SHV- Families

SHV-ESBLs, particularly SHV-2, -5, and -12 are commonly detected in the Middle East and North Africa, albeit they are less frequent than CTX-M ESBLs [66, 79-90] (Table **2**). Similarly SHV-12 and SHV-5 were common in Europe [77]. TEM-4 and TEM-104 have been identified in the Middle East region and North Africa [79, 80], while TEM-3 and TEM-24 remain common ESBLs in Europe [77].

Other ESBLs

PER-ESBLs are class A β-lactamases that are remotely related (25-27% homology) to TEM- and SHV-type ESBLs [91]. These enzymes have been previously detected in *P. aeruginosa* and *A. baumannii* isolates in Turkey [92]. Isolates of *P. aeruginosa* possessing PER ESBLs have been detected in Europe [62] and these enzymes have been more recently detected in *Proteus vulgaris* and *Providencia stuartii* isolates from Algeria [93]. VEB ESBLs are molecular class A enzymes, which are inhibited by clavulanic acid. VEB ESBLs are not related to CTX-M, TEM- or SHV-derived ESBLs, but do share 38% sequence identity with PER-1/PER-2, and 46% identity with the chromosomally encoded class A enzyme, CME-1, of *Chryseobacterium meningosepticum* [94]. They are associated with mobile genetic elements such as plasmids or integrons [95]. VEB ESBLs confer resistance to ceftazidime (MICs $\geq$128 μg/ml) and aztreonam (MICs $\geq$ 32 μg/ml) [95, 96] and have been associated with reduced susceptibility to cefepime in *Enterobacteriaceae* [95] and *Pseudomonas aeruginosa* [97]. The geographic diversity displayed by VEB

ESBLs is remarkable, they have been reported in an *E. coli* isolate from the USA [98], in *P. aeruginosa*, *E. coli*, and *E. cloacae* from Europe [99-101], and in *P. aeruginosa* from Iran [102, 103].

In the Middle East, a VEB-1-like ESBL was identified in *P. aeruginosa* from Kuwait [104]. In North Africa, *bla*$_{VEB-1b}$ was carried on a conjugative plasmid and flanked by repeated elements in a *Providencia stuartii* isolate from Algeria. This was the first report of a *bla*$_{VEB-1b}$ gene cassette not associated with an integron structure [96]. More recently, an *E. cloacae* isolate collected from an Algerian hospital was found to possess *bla*$_{VEB-1}$ [105] (Table **2**). Additional reports on ESBL producing *P. aeruginosa* in the region include OXA-18 [106] and SHV-2a [83, 84] from Tunisia (Table **2**).

Co-Production of CTX-M, TEM- and/or SHV-ESBLs

The description of *K. pneumoniae* and *E. coli* isolates simultaneously coproducing CTX-M ESBLs, TEM-and/or SHV-ESBLs has been reported in the Middle East and North Africa [66, 79, 80, 82, 85, 88, 90, 96, 107] (Table **2**). In their recent review, Coque *et al.* [77] reported the coproduction of TEM- or SHV-ESBLs with CTX-M ESBLs, OXA carbapenemases, a VIM-metallo-β-lactamase and/or the class A KPCs in Europe.

Presence of Genes Encoding Broad Spectrum β-Lactamases Associated With *bla*$_{CTX-M-15}$

Coexistence of the *bla*$_{CTX-M}$ genes with *bla*$_{TEM-1}$ on the same plasmid, and the possible associations with *bla*$_{TEM-2}$, *bla*$_{OXA-1-type}$, and *bla*$_{SHV-type}$ genes have been identified [108, 109]. The broad spectrum class D β-lactamase OXA-1 and the plasmid encoded penicillinase (TEM-1) were co-produced with CTX-M-15 in isolates from Tunisia [69, 82] and Lebanon [107, 110]. An *E. coli* isolate from water samples obtained from fish farms in Egypt was found to possess *bla*$_{CTX-M-15}$ and *bla*$_{OXA-30}$ [80] (Table **2**).

Genetic Background and Mobility of *bla*$_{CTX-M}$ Genes

Plasmids harboring *bla*$_{CTX-M}$ genes are commonly self-transferable plasmids, which helps explain their dissemination [63]. Mobilization of *bla*$_{CTX-M}$ genes is thought to be mediated through IS*Ecp1*-like insertion sequence elements [108, 111]. The *bla*$_{CTX-M}$ gene was carried on plasmids that were self transferable in North African countries [69, 76, 81, 82] and in the UAE [71]. Plasmid characterization classified these plasmids as members of incompatibility FII in Tunisia [88]. A multicenter study in Algeria identified *K. pneumoniae* capable of transferring plasmids [85] Kb that harbored either *bla*$_{CTX-M-15}$ or *bla*$_{CTX-M-3}$. IS*Ecp1B* was found associated with both of the *bla*$_{CTX-M}$ genes [112]. Two studies from Egypt identified the *bla*$_{CTX-M}$ genes and their associated IS*Ecp1* elements mainly in the Enterobacteriaceae [74, 85]. Plasmid transfer by conjugation was documented in *E. coli* producing *bla*$_{CTX-M-15}$ [74] and in *S. typhimurium* producing *bla*$_{CTX-M-14}$ [85].

Clonal Expansion of *E. coli* Producing CTX-M-15

Phylogenetic analysis classified *E. coli* into four phylogenetic groups, A1, B1, B2 and D, while virulent extraintestinal *E. coli* strains fall into groups B2 and D [113]. Phylogenetic grouping is based on genotypic traits such as the presence or absence of a certain gene. A multiplex PCR was used to classify *E. coli* using *chuA* (a gene in enterohemorhagic *E. coli*) and *yiaA* (a chromosomal gene of unknown function) [113]. Nicolas-Chanoine and co-workers [2008] studied *E. coli* isolates from eight countries with respect to their phylogenetic analysis, serotype, genotype using ERIC2 primers, and Multilocus Sequence Typing (MLST). *E. coli* O25:H4 isolates positive for CTX-M-15 and belonging to group B2 from Lebanon, France, Spain, Portugal shared a common sequence type ST131 and the same ERIC2 pattern [114]. CTX-M-15 producing *E. coli* from France, Kuwait, Canada, Portugal, Spain, Switzerland and India were subjected to phylogenetic analysis and those belonging to groups B2 and D were further typed by MLST using standard housekeeping loci (www.mlst.net) [115]. Isolates from Kuwait, France, Canada and India were assigned to groups B2 and sequence type (ST131). The authors concluded that the dissemination of *bla*$_{CTX-M-15}$ gene has been linked to epidemic strains of *E. coli* belonging to phylogenetic group B2 (ST131), and its location on IncF plasmids along with other resistance determinants such as *aac-6'*-lb-cr gene [115]. Interestingly, another study identified *E. coli* carrying the *bla*$_{CTX-M-15}$ gene and belonging to group B2 in France and Tunisia to be linked to the ST131 clone [116].

Phylogenetic analysis and virulence factors determination were used to identify the transfer of a plasmid carrying the $bla_{CTX-M-15}$ from a less virulent *E. coli* clone from Tunisia belonging to group A1 to a more virulent clone belonging to group B2. The authors have suggested that virulence factors such as non-specific adhesins, siderophores, and resistance to phagocytosis enabled the more virulent clone possessing the $bla_{CTX-M-15}$ to spread and persist [69]

Resistance to Cephamycins and pAmpC

Plasmid encoded class AmpC (pAmpC) β-lactamases hydrolyze extended spectrum cephalosporins and cephamycins, but do not hydrolyze cefepime or carbapenems [117]. The nucleotide sequences of plasmid encoded AmpCs are closely related to some chromosomally encoded AmpC β-lactamase. CMY-2 to -7 and LAT-1 are closely related to the chromosomal *ampC* of *C. freundii*, while CMY-1, -8 to -11, and-19 are closely related to the chromosomal *ampC* of *Aeromonas* spp. CMY-2 β-lactamase is the most prevalent worldwide [117]. The nucleotide sequence of the plasmid encoded MIR-1 β-lactamase is closely related to the chromosomal *ampC* of *E. cloacae*, and ACT-1 is related to that of *E. asburiae*. The chromosomal origin of ACC-1 is most likely from *Hafnia alvei*, and the nucleotide sequence of FOX-1 is closely related to the chromosomal *ampC* of *Aeromonas caviae*. Finally, the nucleotide sequence of DHA-1 and -2 are related to the chromosomal ampC of *M. morganii* [117].

In his recent review, Jacoby has mentioned that forty-three CMY alleles are known [http://www.lahey.org/Studies/), and the sequence data for FOX-like; ACC-like; ACT-like; MOX-like and DHA-like enzymes can be found in GenBank [117]. *Klebsiella pneumoniae, Salmonella* spp. and *Proteus* spp. lack chromosomal AmpC β-lactamases, however, pAmpCs have been detected in these isolates [118] [119-123]. Table **2** shows compiled data on Enterobacteriaceae isolates producing ESBLs and pAmpCs [79, 81, 87]. In Algeria, the prevalence of pAmpC producers among Enterobacteriaceae in 3 hospitals was 2.18%. Co-production of β-lactamases has been reported from the isolates collected in this study. The $bla_{CTX-M-15}$ gene was coproduced with bla_{CMY-2} in *K. pneumonia, Serratia marcescens*, and *Proteus mirabilis* isolates from 2 hospitals. One *E. coli* isolate co-produced $bla_{CTX-M-15}$ and bla_{DHA-1}. The bla_{SHV-12} was co-produced with bla_{DHA-1} in an *E. coli* isolate. Other *E. coli* and *P. stuartii* isolates possessed the bla_{CMY-2} gene alone [81]. In addition, CMY-2 was found located on transferable plasmids in *P. stuartii* isolates from Egypt [124], while in an earlier study, CMY-4 was detected in a *K. pneumoniae* isolate collected in a French hospital from a patient originating from Egypt [119].

Carbapenem Resistance

Resistance to carbapenems arises due to the production of hydrolyzing enzymes and/or loss of porin proteins and/or the overproduction of efflux genes [125]. Carbapenemases can be found in 3 out of the 4 molecular classes of β-lactamases, A, B, and D. An example of a class A carbapenemase is KPC which stands for *Klebsiella pneumoniae* carbapenemase. This gene was first identified in the eastern portion of the United States but has quickly spread to other countries in Europe and is a significant problem in Israel. The gene encoding this enzyme can be both chromosomal or plasmid mediated. In most cases, the plasmid version of the gene is located within the 10Kb transposon, Tn4401 [126-128]. The class B enzymes are metallo-β-lactamases and require an active-site zinc ion(s) for activity. Production of these types of enzymes confers resistance to all available β-lactams except aztreonam [129]. The most prevalent and clinically relevant class B β-lactamases are IMP and VIM. In the Middle East, carbapenem resistant *P. aeruginosa* from Saudi Arabia and Tunisia possessed VIM-2 [84, 130-132]. This gene was associated with a class 1 integron [84] [130-132].

OXA β-lactamases are class D enzymes that are capable of hydrolyzing penicillins and oxacillin and are not easily inhibited by clavulanic acid. OXA β-lactamases capable of hydrolyzing carbapenems include subfamilies such as OXA-23, -24, -51, -58 [133]. Most of the OXA-carbapenemases that have been reported were discovered in *A. baumannii* [125]. OXA-23 carbapenemase produced by *A. baumannii* was more frequently reported from Arab countries in the Persian Gulf [134, 135] than from North Africa [136]. OXA-58 and -72 carbapenemases were also reported from Bahrain in the Persian Gulf [134]. Imipenem resistant *A. baumannii* isolates from a Lebanese hospital produced OXA-58. The bla_{OXA-58} gene was harbored on a 29Kb conjugative plasmid flanked by IS18 and ISAba3 [137]. Other studies reported carbapenem resistance in *A. baumannii* from neighboring countries such as Turkey [138] and Iran [139]. In addition, OXA-48 seems to be widespread in the Mediterranean region in Enterobacteriaceae isolates from Turkey, Belgium, Egypt, Tunisia, Lebanon and Israel [140-143]. OXA-48 is located on Tn1999 and confers reduced susceptibility to imipenem, but can not hydrolyze extended spectrum cephalosporins [144]. Reduced susceptibility to imipenem (MICs, 8µg/ml) was seen with transconjugants and clones harboring the KPC gene [126]. Similarly, the MICs of transconjugants/transformants producing OXA-48 show less susceptibility to the carbapenems (MICs, 1µg/ml) much like KPC producers [140, 141]. Since KPCs have only been reported in Israel in the Mediterranean region [145, 146], molecular studies are needed so that laboratories can determine whether carbapenem resistance among clinical isolates is due to OXA-48 or KPCs which could indicate their spread from Israel.

Further studies in the Middle East and North Africa are needed to investigate the molecular mechanisms and epidemiology of carbapenem resistance in *P. aeruginosa* and *A. baumannii* since these isolates represent a threat to successful treatment. Carbapenem resistance in *P. aeruginosa* has been reported in a multicenter study in Minia, Egypt where 22% and 46% of clinical and hospital environmental *P. aeruginosa* isolates; respectively, were resistant to meropenem [20]. The environmental samples were obtained from furniture swabs, medical appliances and surroundings from the same hospitals. In a multicenter pilot survey of resistant bacteria from nine hospitals in France, Tunisia, Morocco and Algeria, carbapenem resistant *A. baumannii* was prevalent in Tunisia but at that time was not found in the other two North African hospitals [42]. Interestingly, resistance to carbapenems in the absence of a carbapenemase can result from the loss of outer membrane porins in *E. coli* and *K. pneumoniae* isolates producing plasmid encoded AmpCs [147, 148]. None of the studies included in this literature search covered porin mutants that produced plasmid encoded AmpC β-lactamases.

Multidrug Resistance to Aminoglycosides, Sulfonamides, Trimethoprim and Tetracyclines

The CTX-M encoding genes are commonly located on plasmids which may also carry genes for resistance to other antibiotics, including aminoglycosides, chloramphenicol, sulfonamide, trimethoprim, and tetracycline [63]. Data from the literature on co-resistance to aminoglycosides, tetracyclines, and trimethoprim in the Middle East and North West Africa indicated that the mechanisms responsible for the resistant phenotypes included *aadA*, *aac(6')*-1b, *aac(3)-II*, *tet*, and *dhfr* (Table **2**) [69, 70, 80, 82, 90, 107, 110]. Some of these genes were harbored on class I integrons [80, 82, 90, 107], while a class II integron was identified in *S. sonnei* harboring resistance genes against trimethoprim and aminoglycosides [149].

Fluoroquinolone Transferable Resistance Genes

Quinolone resistance is traditionally mediated by chromosomal mutations in the target topoisomerase genes encoding DNA gyrase and topoisomerase IV. In addition, changes in efflux pump expression can also contribute to fluoroquinolone resistance [150, 151]. Recently, plasmid associated genes have been implicated in the emergence of fluoroquinolone resistance. *qnr* genes are plasmid mediated and code for a 218-amino-acid protein, which protects DNA gyrase from quinolone binding [152]. The *cr* variant of *aac(6')-Ib* encodes an aminoglycoside acetyltransferase that confers reduced susceptibility to ciprofloxacin by *N*-acetylation of its piperazinyl amine [153].

In Palestine, the transferable quinolone resistance genes *qnrB1* and *aac (6')*-Ib-cr were reported for the first time [90]. In North Africa, *qnr* genes contributed to the reduced susceptibility to fluoroquinolones. *E. coli*, *K. pneumonia*, *E. cloacae*, *K. oxytoca* and *C. freundii* isolates from Tunisia and Egypt carried the genes for *qnrA*, *qnrB*, and *qnrS* [80, 89]. The first report of *qnr* gene in Egypt was in *P. stuartii* isolates from burn patients [154].

The presence of *qnr* facilitates the selection of chromosomal mutations causing high level quinolone resistance [155-157]. *In-vitro* single mutational events in *P. stuartii* isolates possessing *qnr* genes can select isolates with reduced susceptibility to fluoroquinolones to become resistant ones [157]. Similarly, the presence of *aac(6')*-Ib-cr alone increased the frequency of selection of chromosomal mutants upon exposure to ciprofloxacin [153].

Co-Resistance to Fluoroquinolones in CTX-M-15 *E. coli* Producers and Clonal Expansion

Limited information on the co-resistance between fluoroquinolone and β-lactam resistance is available. The co-localization of *bla*CTX-M-15 and *aac(6')*-Ib-cr on the same plasmid was detected in Lebanon [107], and in an *E. coli* isolate from fish farms in Egypt. In addition to these two genes the isolate also carried *bla*OXA-30 [80]. The lack of information combined with the discovery of these important resistant mechanisms in a food source such as fish require the need for aggressive molecular epidemiology studies examining *E. coli* isolates in this region. Furthermore, the sequence type of *E. coli* strains from France, Kuwait, and other European countries was identified as ST131 and carried *bla*CTX-M-15, *bla*OXA-1, *aac(6')*-Ib-cr, and *bla*TEM-1 [115]. In addition to *bla*CTXM-15, other *bla*CTX-M genes and the *aac(6')*-Ib-cr gene were co-localized on conjugative plasmids of >125 Kb. Co-transfer of *qnrB1*, *bla*CTX-M-28, and *aac(6')*-Ib-cr genes has been observed in both a *K. pneumoniae* and an *E. cloacae* isolate from Algeria [76].

Community Acquired Infections Caused by Gram-Negative Bacteria Resistant to Third Generation Cephalosporins or Characterized as ESBL Producers

Gram negative bacteria producing ESBLs and/or imported AmpCs from community sources are a risk for transmission of such resistant determinants to hospitalized patients when infected or colonized patients are admitted [158, 159]. Infections caused by ESBL-producers in the community settings have been studied in many parts of the world. In Canada, a case report on *Citrobacter freundii* obtained from urine cultures of four patients from the community were positive for CTX-M-30 which was carried on a small plasmid lacking *tra* genes; thus the authors have excluded transmission of the *bla*CTX-M gene from other countries and concluded the emergence of the CTX-M-30 variant in the community [160].

Population-based laboratory surveillance studies have been carried out in a large centralized Canadian region where the incidence of disease in the entire population was determined. In these studies, Pitout and co-workers investigated the infections caused by ESBL- and AmpC *E. coli* producers, *Proteus* spp., *Providencia* spp., and *Pseudomonas aeruginosa* and the incidence of healthcare-associated community-onset, and community acquired infections caused by these isolates [161-164]. The Calgary Health Region (CHR) provides all publicly funded healthcare services to the 1.2 million people residing in this large Canadian region covering an area of 37 000 km^2 [165]. In these studies, isolates were obtained from hospitals, nursing homes, physicians' offices and community collection sites. Community-onset isolates were defined as isolates submitted from community-based collection sites or nursing homes, or obtained within 2 days of admission to an acute-care facility [162]. *E. coli* isolates obtained during 2000-2002 caused community onset infections among 71% of the 157 patients from the CHR [161]. The majority of the isolates had positive urine cultures of which 70% were positive for *bla*CTX-M genes [161]. Cefoxitin resistant *E. coli* isolates were obtained from patients in the CHR during 2000-2003, of which 369 isolates were positive for AmpC and 83% of AmpC positive isolates were of community-onset [163]. These AmpC positive *E. coli* isolates were mostly obtained from urine cultures (90% of cases) [163]. Recent surveillance data on ESBL/AmpC positive bacteria from outpatient clinics and nursing homes in Omaha, Nebraska in USA have shown that nursing homes were an important source of infections caused by ESBL/AmpC producers, where 70-79% of AmpC and ESBL producers; respectively came from nursing homes and 20-21% were obtained from outpatient clinics [166].

Resistance to 3rd generation cephalosporins among *E. coli* isolates causing community acquired urinary tract infections were reported in Lebanon and Saudi Arabia [61, 167]. Infections presented on admission or those occurring within 48h-72h of admission were considered community acquired [61, 167]. The *E. coli* isolates in the Saudi study were found to possess ESBLs. Generally, the proportion of resistant bacteria and/or ESBL producers was less among isolates obtained from outpatients (4.5%) compared to those obtained from inpatients (15.4%) [61]. During a 6 year retrospective study in a hospital in Saudi Arabia, the susceptibility of *K. pneumoniae* from inpatients and outpatients was analyzed [168]. Resistance to ceftriaxone and ceftazidime was reported with higher rates of resistance among the hospital pathogens. Additionally, *K. pneumoniae* isolates obtained from malnourished children from Jordan were found to possess ESBLs which did not appear to be clonal as the isolates had different Random Amplified Polymorphic DNA (RAPD) fingerprint patterns [169].

A survey was carried out in Sweden to identify ESBL producing *E. coli* isolates obtained from stool samples of patients with travelers' diarrhea [170]. Out of the 242 isolates, 58 *E. coli* produced ESBLs. Of these, 3% were isolated from patients who traveled in Europe, while 50% and 22% were obtained from patients who traveled to Egypt and Thailand; respectively [170]. The dissemination of multidrug resistant *P. aeruginosa* from environmental sources was investigated in Jordan. *P. aeruginosa* isolated from drinking water and stool specimens of outpatients and inpatients were found to share common serotypes and biotypes. Isolates from stool specimens were more resistant to antibiotics than those from water samples. However, 10-20% of the *P. aeruginosa* isolated from water samples were resistant to ceftazidime, piperacillin-tazobactam, aztreonam, and imipenem [171]. One year later, Shehabi *et al.* (2006) published data on resistant *E. coli* isolates from drinking water and human stool specimens collected from Jordan [172]. As expected, the *E. coli* isolates from human stool were more resistant to ampicillin, trimethoprim/sulfamethoxazole, nalidixic acid, cefuroxime, tetracycline, gentamicin and norfloxacin. All *E. coli* transconjugants possessed class I integrons and were mostly associated with three transferable resistance determinants, to ampicillin, sulfamethoxazole and tetracycline [172].

Animal-to-Human Transfer of Resistance

The use of veterinary β-lactams can select for indigenous ESBL-producing *E. coli* in animal intestines and may facilitate the acquisition of ESBLs in bacterial strains through horizontal transfer [77]. The transmission of bacteria possessing resistance genes from animals to humans through consumption can result in colonization of human bowel flora [46]. In his review on the molecular epidemiology of antibiotic resistance genes, Hawkey has outlined the possible means of transmission of antibiotic resistance genes in *E. coli* through animal consumption, soil, sewage and clinical settings [46]. Multidrug resistant *Salmonella enterica* serovar Typhimurium and Enteritidis were isolated from diarrheal calves from Egypt. The isolates produced bla_{SHV-12} and the plasmid encoded bla_{CMY-2} [87]. Class 1 integrons possessed gene cassettes conferring resistance to aminoglycosides (*aadA1*, *aadA2* and *aadA5*), and trimethoprim (*dfrA1* and *dfrA15*). A class 2 integron harboring *dfrA1-sat2-aadA1* gene cassettes was identified in only one isolate of *S. enterica* serovar Enteritidis The plasmid-mediated quinolone resistance genes, *qnrB*, *qnrS* and *aac(6')*-Ib-cr were also identified from these calf isolates [87]. Thus it may not be uncommon that multidrug resistant pathogens are transferred to humans. Transmission of *S. enterica* among other enteric pathogens from calves to humans was documented in farm day camp in the USA where children came into direct contact with ill calves [173].

Similarly, antimicrobial use in aquaculture is thought to create a reservoir of transferable resistance genes in bacteria in aquatic environments from which such genes can be disseminated by horizontal gene transfer to other bacteria and reach human pathogens [174]. Very recently, isolates of the Enterobacteriaceae family possessing the ESBL genes $bla_{CTX-M-15}$, $bla_{TEM-104}$, and bla_{SHV-89} were isolated from water samples taken from fish farms in Northern Egypt [80]. Detection of resistant determinants in extraintestinal clinical isolates from companion animals has been thoroughly studied by Darren Trott and his research team from Australia. Multidrug resistant *E. coli* (MDREC) isolates positive for CMY-7 were obtained from hospitalized dogs with opportunistic infections in veterinary hospitals in Australia [175]. Based on restriction endonucleases digestion patterns and plasmid profiles, the MDREC isolates were grouped into 2 clonal groups. Clonal group 1 (CG1) possessed a large plasmid (~ 170 Kb) that carried bla_{TEM}, *catA1* and class 1 integron-associated *dfrA17-aadA5* genes. CG2 isolates possessed a second ~93 kb plasmid which harbored bla_{TEM} and unidentified class 1 integron genes [175].

This cluster of extraintestinal infection with MDREC initiated a 1-year infection control study where MDREC isolates were cultured from canine rectal swabs, hospital environmental samples and human rectal swabs from hospital employees [176]. MDREC isolates belonging to CG1 were obtained from clinical cases of extraintestinal infection and rectal swabs from hospitalized dogs and from the hospital environment. CG2 isolates were obtained from clinical cases, canine rectal swabs as well as from human rectal swabs of 2 hospital employees. Thus MDREC isolates belonging to CG2 were confirmed to colonize both humans and dogs. Possible transfer of MDREC between dogs and humans may occur by the faecal-oral route [176]; especially since evidence of clonal relationship between canine fecal *E. coli* and human clinical *E. coli* isolates has been reported [177, 178].

Table 2: ESBLs and Other Plasmid-Encoded Resistance Determinants Detected. I-North Africa (Algeria).

ESBLs	Species	IS Elements	Integron	Integron Associated Genes	Other Resistant Determinants	Plasmid Characterization**	Country	Reference
$bla_{CTX-M-15}$ $bla_{CTX-M-3}$	*K. pneumonia*	ISEcp1B	Class I	N/A	bla_{TEM-1}	ST pl 85Kb (bla_{TEM-1}, $bla_{CTX-M-15}$, $bla_{CTX-M-3}$, AM^r, sul^r	Algeria	Messai *et al.*, 2008 [112]
$bla_{CTX-M-28}$	*Enterobacteriaceae*	N/A	N/A	N/A	bla_{TEM-1}, qnrB1 aac (6')-Ib aac (6')-Ib-cr	ST pl high Mwt Co-transfer of qnrB1, $bla_{CTX-M-28}$, aac (6')-Ib-cr	Algeria	Meradi *et al.*, 2009 [76]
$bla_{CTX-M-15}$ $bla_{CTX-M-3}$	*K. pneumonia* *E. cloacae, E. coli*	N/A	N/A	N/A	bla_{TEM-1} bla_{SHV-1}[a]	Co-transfer of $bla_{CTX-M-15}$ and AM^r in *E. coli* isolates	Algeria	Touati *et al.*, 2006 [67]
$bla_{CTX-M-15}$, bla_{SHV-12}	Enterobacteriaceae	N/A	N/A	N/A	bla_{CMY-2} bla_{DHA-1}	ST pl harboring $bla_{CTX-M-15}$, bla_{SHV-12}, bla_{CMY-2}	Algeria	Iabadene *et al.*, 2009 [81]
bla_{PER-1}	*Proteus vulgaris* *Providencia stuartii*	ISPa12	N/A	N/A	N/A	ST pl 100 Kb Co-transfer of bla_{PER-1}, AM^r, sul^r, tmp^r in *P. vulgaris*	Algeria	Iabadene *et al.*, 2009 [93]
$bla_{CTX-M-14}$	*S. enterica* serotype Kedougou	ISEcp1	N/A	N/A	aac(3)-II bla_{TEM-1}	$bla_{CTX-M-14}$ not transferable	Algeria	Iabadene *et al.*, 2009 [179]
$bla_{CTX-M-15}$ $bla_{CTX-M-3}$ bla_{SHV-12} bla_{VEB-1}	*E. cloacae*	N/A	N/A	N/A	qnrS1 qnrB1 qnrB4	ST pl 85 - >100 Kb	Algeria	Iabadene *et al.*, 2008 [105]
bla_{VEB-1} bla_{SHV-2}	*P. stuartii*	N/A	Repeated elements (Re 1,2,3) instead	N/A	bla_{TEM-2}	ST pl 160 Kb (bla_{VEB-1}, bla_{SHV-2}, bla_{TEM-2})	Algeria	Aubert *et al.*, 2005 [96]

[a] Genes are chromosomally encoded in *K. pneumonia*   N/A: data not available.

tmp^r: trimethoprim resistance determinant.

sul^r: sulfonamide resistance determinant.

AM^r: aminoglycoside resistance determinant.

ST pl: self transferable plasmid. Genes showed between parentheses are those transferred during conjugation.

Table 2: *cont.* I-North Africa (Tunisia).

ESBLs	Species	IS Elements Upstream bla_{CTX-M} genes	Integrons	Integron Associated Genes	Other Resistant Determinants Coproduced	Plasmid Characterization	Country	Reference
$bla_{CTX-M-15}$ bla_{SHV-11} bla_{SHV-27} $bla_{SHV-103}$	*E. coli* *K. pneumonia*	ISEcp1	Class 1	dfrA5 + ereA2 aadA	bla_{OXA-1} bla_{TEM-1b}	ST pl 70Kb ($bla_{CTX-M-15}$, bla_{OXA-1}, bla_{TEM-1b})	Tunisia	Abbassi *et al.*, 2008 [82]

Table 2: cont....

$bla_{CTX-M-15}$ $bla_{CTX-M-16}$	E. coli K. pneumonia	N/A	N/A	N/A	bla_{OXA-1} bla_{TEM-1} tetA, sul2 aac(6')-1b aac(3)-II sul1	ST pl	Tunisia	Mamlouk et al., 2006 [69]
$bla_{CTX-M-15}$	E. coli	ISEcp1	N/A	N/A	bla_{OXA-1} aac(6')-1b aac(3)-II	IncFII	Tunisia	Lavollay et al., 2006 [70]
bla_{SHV-2a} bla_{TEM-4}	S. enterica serotype Mbandaka	N/A	N/A	N/A	bla_{ACC}	ST pl 110-140 Kb (bla_{SHV-2a}, bla_{TEM-4}, AM^r, sul^r)	Tunisia	Makanera et al., 2003 [79]
$bla_{CTX-M-27}$	S. enterica serotype Livingstone	ISEcp1	Class 1	dfrA21	N/A	ST pl 40Kb ($bla_{CTX-M-27}$)	Tunisia	Bouallegue-Godet et al., 2005 [180]
$bla_{CTX-M-28}$	K. pneumonia	N/A	N/A	N/A	N/A	ST pl 50Kb ($bla_{CTX-M-28}$)	Tunisia	Ben Achour et al., 2009 [75]

N/A: data not available

IncFII: plasmid incompatibility grouping using PCR based replicon typing (Lavollay *et al.*, 2006)

ST pl: self transferable plasmid. Genes showed between parentheses are those transferred during conjugation

sul^r: sulfonamide resistance determinant

AM^r: aminoglycoside resistance determinant

Table 2: *cont.* I-North Africa (Tunisia).

ESBLs	Species	IS Elements Upstream bla_{CTX-M} Genes	Integrons	Integron Associated Genes	Other Resistant Determinants Coproduced	Plasmid Characterization	Country	Reference
$bla_{CTX-M-15}$ $bla_{CTX-M-14}$ $bla_{CTX-M-27}$ bla_{SHV-12} bla_{SHV-2a}	K. pneumonia	[a]ISEcpI [b]IS26	N/A	N/A	bla_{TEM-1}	[c]IncFII and IncL/M [d]Hl2 replicon	Tunisia	ElHani et al., 2010 [88]
$bla_{CTX-M-15}$ bla_{SHV-12} bla_{SHV-28}	Enterobacteriaceae	ISEcl2[e]	Class 1	qnrB2	qnrB1,qnrB2, qnrA6, qnrS1	55-150 Kb	Tunisia	Dahmen et al., 2009 [89]
N/A	A. baumannii	[f]ISAba1	N/A	N/A	bla_{OXA-23}[g]	35 Kb	Tunisia	Mansour et al., 2008 [136]
N/A	P. aeruginosa	N/A	Class 1	bla_{VIM-2}	N/A	N/A	Tunisia	Mansour, et al 2009 [131]

Table 2: cont….

bla_{OXA-18}	P. aeruginosa	N/A	N/A	N/A	bla_{SHV-1} bla_{TEM-1}	No detected plasmid	Tunisia	Kalai Blagui *et al.*, 2007 [106]
^{h} bla_{SHV-2a}	P. aeruginosa	IS26	N/A	N/A	N/A	N/A	Tunisia	Mansour, *et al* 2009 [83]
bla_{SHV-2a}	P. aeruginosa	N/A	Class 1	bla_{VIM-2}	N/A	N/A	Tunisia	Hammami *et al.*, 2010 [84]

^{a} IS*EcpI* upstream bla_{CTX-M} genes ^{b} IS*26* upstream bla_{SHV}, promoter in the opposite direction.

^{c} Plasmids carrying $bla_{CTX-M-15}$/bla_{SHV-2a} ^{d} Plasmid carrying $bla_{SHV-12.}$

^{e} *qnrS1* gene was located downstream of an IS*Ecl2* element on plasmids.

^{f} IS*Aba1* upstream of the bla_{OXA-23} gene chromosomally located since plasmid hybridization was negative.

^{g} Gene is chromosomally encoded (no hybridization of bla_{OXA-23} with plasmid DNA).

^{h} Gene is chromosomally encoded.

N/A: data not available.

Inc: plasmid incompatibility grouping using PCR based replicon typing [ElHani *et al.*, 2010].

ST pl: self transferable plasmid. Genes showed between parentheses are those transferred during conjugation.

Table 2: *cont.* I-North Africa (Egypt).

ESBLs	Species	IS Elements Upstream bla_{CTX-M} Genes	Integrons	Integron Associated Genes	Otherresistant Determinants Coproduced	Plasmid Characterization	Country	Reference
$bla_{CTX-M-1-}$ Group $bla_{CTX-M-9-}$ Group	E. coli	N/A	N/A	N/A	N/A	N/A	Egypt	Tham *et al.*, 2010 [170]
$bla_{CTX-M-15}$ $bla_{CTX-M-14}$ $bla_{CTX-M-27}$	E. coli	N/A	N/A	N/A	aac3-IIc, aac6'-Ib ant3'-Ia aph3-Ia strA, strB	<8 Kb to >160 Kb	Egypt	AlAgamy *et al.*, 2006 [68]
$bla_{CTX-M-15}$ $bla_{CTX-M-14}$	E. coli E. cloacae K. pneumonia	IS*Ecp1*	N/A	N/A	$bla_{TEM-1-like}$ $bla_{SHV-1-like}$	ST pl($bla_{CTX-M-15}$)	Egypt	Khalaf *et al.*, 2009 [74]
$bla_{CTX-M-14}$ bla_{SHV-12}	S. typhimurium	IS*Ecp1*	N/A	N/A	bla_{OXA-1} $bla_{TEM-1-like}$	ST pl($bla_{CTX-M-14}$)	Egypt	AbdElGhany *et al.*, 2010 [85]
bla_{SHV-2}	K. pneumonia	N/A	N/A	N/A	bla_{SHV-1}	N/A	Egypt	Abdel Hady *et al.*, 2008 [86]
$bla_{CTX-M-15}$ $bla_{TEM-104}$ bla_{SHV-89}	E. coli E. cloacae K. pneumonia	N/A	Class 1	dfrA, aad, aac(3)-Id, catB3,	bla_{TEM-1} bla_{OXA-30} tetA, B, C, D qnrA, qnr B, qnr S, aac(6')-Ib-cr	N/A	Egypt-Fish farms	Ishida *et al.*, 2010 [80]
$bla_{CTX-M-1}$	K. pneumonia	N/A	N/A	N/A	bla_{TEM} bla_{SHV}	N/A	Egypt	Ahmed *et al.*, 2009 [181]

ST pl: self transferable plasmid. Genes showed between parentheses are those transferred during conjugation.
N/A: data not available.

Table 2: *cont.* II- Middle East.

ESBLs	Species	IS Elements Upstream *bla*CTX-M Genes	Integron	Integron Associated Genes	Other Resistant Determinants Coproduced	Plasmid Characterization	Country	Reference
*bla*SHV-12	*S. enterica*	N/A	Class 1	*aad, dfrA,*	*bla*TEM-1, *bla*CMY-2 *qnrB, qnrS, aac(6')-Ib-cr*	N/A	Egypt	Ahmed *et al.,* 2009 [87]
			Class 2	*dfrA1-sat2-aadA1*				
N/A	*K. pneumonia*	N/A	N/A	N/A	*bla*CMY-4	ST pl >130 Kb (*bla*CMY-4,AM^r, *sul^r*)	Egypt	Decre *et al.,* 2002 [119]
N/A	*Providencia stuartii*	N/A	Class 1	*aac(6')-Ib ant(2")-Ia*	*bla*CMY-2 *bla*TEM-1 *aph(3)-I, aac(3)-IIc*	ST pl (*bla*CMY-2, *aac(6')-Ib, ant(2")-Ia*)	Egypt	Khalaf *et al.,* 2004 [124]
*bla*CTX-M-15 *bla*SHV-5a	*E. coli K. pneumonia C. freundii E. cloacae*	N/A	N/A	N/A	*bla*TEM-1 *bla*OXA-1	N/A	Lebanon	Moubareck *et al.,* 2005 [66]
*bla*CTX-M-15	*E. coli K. pneumonia*	ISEcp1	Class 1	N/A	*bla*OXA-1, *bla*SHV *bla*TEM-1 *aac(6')-Ib-cr*	Inc FII plasmid ST pl 90KB (*bla*CTX-M-15, *aac(6')-Ib-cr*)	Lebanon	Kanj *et al.,* 2008 [107]
*bla*CTX-M-15	*S. sonnei*	ISEcp1	Class 2	*dhfr1, aadA1 sat1*	*bla*TEM-1	70Kb plasmid harboring *bla*CTX-M-15	Lebanon	Matar *et al.,* 2007 [149]
*bla*CTX-M-15	*S. enterica*	ISEcp1	N/A	N/A	*bla*OXA-30 *bla*TEM-1	ST pl (AM^r, *sul^r*, *tet^r*, *bla*CTX-M-15, *bla*TEM-1, *bla*OXA-30)	Lebanon	Weill *et al.,* 2004 [110]
*bla*CTX-M-15 *bla*CTX-M-56 *bla*SHV-12 *bla*SHV-32	Gram negative bacteria	N/A	Class 1	*dfrA, qnrB2,aad,aac(6')-Ib, cmlA*	*bla*OXA-1, *bla*SHV-1, *bla*TEM-1, *aac(6')-Ib-cr, qnrB*	N/A	Palestine	Hussein *et al.,* 2009 [90]
			Class 2	N/A				

N/A: data not available.

IncFII: plasmid incompatibility grouping using PCR based replicon typing (Kanj *et al.,* 2008].

ST pl: self transferable plasmid. Genes showed between parentheses are those transferred during conjugation.

sul^r: sulfonamide resistance determinant AM^r: aminoglycoside resistance determinant   *tet^r*: tetracycline resistance determinant.

Table 2: *cont.* III- Persian Gulf.

ESBLs	Species	IS Elements Upstream *bla*CTX-M Genes	Integrons	Integron Associated Genes	Other Resistant Determinants Coproduced	Plasmid Characterization	Country	Reference
N/A	*A. baumannii*	^{a}ISAba1 ^{b}ISAba3	N/A	N/A	*bla*OXA-23 *bla*OXA-58 *bla*OXA-72	ST pl 130 Kb (*bla*OXA-23 only)	Bahrain	Mugnier *et al.,* 2009 [134]
N/A	*A. baumannii*	^{d}N/A	N/A	N/A	*bla*OXA-23	ST pl 70 Kb (*bla*OXA-23) in one isolate only	UAE	Mugnier *et al.,* 2008 [135]
*bla*CTX-M-15	*E. coli K. pneumonia*	N/A	N/A	N/A	N/A	N/A	Kuwait	Ensor *et al.,* 2009 [182]

Table 2: cont....

bla	organism	IS	col4	col5	bla	plasmid	country	ref
bla_CTX-M-15	*Salmonella* spp.	IS*Ecp1*	ND	ND	bla_TEM	ND	Kuwait	Rotimi *et al.*, 2008 [73]
bla_CTX-M-15	EAEC	IS*Ecp1*	ND	ND	bla_TEM-1	ST pl 95 Kb (bla_TEM-1, bla_CTX-M-15)	UAE	Sonnevend *et al.*, 2006 [71]
bla_CTX-M-1-like, bla_CTX-M-9-like,	*K. pneumonia*	[c]IS*Ecp1*	ND	ND	bla_TEM bla_SHV	N/A	Saudi Arabia	AlAgamy *et al.*, 2009 [183]
N/A	*P. aeruginosa*	ND	Class 1	bla_VIM-2	N/A	Plasmid analysis didn't reveal any plasmid. Conjugation experiments failed to transfer bla_VIM-2	Saudi Arabia	Guerin *et al.*, 2005 [132]
N/A	*P. aeruginosa*	ND	Class 1	bla_VIM-2	N/A	Conjugation experiments failed to transfer bla_VIM-2	Saudi Arabia	AlAgamy *et al.*, 2009 [130]

[a]IS*Aba1* was upstream the bla_OXA-23 gene   [b]IS*Aba3* was upstream the bla_OXA-58 gene.

[c] 10% of isolates possessed IS*Ecp1* [AlAgamy *et al.*, 2009][183].

[d] The four clonally related isolates harbored chromosomally located bla_OXA-23 within a Tn006.

UAE: United Arab Emirates.

ST pl: self transferable plasmid. Genes showed between parentheses are those transferred during conjugation.

N/A: data not available.

General Table Notes

The compiled data obtained from the literature search on reported ESBLs in this table does not represent all studies in the literature on ESBLs in the region. Data are based on referenced studies in the text.

INFECTION CONTROL PROGRAMS AND OTHER INTERVENTIONS

Infection control efforts are mainly concerned with the control of nosocomial/healthcare associated infections. Some studies have thoroughly investigated the modes of transmission and threats of viral blood borne infections in the region especially health related infections such as HIV, hepatitis B and C [184-186]. In Egypt, a national infection control program was primarily launched to prevent transmission of hepatitis B and C but an added benefit of this surveillance program was a decrease in the rates nosocomial infections [187]. This section will address studies that identified the modes of spread of nosocomial infections, how infection control teams faced outbreaks and how they attempted to control endemic and epidemic nosocomial pathogens. A national Infection Control program that was launched in Egypt in 2001 will be exemplified. The current situation in the region on the level of healthcare intervention to limit nosocomial pathogens will be discussed.

Within a hospital setting, genetically similar resistant organisms disseminate through horizontal patient-to-patient transfer. Some studies investigated the clonal outbreak of a single bacterial strain using molecular typing methods, and detected self-transferable plasmids that have also contributed to the spread of resistance. One study compiling 6 years and 5 months (1999-2005) of data from hospitalized patients in a university hospital in Tunisia used Multilocus Sequence Typing (MLST) to demonstrate that specific clones (ST101 and ST107) of the CTX-M-15 producing *K. pneumoniae* isolates disseminated within the ICU ward, and the ST147 clone was detected in both the ICU and Pediatric unit [88]. Three *K. pneumoniae* isolates producing CTX-M-15 coproduced SHV-12 ESBLs and shared the same sequence type (ST107) [88]. A study that covered 3 urban hospitals in Algiera during the years 2003-2007, revealed the genetic relatedness among *E. coli* isolates producing CMY-2 obtained from one hospital [81], using ERIC PCR (Enterobacteriaceae Repetitive Intergenic Consesus) [188]. The same study identified similar ERIC PCR patterns among *Providencia stuartii* CMY-2 producers from another hospital [81]. Interestingly, plasmids harboring the bla_{CMY-2} and bla_{CTX-M} genes from both studies were self transferable [81, 88]. Hence, the spread of resistance to β-lactams was due to clonal expansion of isolates which disseminated through horizontal patient-to-patient transfer besides the movement of plasmids harboring the respective gene [81, 88].

Results from other studies have shown that self transferable plasmids harboring ESBL-encoding genes were well established under selective pressure by using similar drugs in hospitals. Clonal spread of a strain possessing ESBL-encoding genes was excluded in these studies because of the multiple genetic profiles exhibited by strain typing [107, 112, 189]. Typing of *K. pneumoniae* isolates (39 isolates) obtained from Algerian hospitals and producing CTX-M-3 and -15 ESBLs resulted in thirty-seven genotypes. The bla_{CTX-M} genes and the upstream IS*Ecp1* element were transferred by conjugation [112]. In another study, *E. cloacae* isolates were collected during 2003-2007, from eight hospitals that were located in distant areas of Algeria [105]. Twenty-five out of the 141 isolates collected were identified as ESBL producers and subjected further to ERIC- PCR typing. Heterogeneity in isolates' genetic profile was observed when 20 different genotypes were identified. Self transferable plasmids of ~85-150 Kb transferred $bla_{CTX-M-15}$, $bla_{CTX-M-3}$ and bla_{SHV-12} genes [105]. In Lebanon, multiple genotypes were identified when *E. coli* and *K. pneumoniae* producing CTX-M-15 were typed using Random Amplified Polymorphic DNA (RAPD) PCR during 1997-2002, and 2004-2005 [107]. The RAPD technique uses PCR and single short arbitrary oligonucleotide primers to amplify DNA, producing characteristic fingerprints of a particular strain [190]. By using this technique it was established that resistance transfer was due to a large conjugative plasmid (90Kb) harboring the $bla_{CTX-M-15}$ and *aac-6'-Ib-cr* genes [107].

Infection control teams are dependent on molecular typing assays in order to identify multiple clones causing infection and take appropriate measures to control the outbreak. A polyclonal outbreak was reported in 2001 in a University hospital in Cairo, Egypt [68]. *E. coli* isolates producing $bla_{CTX-M-14, -15 \text{ and } -27}$ were obtained from inpatients suffering from urinary tract infections. Seven different clones were identified; in each clone, isolates shared an identical PFGE pattern, similar susceptibility patterns and similar plasmid profiles [68]. In Lebanon, the spread of hospital- and community acquired ESBL producers were investigated in 2003. *E. coli* isolates producing CTX-M-15 or SHV-5a were obtained from fecal samples from inpatients and healthcare workers in five hospitals [66]. The spread of community acquired ESBL producers was investigated by obtaining fecal samples from healthy candidates. Pulsed field gel electrophoresis revealed diverse patterns of *E. coli* isolates. A common genotype was shared by three epidemiologically unrelated isolates from inpatients in 3 different hospitals, while two isolates sharing the same pulsed field pattern were obtained from inpatients in the same hospital ward. Two isolates obtained from healthy subjects belonged to the same genotype. Interestingly, an isolate obtained from an inpatient in a hospital shared the same genotype of another isolate from a healthcare worker in the same hospital ward [66].

Outbreaks caused by clonally unrelated Gram positive cocci were identified using genotypic methods in this geographical region. *S. epidermidis* isolates in a hospital in Lebanon were typed using RAPD PCR. Strain diversity was evident when the 40 *S. epidermidis* isolates from inpatient clinical specimens were typed into 12 patterns, indicating that various clusters of infection or colonization occurred in the medical center [191]. Specific MRSA clones within hospital wards were identified using PFGE in Saudi Arabia [192]. Multiple clusters of infections caused by *S. aureus* and coagulase negative staphylococci were identified using RAPD and PFGE techniques in a hospital in Morocco [193].

Epidemic Outbreak and Intervention

A two month outbreak in 2001 was due to contamination of IV fluids in a NICU in a large tertiary teaching hospital in Cairo [54]. *K. pneumoniae* was the most common pathogen (70%) isolated followed by *E. cloacae* (10%), *E. coli* (6%) and *A. baumannii* (3%). Fifty-eight percent of the *K. pneumoniae* isolates produced ESBLs [54]. The investigating team noticed malpractice of infection control procedures such as lack of hand hygiene, absence of soap and paper towels at sinks; alcohol-based hand rub was seldom used. The IV fluids were delivered in their original containers and were prepared by NICU nurses, containers were left by the bed side until empty, cloth tape was used to seal the top of preservative-free ampoules, and multidose IV containers were available at the pharmacy and were used until empty. Nurses repeatedly inserted syringes into tops of bottles and mixed IV fluids using old bottles stored for several days with newly delivered bottles. Open partially used bottles were used for several days until empty [54]. The investigating team took steps to prevent contamination. Large 500ml IV fluids were replaced by smaller 250ml bottles, each infant had its own IV fluid bottle that was stored in the refrigerator and discarded within 24 h. NICU nurses received training on aseptic IV fluid and medication preparation. The intervention was supported by the clinical laboratory, although ongoing laboratory-based surveillance was required to monitor the impact of changes in infection control practices [54]. The risk of umbilical catheter-associated bloodstream infection in a NICU in a hospital in Saudi Arabia was examined during 2006 and 2007 [194]. The implementation of strict infection control practices was effective in reducing rates of blood stream infections.

Endemic Outbreak and Infection Control Measures

Nosocomial pathogens are frequently contaminating environmental surfaces, ultrasonic gels, and ventilators thus creating an endemic source of infection. In their review, Paterson and Bonomo have suggested infection control measures should include the detection of colonization and infection, contact isolation by the use of gowns and gloves, and identifying environmental source of infection to control endemic nosocomial pathogens [62].

Changes in antibiotic policy will also help reduce the selection of resistant pathogens. Gad and co-workers (2007)[20] hypothesized that the resistant phenotype observed for *P. aeruginosa* isolates in Minia hospitals was mainly due to antibiotic pressure and they recommended to decrease the use of fluoroquinolones and suggested the use of combination therapy [20]. Another study from Egypt addressed the problem of ESBL producers in their hospital and argued that restricting the use of antibiotics may not be the solution, but recommended the use of aminoglycosides/imipenem combination and deescalation to a narrow spectrum antibiotic [55]. Moreover, the author pointed out the need to control cross contamination and monitor resistance patterns in Gram negative pathogens and to modify institutional antibiotic formularies [55]. Studies from neighboring countries in the region have also recommended the prudent use of antibiotics to reduce pressure on sensitive strains and to control the incidence of resistant strains [195]. Combination therapy of meropenem and vancomycin was effective but a periodic antimicrobial susceptibility survey was required to determine the most appropriate treatment regimen in ICUs in a Persian hospital [195]. Kader and Kumar [60] suggested restricted antibiotic use and implementation of infection control measures to limit nosocomial infections by ESBL *E. coli* and *K. pneumoniae* producers in Saudi hospitals. Infections caused by these pathogens were treatable by carbapenems and piperacillin/tazobactam [60].

Ahmed and co-workers displayed the risk factors associated with the acquisition of nosocomial Blood Stream Infections (BSI) such as previous antibiotic therapy, and mechanical ventilation in Assuit hospitals in Egypt during the year 2006 [181]. Environmental contamination rate with BSI pathogens was seen highest in trauma ICU (82%), followed by chest ICU (77.8%) and post-operative ICUs (75%); mainly caused by *S. aureus*, *K. pneumoniae* and *E. coli*. Nosocomial *K. pneumoniae* isolates positive for CTX-M-1, SHV- and TEM β-lactamases, and hospital environmental *K. pneumoniae* isolates were typed with RAPD PCR. Fifty RAPD genotypes were identified among the 54 *K. pneumoniae* isolates studied. In the trauma ICU, 2 environmental and one clinical *K. pneumoniae* isolates shared the same genotype; suggesting the transmission of environmental samples to the patient. The authors have stressed the need to improve hospital hygiene and the adoption of new antibiotic policies [181].

National Infection Control Program in Egypt

The rapid population growth in Egypt and the ongoing development of the Healthcare system posed challenges to the Egyptian health care system that required the implementation of a National Infection Control Program in 2001. It would be helpful to the reader to understand the healthcare structure in Egypt. The health care system within the Ministry of Health and Population (MOHP) in Egypt is composed of a network of different types and levels of health care facilities that vary from small primary rural health care units to large tertiary care hospitals. In each of the 27 governorates in Egypt, there are 10 to 20 large hospitals and approximately 200 primary rural health care units. Medical services are free in University and MOHP hospitals. Other types of hospitals include private hospitals, military hospitals and hospitals affiliated with other ministries [187]. Collaborative work between the Egyptian Ministry of health (MOHP), the WHO and the US Naval Medical Research Unit no. 3 (NAMRU) initiated an Infection Control (IC) program that started in 2001. From 2001-2006, the program was implemented in 72 hospitals in 13 governorates in the country with the outcome of training 235 Infection Control professionals [187].

The IC program started with an advisory group which stated the job description for each member of an IC team at each level of health care service. Infection control units were established in every health care unit (central, governorate and facility levels). In 2002, Infection Control guidelines were developed and comprised 2 parts, I: Standard precautions and II: Practices in special care settings (www.ems.org.eg). A training plan was developed for hospitals and health care facilities. In each targeted facility, an IC team, comprised of a physician and two nurses, formulated IC policies, trained facility employees to implement safe practices, investigated outbreaks, and monitored daily practices of patient care in the facility [187]. It was planned to expand the IC program to cover all 27 governorates in the country by 2008 and to start a national surveillance system for hospital acquired infections [187].

The Current Situation on Infection Control in the Region

During February 2005, information on infection control activities in the region was obtained from questionnaires that were sent to 45 participating secondary or tertiary hospitals in southern (Algeria, Morocco, Libiya, and Malta) and eastern Mediterranean countries (Egypt, Lebanon, Cyprus, Turkey, and Jordan). The questionnaires were answered by infection control personnel in the respective hospitals [196]. All but one participating hospital from southern Mediterranean countries and 75% of hospitals from eastern Mediterranean countries were university hospitals. Eastern Mediterranean countries reported the availability of infection control doctors and infection control nurses. A low percentage of participating hospitals from southern and eastern Mediterranean countries adopted hospital treatment guidelines (35% and 25%; respectively) [196]. Evaluation of questionnaires revealed that only 38-41% of hospitals from southern and eastern countries adhered to hospital antibiotic policies, surveillance activities, and reported resistance data to prescribers [196].

In 2006, the situation on infection control was evaluated in 78% of hospitals participating in the ARMed study [40]. A questionnaire covering Infection Control practices such as patient isolation and hand hygiene was sent to participating hospitals. The evaluation of questionnaires revealed the lack of convenient distance of sinks from patients' beds. The use of soap bars was reported in 29% of participating hospitals and use of cloth towels was reported in 38% of participating hospitals. During the same year, the assessment of knowledge of hand hygiene and the extent of hand hygiene practices was simultaneously investigated by members of the Infection Control team in Ain Shams University hospitals in Egypt [197]. Physicians were more compliant to hand washing practices (37%) than other healthcare workers. Routine handwashing was commonly employed (64.2%), while the use of antiseptic was less common (3.9%). Problems encountered with routine handwashing were the unavailability of paper towels, and problems leading to ineffective hand hygiene were improper hand drying and short contact time after the use of antiseptic [197].

In the study evaluating infection control practices in ARMed participating hospitals, healthcare professionals faced some problems such as over crowdedness in 60% of participating hospitals, especially in ICUs [40]. Policies developed to control MRSA were present in 80% of the hospitals, while those for Vancomycin resistant Enterococci and ESBL producers were less frequently implemented (in 46% of hospitals). Patients presenting with infections caused by multidrug resistant organisms were isolated in 70% of hospitals. Some of these hospitals adopted single rooms for patient isolation while others used patient cohorting [40]. These data reflect that although the practices introduced by the IC programs clearly had an impact, compliance is not 100% and therefore inadequate. It is therefore imperitive that more support be given to IC programs to carryout and expand the existing IC programs. It is evident that we have a long way to go to address all the problems associated with healthcare infections. But these problems present an economic burden on the healthcare system in the countries of this region and the IC program is a cost-effective program in which to tackle the enormous problem of antibiotic resistance in resource-limited countries as well as countries in which the resources are not as limited [196].

This chapter has pointed out that antibiotic resistance is a problem which is multifaceted and that is one of the reasons it is hard to control. As the reader can now understand the multifaceted aspects of antibiotic resistance, including the bugs and resistance mechanisms themselves as well as use and availability of antibiotics, are all important in the overall outcome in this resistance fight.

REFERENCES

[1]   Raymond DP, Pelletier SJ, Crabtree TD, *et al.* Impact of antibiotic-resistant Gram-negative bacilli infections on outcome in hospitalized patients. Crit Care Med 2003; 31(4): 1035-41.

[2]   Laxminarayan R, Zulfiqar B, Adrian D, *et al.* Drug Resistance. In: Jamison, editor. Disease Control Priorities in Developing Countries. New York: Oxford University Press; 2006. p. 1034-51.

[3]   Yalcin AN, Hayran M, Unal S. Economic analysis of nosocomial infections in a Turkish university hospital. J Chemother 1997; 9(6): 411-14.

[4]   Llor C, Cots JM. The sale of antibiotics without prescription in pharmacies in Catalonia, Spain. Clin Infect Dis 2009 15; 48(10): 1345-9.

[5]   Grigoryan L, Haaijer-Ruskamp FM, Burgerhof JG, *et al.* Self-medication with antimicrobial drugs in Europe. Emerg Infect Dis 2006; 12(3): 452-59.

[6]   Goossens H, Guillemot D, Ferech M, *et al.* National campaigns to improve antibiotic use. Eur J Clin Pharmacol 2006; 62(5): 373-79.

[7]   Sabuncu E, David J, Bernede-Bauduin C, *et al.* Significant reduction of antibiotic use in the community after a nationwide campaign in France, 2002-2007. PLoS Med 2009; 6(6): e1000084.

[8]   Awad A, Eltayeb I, Matowe L, *et al.* Self-medication with antibiotics and antimalarials in the community of Khartoum State, Sudan. J Pharm Pharm Sci 2005; 8(2): 326-31.

[9]   Mwambete KD. Irrational antibiotic usage in boarding secondary school settings in Dar es Salaam. East Afr J Public Health 2009; 6(2):200-4.

[10]   Abasaeed A, Vlcek J, Abuelkhair M, *et al.* Self-medication with antibiotics by the community of Abu Dhabi Emirate, United Arab Emirates. J Infect Dev Ctries 2009; 3(7): 491-97.

[11]   Al-Azzam SI, Al-Husein BA, Alzoubi F, *et al.* Self-medication with antibiotics in Jordanian population. Int J Occup Med Environ Health. 2007; 20(4): 373-80.

[12]   Al-Bakri AG, Bustanji Y, Yousef AM. Community consumption of antibacterial drugs within the Jordanian population: sources, patterns and appropriateness. Int J Antimicrob Agents 2005; 26(5): 389-95.

[13]   Earnshaw S, Monnet DL, Duncan B, *et al.* European Antibiotic Awareness Day, 2008 - the first Europe-wide public information campaign on prudent antibiotic use: methods and survey of activities in participating countries. Euro Surveill 2009; 14(30): 19280.

[14]   Nsubuga P, Mark EW, Stephen BT, *et al.* Public Health Surveillance: A Tool for Targeting and Monitoring Interventions. In: Jamison, editor. Disease Control Priorities in Developing Countries: New York: Oxford University press 2006; pp. 997-1015.

[15]   El Kholy A, Baseem H, Hall GS, *et al.* Antimicrobial resistance in Cairo, Egypt 1999-2000: a survey of five hospitals. J Antimicrob Chemother 2003; 51(3): 625-30.

[16]   Bouchillon SK, Johnson BM, Hoban DJ, *et al.* Determining incidence of extended spectrum beta-lactamase producing Enterobacteriaceae, vancomycin-resistant Enterococcus faecium and methicillin-resistant Staphylococcus aureus in 38 centres from 17 countries: the PEARLS study 2001-2002. Int J Antimicrob Agents. 2004; 24(2): 119-24.

[17]   Borg MA, Scicluna E, de Kraker M, *et al.* Antibiotic resistance in the southeastern Mediterranean--preliminary results from the ARMed project. Euro Surveill. 2006; 11(7): 164-67.

[18]   Borg MA, de Kraker M, Scicluna E, *et al.* Prevalence of methicillin-resistant Staphylococcus aureus (MRSA) in invasive isolates from southern and eastern Mediterranean countries. J Antimicrob Chemother 2007; 60(6): 1310-15.

[19]   Borg MA, van de Sande-Bruinsma N, Scicluna E, *et al.* Antimicrobial resistance in invasive strains of Escherichia coli from southern and eastern Mediterranean laboratories. Clin Microbiol Infect 2008; 14(8): 789-96.

[20] Gad GF, El-Domany RA, Zaki S, *et al.* Characterization of Pseudomonas aeruginosa isolated from clinical and environmental samples in Minia, Egypt: prevalence, antibiogram and resistance mechanisms. J Antimicrob Chemother 2007; 60(5): 1010-17.

[21] Ramdani-Bouguessa N, Bes M, Meugnier H, *et al.* Detection of methicillin-resistant Staphylococcus aureus strains resistant to multiple antibiotics and carrying the Panton-Valentine leukocidin genes in an Algiers hospital. Antimicrob Agents Chemother 2006; 50(3): 1083-85.

[22] Ben Jemaa Z, Mahjoubi F, Ben Haj H'mida Y, *et al.* Antimicrobial susceptibility and frequency of occurrence of clinical blood isolates in Sfax-Tunisia (1993-1998). Pathol Biol (Paris). 2004; 52(2): 82-8.

[23] Al-Zu'bi E, Bdour S, Shehabi AA. Antibiotic resistance patterns of mecA-positive Staphylococcus aureus isolates from clinical specimens and nasal carriage. Microb Drug Resist 2004; 10(4): 321-4.

[24] Kanj SS, Ghaleb PA, Araj GF. Glycopeptide and oxacillin activity against Staphylococcus aureus isolates at a tertiary care center in Lebanon. J Med Liban 2004; 52(1): 8-12.

[25] Ahmed MM, Bahlas S. Bacteriological profile and antimicrobial resistance patterns of clinical bacterial isolates in a University Hospital. Travel Med Infect Dis 2009; 7(4): 235-8.

[26] Utsui Y, Yokota T. Role of an altered penicillin-binding protein in methicillin- and cephem-resistant Staphylococcus aureus.. Antimicrob Agents Chemother 1985; 28: 397-403.

[27] Ma XX, Ito T, Tiensasitorn C, *et al.* Novel type of staphylococcal cassette chromosome mec identified in community-acquired methicillin-resistant Staphylococcus aureus strains. Antimicrob Agents Chemother 2002; 46: 1147-52.

[28] Deurenberg RHCV, Kalenic S, Friedrich AW, *et al.* The molecular evolution of methicillin-resistant Staphylococcus aureus. Clin Microbiol Infect 2007; 13: 222-35.

[29] Wisplinghoff H, Rosato AE, Enright MC, *et al.* Related clones containing SCCmec type IV predominate among clinically significant Staphylococcus epidermidis isolates. Antimicrob Agents Chemother 2003; 47(11): 3574-9.

[30] Boucher HW, Corey GR. Epidemiology of methicillin-resistant Staphylococcus aureus. Clin Infect Dis 2008 1; 46 Suppl 5: S344-9.

[31] Vandenesch F, Naimi T, Enright MC, *et al.* Community-acquired methicillin-resistant Staphylococcus aureus carrying Panton-Valentine leukocidin genes: worldwide emergence. Emerg Infect Dis 2003; 9(8): 978-84.

[32] Enany S, Higuchi W, Okubo T, *et al.* Brain abscess caused by Panton-Valentine leukocidin-positive community-acquired methicillin-resistant Staphylococcus aureus in Egypt, April 2007. Euro Surveill 2007; 12(9): E070927.2.

[33] Enany S, Yaoita E, Yoshida Y, *et al.* Molecular characterization of Panton-Valentine leukocidin-positive community-acquired methicillin-resistant Staphylococcus aureus isolates in Egypt. Microbiol Res 2010; 165(2): 152-62.

[34] El-Sharif A, Ashour HM. Community-acquired methicillin-resistant Staphylococcus aureus (CA-MRSA) colonization and infection in intravenous and inhalational opiate drug abusers. Exp Biol Med (Maywood). 2008; 233(7):874-80.

[35] Chongtrakool P, Ito T, Ma XX, *et al.* Staphylococcal cassette chromosome mec (SCCmec) typing of methicillin-resistant Staphylococcus aureus strains isolated in 11 Asian countries: a proposal for a new nomenclature for SCCmec elements. Antimicrob Agents Chemother 2006; 50(3): 1001-12.

[36 Monnet DL, MacKenzie FM, Lopez-Lozano JM, *et al.* Antimicrobial drug use and methicillin-resistant Staphylococcus aureus, Aberdeen, 1996-2000. Emerg Infect Dis 2004; 10(8): 1432-41.

[37] Gur D, Unal S. Resistance to antimicrobial agents in Mediterranean countries. Int J Antimicrob Agents 2001; 17(1):21-6.

[38] Borg MA, Zarb P, Ferech M, *et al.* Antibiotic consumption in southern and eastern Mediterranean hospitals: results from the ARMed project. J Antimicrob Chemother 2008; 62(4): 830-6.

[39] Raveh D, Levy Y, Schlesinger Y, *et al.* Longitudinal surveillance of antibiotic use in the hospital. Qjm. 2001; 94(3):141-52.

[40] Borg MA, Cookson BD, Gur D, *et al.* Infection control and antibiotic stewardship practices reported by south-eastern Mediterranean hospitals collaborating in the ARMed project. J Hosp Infect 2008; 70(3): 228-34.

[41] Narasimhan V, Brown H, Pablos-Mendez A, *et al.* Responding to the global human resources crisis. Lancet. 2004; 363(9419): 1469-72.

[42] Amazian K, Fendri C, Missoum MF, *et al.* Multicenter pilot survey of resistant bacteria in the Mediterranean area. Eur J Clin Microbiol Infect Dis 2006; 25(5): 340-3.

[43] Livermore DM. beta-Lactamases in laboratory and clinical resistance. Clin Microbiol Rev. 1995; 8(4):557-84.

[44]   Ambler RP, Coulson AF, Frere JM, *et al.* A standard numbering scheme for the class A beta-lactamases. Biochem *J* 1991 15; 276 (Pt 1): 269-70.

[45]   Bush K, Jacoby GA, Medeiros AA. A functional classification scheme for beta-lactamases and its correlation with molecular structure. Antimicrob Agents Chemother 1995; 39(6): 1211-33.

[46]   Hawkey PM. Molecular epidemiology of clinically significant antibiotic resistance genes. Br J Pharmac*ol* 2008; 153 Suppl 1: S406-13.

[47]   Giske CG, Sundsfjord AS, Kahlmeter G, *et al.* Redefining extended-spectrum beta-lactamases: balancing science and clinical need. J Antimicrob Chemother 2009; 63(1): 1-4.

[48]   Poirel L, Girlich D, Naas T, *et al.* OXA-28, an extended-spectrum variant of OXA-10 beta-lactamase from Pseudomonas aeruginosa and its plasmid- and integron-located gene. Antimicrob Agents Chemother 2001; 45(2): 447-53.

[49]   Naas T, Sougakoff W, Casetta A, *et al.* Molecular characterization of OXA-20, a novel class D beta-lactamase, and its integron from Pseudomonas aeruginosa. Antimicrob Agents Chemother 1998; 42(8): 2074-83.

[50]   Toleman MA, Rolston K, Jones RN, *et al.* Molecular and biochemical characterization of OXA-45, an extended-spectrum class 2d' beta-lactamase in Pseudomonas aeruginosa. Antimicrob Agents Chemother 2003; 47(9): 2859-63.

[51]   Danel F, Hall LM, Gur D, *et al.* OXA-15, an extended-spectrum variant of OXA-2 beta-lactamase, isolated from a Pseudomonas aeruginosa strain. Antimicrob Agents Chemother 1997; 41(4): 785-90.

[52]   Poirel L, Gerome P, De Champs C, *et al.* Integron-located oxa-32 gene cassette encoding an extended-spectrum variant of OXA-2 beta-lactamase from Pseudomonas aeruginosa. Antimicrob Agents Chemother 2002; 46(2): 566-69.

[53]   Philippon LN, Naas T, Bouthors AT, *et al.* OXA-18, a class D clavulanic acid-inhibited extended-spectrum beta-lactamase from Pseudomonas aeruginosa. Antimicrob Agents Chemother 1997; 41(10): 2188-95.

[54]   Moore KL, Kainer MA, Badrawi N, *et al.* Neonatal sepsis in Egypt associated with bacterial contamination of glucose-containing intravenous fluids. Pediatr Infect Dis J 2005; 24(7): 590-94.

[55]   Zaki Mel S. Extended spectrum beta-lactamases among gram-negative bacteria from an Egyptian pediatric hospital: a two-year experience. J Infect Dev Ctries 2007; 1(3): 269-74.

[56]   Shehabi AA, Baadran, I. Microbial infection and antibiotic resistance patterns among Jordanian intensive care patients. Eastern Mediterran Health J 1996; 2: 515-20.

[57]   Shehabi AA, Mahafzah A, Baadran I, *et al.* High incidence of Klebsiella pneumoniae clinical isolates to extended-spectrum B-lactam drugs in intensive care units. Diagn Microbiol Infect Dis 2000; 36(1): 53-56.

[58]   Panhotra BR, Saxena AK, Al-Ghamdi AM. Extended-spectrum beta-lactamase-producing Klebsiella pneumoniae hospital acquired bacteremia. Risk factors and clinical outcome. Saudi Med J 2004; 25(12):1871-76.

[59]   El-Khizzi NA, Bakheshwain SM. Prevalence of extended-spectrum beta-lactamases among Enterobacteriaceae isolated from blood culture in a tertiary care hospital. Saudi Med J 2006; 27(1): 37-40.

[60]   Kader AA, Kumar A. Prevalence and antimicrobial susceptibility of extended-spectrum beta-lactamase-producing Escherichia coli and Klebsiella pneumoniae in a general hospital. Ann Saudi Med 2005; 25(3): 239-42.

[61]   Khanfar HS, Bindayna KM, Senok AC, *et al.* Extended spectrum beta-lactamases (ESBL) in Escherichia coli and Klebsiella pneumoniae: trends in the hospital and community settings. J Infect Dev Ctries 2009; 3(4): 295-99.

[62]   Paterson DL, Bonomo RA. Extended-spectrum beta-lactamases: a clinical update. Clin Microbiol Rev 2005; 18(4): 657-86.

[63]   Bonnet R. Growing group of extended-spectrum beta-lactamases: the CTX-M enzymes. Antimicrob Agents Chemother 2004; 48(1):1-14.

[64]   Poirel L, Gniadkowski M, Nordmann P. Biochemical analysis of the ceftazidime-hydrolysing extended-spectrum beta-lactamase CTX-M-15 and of its structurally related beta-lactamase CTX-M-3. J Antimicrob Chemother 2002; 50(6): 1031-34.

[65]   Pitout JD, Hossain A, Hanson ND. Phenotypic and molecular detection of CTX-M-beta-lactamases produced by Escherichia coli and Klebsiella spp. J Clin Microbiol 2004; 42(12): 5715-21.

[66]   Moubareck C, Daoud Z, Hakime NI, *et al.* Countrywide spread of community- and hospital-acquired extended-spectrum beta-lactamase (CTX-M-15)-producing Enterobacteriaceae in Lebanon. J Clin Microbiol 2005; 43(7): 3309-13.

[67]   Touati A, Benallaoua S, Forte D, *et al.* First report of CTX-M-15 and CTX-M-3 beta-lactamases among clinical isolates of Enterobacteriaceae in Bejaia, Algeria. Int J Antimicrob Agents 2006; 27(5): 397-402.

[68]   Mohamed Al-Agamy MH, El-Din Ashour MS, Wiegand I. First description of CTX-M beta-lactamase-producing clinical Escherichia coli isolates from Egypt. Int J Antimicrob Agents 2006; 27(6): 545-8.

[69]   Mamlouk K, Boutiba-Ben Boubaker I, Gautier V, *et al.* Emergence and outbreaks of CTX-M beta-lactamase-producing Escherichia coli and Klebsiella pneumoniae strains in a Tunisian hospital. J Clin Microbiol 2006; 44(11): 4049-56.

[70]   Lavollay M, Mamlouk K, Frank T, *et al.* Clonal dissemination of a CTX-M-15 beta-lactamase-producing Escherichia coli strain in the Paris area, Tunis, and Bangui. Antimicrob Agents Chemother 2006; 50(7): 2433-8.

[71]   Sonnevend A, Al Dhaheri K, Mag T, *et al.* CTX-M-15-producing multidrug-resistant enteroaggregative Escherichia coli in the United Arab Emirates. Clin Microbiol Infect 2006; 12(6): 582-85.

[72]   Moubareck C, Doucet-Populaire F, Hamze M, *et al.* First extended-spectrum-beta-lactamase (CTX-M-15)-producing Salmonella enterica serotype typhimurium isolate identified in Lebanon. Antimicrob Agents Chemother 2005; 49(2): 864-65.

[73]   Rotimi VO, Jamal W, Pal T, *et al.* Emergence of CTX-M-15 type extended-spectrum beta-lactamase-producing Salmonella spp. in Kuwait and the United Arab Emirates. J Med Microbiol 2008; 57(Pt 7): 881-86.

[74]   Khalaf NG, Eletreby MM, Hanson ND. Characterization of CTX-M ESBLs in Enterobacter cloacae, Escherichia coli and Klebsiella pneumoniae clinical isolates from Cairo, Egypt. BMC Infect Dis 2009; 9: 84.

[75]   Ben Achour N, Mercuri PS, Power P, *et al.* First detection of CTX-M-28 in a Tunisian hospital from a cefotaxime-resistant Klebsiella pneumoniae strain. Pathol Biol (Paris) 2009; 57(5): 343-48.

[76]   Meradi L, Djahoudi A, Abdi A, *et al.* Qnr and aac (6')-Ib-cr types quinolone resistance among Enterobacteriaceae isolated in Annaba, Algeria. Pathol Biol (Paris). 2009 Nov 4.

[77]   Coque TM, Baquero F, Canton R. Increasing prevalence of ESBL-producing Enterobacteriaceae in Europe. Euro Surveill 2008 20; 13(47): pii: 19044.

[78]   Livermore DM, Canton R, Gniadkowski M, *et al.* CTX-M: changing the face of ESBLs in Europe. J Antimicrob Chemother 2007; 59(2): 165-74.

[79]   Makanera A, Arlet G, Gautier V, *et al.* Molecular epidemiology and characterization of plasmid-encoded beta-lactamases produced by Tunisian clinical isolates of Salmonella enterica serotype Mbandaka resistant to broad-spectrum cephalosporins. J Clin Microbiol 2003; 41(7): 2940-5.

[80]   Ishida Y, Ahmed AM, Mahfouz NB, *et al.* Molecular Analysis of Antimicrobial Resistance in Gram-Negative Bacteria Isolated from Fish Farms in Egypt. J Vet Med Sci 2010; 72(6): 727-34.

[81]   Iabadene H, Messai Y, Ammari H, *et al.* Prevalence of plasmid-mediated AmpC beta-lactamases among Enterobacteriaceae in Algiers hospitals. Int J Antimicrob Agents 2009; 34(4): 340-2.

[82]   Abbassi MS, Torres C, Achour W, *et al.* Genetic characterisation of CTX-M-15-producing Klebsiella pneumoniae and Escherichia coli strains isolated from stem cell transplant patients in Tunisia. Int J Antimicrob Agents 2008; 32(4): 308-14.

[83]   Mansour W, Dahmen S, Poirel L, *et al.* Emergence of SHV-2a extended-spectrum beta-lactamases in clinical isolates of Pseudomonas aeruginosa in a university hospital in Tunisia. Microb Drug Resist. 2009; 15(4): 295-301.

[84]   Hammami S, Gautier V, Ghozzi R, *et al.* Diversity in VIM-2-encoding class 1 integrons and occasional blaSHV2a carriage in isolates of a persistent, multidrug-resistant Pseudomonas aeruginosa clone from Tunis. Clin Microbiol Infect 2010; 16(2): 189-93.

[85]   AbdelGhani SM, Moland ES, Black JA, *et al.* First report of CTX-M-14 producing clinical isolates of Salmonella serovar Typhimurium from Egypt. J Infect Dev Ctries. 2009; 4(1): 58-60.

[86]   Abdel-Hady H, Hawas S, El-Daker M, *et al.* Extended-spectrum beta-lactamase producing Klebsiella pneumoniae in neonatal intensive care unit. J Perinatol 2008; 28(10): 685-90.

[87]   Ahmed AM, Younis EE, Ishida Y, *et al.* Genetic basis of multidrug resistance in Salmonella enterica serovars Enteritidis and Typhimurium isolated from diarrheic calves in Egypt. Acta Trop. 2009; 111(2): 144-49.

[88]   Elhani D, Bakir L, Aouni M, *et al.* Molecular epidemiology of extended-spectrum beta-lactamase-producing Klebsiella pneumoniae strains in a university hospital in Tunis, Tunisia, 1999-2005. Clin Microbiol Infect 2010; 16(2): 157-64.

[89]   Dahmen S, Poirel L, Mansour W, *et al.* Prevalence of plasmidmediated quinolone resistance determinants in Enterobacteriaceae from Tunisia. Clin Microbiol Infect 2009; 16(7): 1019-23.

[90]   Hussein AI, Ahmed AM, Sato M, *et al.* Characterization of integrons and antimicrobial resistance genes in clinical isolates of Gram-negative bacteria from Palestinian hospitals. Microbiol Immunol 2009; 53(11): 595-602.

[91]   Nordmann P, Naas T. Sequence analysis of PER-1 extended-spectrum beta-lactamase from Pseudomonas aeruginosa and comparison with class-A beta-lactamases. Antimicrob Agents Chemother 1994; 38(1): 104-14.

[92]   Vahaboglu H, Ozturk R, Aygun G, *et al.* Widespread detection of PER-1-type extended-spectrum beta-lactamases among nosocomial Acinetobacter and Pseudomonas aeruginosa isolates in Turkey: a nationwide multicenter study. Antimicrob Agents Chemother 1997; 41(10): 2265-69.

[93]   Iabadene H, Dallenne C, Messai Y, *et al.* Emergence of extended-spectrum beta-lactamase PER-1 in Proteus vulgaris and Providencia stuartii isolates from Algiers, Algeria. Antimicrob Agents Chemother 2009; 53(9): 4043-44.

[94]   Rossolini GM, Franceschini N, Lauretti L, *et al.* Cloning of a Chryseobacterium (Flavobacterium) meningosepticum chromosomal gene (blaA (CME)) encoding an extended-spectrum class A beta-lactamase related to the Bacteroides cephalosporinases and the VEB-1 and PER beta-lactamases. Antimicrob Agents Chemother 1999; 43(9): 2193-99.

[95]   Poirel L, Naas T, Guibert M, *et al.* Molecular and biochemical characterization of VEB-1, a novel class A extended-spectrum beta-lactamase encoded by an Escherichia coli integron gene. Antimicrob Agents Chemother 1999; 43(3): 573-81.

[96]   Aubert D, Naas T, Lartigue MF, *et al.* Novel genetic structure associated with an extended-spectrum beta-lactamase blaVEB gene in a Providencia stuartii clinical isolate from Algeria. Antimicrob Agents Chemother 2005; 49(8): 3590-92.

[97]   Girlich D, Naas T, Leelaporn A, *et al.* Nosocomial spread of the integron-located veb-1-like cassette encoding an extended-pectrum beta-lactamase in Pseudomonas aeruginosa in Thailand. Clin Infect Dis 2002 1; 34(5): 603-11.

[98]   Khalaf NG, Moland,E.S., Thomson, *et al.* Production of a Novel Extended Spectrum Beta Lactamase, VEB-5 in an E. coli Isolate from the United States.; GenBank Accession number EF420108. 2007.

[99]   Woodford N, Zhang J, Kaufmann ME, *et al.* Detection of Pseudomonas aeruginosa isolates producing VEB-type extended-spectrum beta-lactamases in the United Kingdom. J Antimicrob Chemother 2008; 62(6): 1265-68.

[100]   Mammeri H, Van De Loo M, Poirel L, *et al.* Emergence of plasmid-mediated quinolone resistance in Escherichia coli in Europe. Antimicrob Agents Chemother 2005; 49(1): 71-76.

[101]   Poirel L, Van De Loo M, Mammeri H, *et al.* Association of plasmid-mediated quinolone resistance with extended-spectrum beta-lactamase VEB-1. Antimicrob Agents Chemother 2005; 49(7): 3091-94.

[102]   Shahcheraghi F, Badmasti F, Feizabadi MM. Molecular characterization of class 1 integrons in MDR Pseudomonas aeruginosa isolated from clinical settings in Iran, Tehran. FEMS Immunol Med Microbiol 2010; 58(3): 421-25.

[103]   Mirsalehian A, Feizabadi M, Nakhjavani FA, *et al.* Detection of VEB-1, OXA-10 and PER-1 genotypes in extended-spectrum beta-lactamase-producing Pseudomonas aeruginosa strains isolated from burn patients. Burns 2010; 36(1): 70-74.

[104]   Poirel L, Rotimi VO, Mokaddas EM, *et al.* VEB-1-like extended-spectrum beta-lactamases in Pseudomonas aeruginosa, Kuwait. Emerg Infect Dis 2001; 7(3): 468-70.

[105]   Iabadene H, Messai Y, Ammari H, *et al.* Dissemination of ESBL and Qnr determinants in Enterobacter cloacae in Algeria. J Antimicrob Chemother 2008; 62(1): 133-6.

[106]   Kalai BS, Achour W, Abbassi MS, *et al.* Nosocomial outbreak of OXA-18-producing Pseudomonas aeruginosa in Tunisia. Clin Microbiol Infect 2007; 13(8): 794-800.

[107]   Kanj SS, Corkill JE, Kanafani ZA, *et al.* Molecular characterisation of extended-spectrum beta-lactamase-producing Escherichia coli and Klebsiella spp. isolates at a tertiary-care centre in Lebanon. Clin Microbiol Infect 2008; 14(5): 501-04.

[108]   Karim A, Poirel L, Nagarajan S, *et al.* Plasmid-mediated extended-spectrum beta-lactamase (CTX-M-3 like) from India and gene association with insertion sequence ISEcp1. FEMS Microbiol Lett 2001 24; 201(2): 237-41.

[109]   Sabate M, Tarrago R, Navarro F, *et al.* Cloning and sequence of the gene encoding a novel cefotaxime-hydrolyzing beta-lactamase (CTX-M-9) from Escherichia coli in Spain. Antimicrob Agents Chemother 2000; 44(7): 1970-73.

[110]   Weill FX, Perrier-Gros-Claude JD, Demartin M, *et al.* Characterization of extended-spectrum-beta-lactamase (CTX-M-15)-producing strains of Salmonella enterica isolated in France and Senegal. FEMS Microbiol Lett 2004 15; 238(2): 353-58.

[111]   Poirel L, Lartigue MF, Decousser JW, *et al.* ISEcp1B-mediated transposition of blaCTX-M in Escherichia coli. Antimicrob Agents Chemother 2005; 49(1): 447-50.

[112] Messai Y, Iabadene H, Benhassine T, *et al.* Prevalence and characterization of extended-spectrum beta-lactamases in Klebsiella pneumoniae in Algiers hospitals (Algeria). Pathol Biol (Paris) 2008; 56(5): 319-25.

[113] Clermont O, Bonacorsi S, Bingen E. Rapid and simple determination of the Escherichia coli phylogenetic group. Appl Environ Microbiol 2000; 66(10): 4555-58.

[114] Nicolas-Chanoine MH, Blanco J, Leflon-Guibout V, *et al.* Intercontinental emergence of Escherichia coli clone O25:H4-ST131 producing CTX-M-15. J Antimicrob Chemother 2008; 61(2): 273-81.

[115] Coque TM, Novais A, Carattoli A, *et al.* Dissemination of clonally related Escherichia coli strains expressing extended-spectrum beta-lactamase CTX-M-15. Emerg Infect Dis 2008; 14(2): 195-200.

[116] Clermont O, Lavollay M, Vimont S, *et al.* The CTX-M-15-producing Escherichia coli diffusing clone belongs to a highly virulent B2 phylogenetic subgroup. J Antimicrob Chemother 2008; 61(5): 1024-28.

[117] Jacoby GA. AmpC beta-lactamases. Clin Microbiol Rev 2009; 22(1): 161-82.

[118] Hanson ND, Thomson KS, Moland ES, *et al.* Molecular characterization of a multiply resistant Klebsiella pneumoniae encoding ESBLs and a plasmid-mediated AmpC. J Antimicrob Chemother 1999; 44(3): 377-80.

[119] Decre D, Verdet C, Raskine L, *et al.* Characterization of CMY-type beta-lactamases in clinical strains of Proteus mirabilis and Klebsiella pneumoniae isolated in four hospitals in the Paris area. J Antimicrob Chemother 2002; 50(5): 681-88.

[120] Moland ES, Hanson ND, Black JA, *et al.* Prevalence of newer beta-lactamases in gram-negative clinical isolates collected in the United States from 2001 to 2002. J Clin Microbiol 2006; 44(9): 3318-24.

[121] Hanson ND, Moland ES, Hossain A, *et al.* Unusual Salmonella enterica serotype Typhimurium isolate producing CMY-7, SHV-9 and OXA-30 beta-lactamases. J Antimicrob Chemother 2002; 49(6): 1011-14.

[122] Pitout JD, Reisbig MD, Mulvey M, *et al.* Association between handling of pet treats and infection with Salmonella enterica serotype newport expressing the AmpC beta-lactamase, CMY-2. J Clin Microbiol 2003; 41(10): 4578-82.

[123] Moland ES, Black JA, Ourada J, *et al.* Occurrence of newer beta-lactamases in Klebsiella pneumoniae isolates from 24 U.S. hospitals. Antimicrob Agents Chemother 2002; 46(12): 3837-42.

[124] Khalaf N, Wiegand, I, Wiedemann B. Detection of CMY-2 beta-lactamases in clinical P. stuartii isolates from Egypt. R1962 ECCMID Prague; 2004.

[125] Queenan AM, Bush K. Carbapenemases: the versatile beta-lactamases. Clin Microbiol Rev 2007; 20(3): 440-58.

[126] Yigit H, Queenan AM, Anderson GJ, *et al.* Novel carbapenem-hydrolyzing beta-lactamase, KPC-1, from a carbapenem-resistant strain of Klebsiella pneumoniae. Antimicrob Agents Chemother 2001; 45(4): 1151-61.

[127] Yigit H, Queenan AM, Rasheed JK, *et al.* Carbapenem-resistant strain of Klebsiella oxytoca harboring carbapenem-hydrolyzing beta-lactamase KPC-2. Antimicrob Agents Chemother 2003; 47(12): 3881-89.

[128] Naas T, Cuzon G, Villegas MV, *et al.* Genetic structures at the origin of acquisition of the beta-lactamase bla KPC gene. Antimicrob Agents Chemother 2008; 52(4): 1257-63.

[129] Nordmann P, Poirel L. Emerging carbapenemases in Gram-negative aerobes. Clin Microbiol Infect 2002; 8(6): 321-31.

[130] Al-Agamy MH, Shibl AM, Tawfik AF, *et al.* High prevalence of metallo-beta-lactamase-producing Pseudomonas aeruginosa from Saudi Arabia. J Chemother 2009; 21(4): 461-62.

[131] Mansour W, Poirel L, Bettaieb D, *et al.* Metallo-beta-lactamase-producing Pseudomonas aeruginosa isolates in Tunisia. Diagn Microbiol Infect Dis 2009; 64(4): 458-61.

[132] Guerin F, Henegar C, Spiridon G, *et al.* Bacterial prostatitis due to Pseudomonas aeruginosa harbouring the blaVIM-2 metallo-{beta}-lactamase gene from Saudi Arabia. J Antimicrob Chemother 2005; 56(3): 601-02.

[133] Walther-Rasmussen J, Hoiby N. OXA-type carbapenemases. J Antimicrob Chemother 2006; 57(3): 373-83.

[134] Mugnier PD, Bindayna KM, Poirel L, *et al.* Diversity of plasmid-mediated carbapenem-hydrolysing oxacillinases among carbapenem-resistant Acinetobacter baumannii isolates from Kingdom of Bahrain. J Antimicrob Chemother 2009; 63(5):1071-73.

[135] Mugnier P, Poirel L, Pitout M, *et al.* Carbapenem-resistant and OXA-23-producing Acinetobacter baumannii isolates in the United Arab Emirates. Clin Microbiol Infect 2008; 14(9): 879-82.

[136] Mansour W, Poirel L, Bettaieb D, *et al.* Dissemination of OXA-23-producing and carbapenem-resistant Acinetobacter baumannii in a University Hospital in Tunisia. Microb Drug Resist 2008; 14(4): 289-92.

[137] Zarrilli R, Vitale D, Di Popolo A, *et al.* A plasmid-borne blaOXA-58 gene confers imipenem resistance to Acinetobacter baumannii isolates from a Lebanese hospital. Antimicrob Agents Chemother 2008; 52(11): 4115-20.

[138] Gur D, Korten V, Unal S, *et al.* Increasing carbapenem resistance due to the clonal dissemination of oxacillinase (OXA-23 and OXA-58)-producing Acinetobacter baumannii: report from the Turkish SENTRY Program sites. J Med Microbiol 2008; 57(Pt 12): 1529-32.

[139] Feizabadi MM, Fathollahzadeh B, Taherikalani M, *et al.* Antimicrobial susceptibility patterns and distribution of blaOXA genes among Acinetobacter spp. Isolated from patients at Tehran hospitals. Jpn J Infect Dis 2008; 61(4): 274-78.

[140] Cuzon G, Naas T, Bogaerts P, *et al.* Plasmid-encoded carbapenem-hydrolyzing beta-lactamase OXA-48 in an imipenem-susceptible Klebsiella pneumoniae strain from Belgium. Antimicrob Agents Chemother 2008; 52(9): 3463-64.

[141] Cuzon G, Naas T, Lesenne A, *et al.* Plasmid-mediated carbapenem-hydrolysing OXA-48 beta-lactamase in Klebsiella pneumoniae from Tunisia. Int J Antimicrob Agents 2010; 36(1):91-93.

[142] Carrer A, Poirel L, Yilmaz M, *et al.* Spread of OXA-48-encoding plasmid in Turkey and beyond. Antimicrob Agents Chemother 2010; 54(3): 1369-73.

[143] Matar GM, Dandache I, Carrer A, *et al.* Spread of OXA-48-mediated resistance to carbapenems in Lebanese Klebsiella pneumoniae and Escherichia coli that produce extended spectrum beta-lactamase. Ann Trop Med Parasitol; 104(3): 271-74.

[144] Aubert D, Naas T, Heritier C, *et al.* Functional characterization of IS1999, an IS4 family element involved in mobilization and expression of beta-lactam resistance genes. J Bacteriol 2006; 188(18): 6506-14.

[145] Navon-Venezia S, Chmelnitsky I, Leavitt A, *et al.* Plasmid-mediated imipenem-hydrolyzing enzyme KPC-2 among multiple carbapenem-resistant Escherichia coli clones in Israel. Antimicrob Agents Chemother 2006; 50(9): 3098-101.

[146] Chmelnitsky I, Navon-Venezia S, Strahilevitz J, *et al.* Plasmid-mediated qnrB2 and carbapenemase gene bla(KPC-2) carried on the same plasmid in carbapenem-resistant ciprofloxacin-susceptible Enterobacter cloacae isolates. Antimicrob Agents Chemother 2008; 52(8):2962-65.

[147] Stapleton PD, Shannon KP, French GL. Carbapenem resistance in Escherichia coli associated with plasmid-determined CMY-4 beta-lactamase production and loss of an outer membrane protein. Antimicrob Agents Chemother 1999; 43(5): 1206-10.

[148] Bradford PA, Urban C, Mariano N, *et al.* Imipenem resistance in Klebsiella pneumoniae is associated with the combination of ACT-1, a plasmid-mediated AmpC beta-lactamase, and the foss of an outer membrane protein. Antimicrob Agents Chemother 1997; 41(3): 563-69.

[149] Matar GM, Jaafar R, Sabra A, *et al.* First detection and sequence analysis of the bla-CTX-M-15 gene in Lebanese isolates of extended-spectrum-beta-lactamase-producing Shigella sonnei. Ann Trop Med Parasitol 2007; 101(6): 511-17.

[150] Hooper DC. Mechanisms of fluoroquinolone resistance. Drug Resist Updat 1999; 2(1): 38-55.

[151] Hooper DC. Mechanisms of action and resistance of older and newer fluoroquinolones. Clin Infect Dis 2000; 31 Suppl 2: S24-28.

[152] Tran JH, Jacoby GA. Mechanism of plasmid-mediated quinolone resistance. Proc Natl Acad Sci U S A. 2002 Apr 16; 99(8): 5638-42.

[153] Robicsek A, Strahilevitz J, Jacoby GA, *et al.* Fluoroquinolone-modifying enzyme: a new adaptation of a common aminoglycoside acetyltransferase. Nat Med 2006; 12(1): 83-88.

[154] Wiegand I, Khalaf N, Al-Agamy MHM, *et al.* First detection of the transferable quinolone resistance determinant in clinical Providencia stuartii strains in Egypt. O347 ECCMID. Prague; 2004.

[155] Martinez-Martinez L, Pascual A, Jacoby GA. Quinolone resistance from a transferable plasmid. Lancet. 1998 14; 351(9105): 797-99.

[156] Jacoby GA, Chow N, Waites KB. Prevalence of plasmid-mediated quinolone resistance. Antimicrob Agents Chemother 2003; 47(2): 559-62.

[157] Wiegand I, Luhmer-Becker I, Wiedemann B. Effect of the plasmid encoded quinolone resistance determinant in P. stuartii on the selection of strains with clinical resistance to ciprofloxacin. P1417 ECCMID. Copenhagen; 2005.

[158] Rice LB, Willey SH, Papanicolaou GA, *et al.* Outbreak of ceftazidime resistance caused by extended-spectrum beta-lactamases at a Massachusetts chronic-care facility. Antimicrob Agents Chemother 1990; 34(11): 2193-9.

[159] Wiener J, Quinn JP, Bradford PA, *et al.* Multiple antibiotic-resistant Klebsiella and Escherichia coli in nursing homes. Jama. 1999 10; 281(6): 517-23.

[160] Abdalhamid B, Pitout JD, Moland ES, *et al.* Community-onset disease caused by Citrobacter freundii producing a novel CTX-M beta-lactamase, CTX-M-30, in Canada. Antimicrob Agents Chemother 2004; 48(11): 4435-7.

[161] Pitout JD, Hanson ND, Church DL, *et al.* Population-based laboratory surveillance for Escherichia coli-producing extended-spectrum beta-lactamases: importance of community isolates with blaCTX-M genes. Clin Infect Dis 2004 15; 38(12): 1736-41.

[162] Laupland KB, Parkins MD, Ross T, *et al*. Population-based laboratory surveillance for tribe Proteeae isolates in a large Canadian health region. Clin Microbiol Infect 2007; 13(7): 683-8.

[163] Pitout JD, Gregson DB, Church DL, *et al*. Population-based laboratory surveillance for AmpC beta-lactamase-producing Escherichia coli, Calgary. Emerg Infect Dis 2007; 13(3): 443-8.

[164] Parkins MD, Gregson DB, Pitout JD, *et al*. Population-based study of the epidemiology and the risk factors for Pseudomonas aeruginosa bloodstream infection. Infection 2010; 38(1): 25-32.

[165] Pitout JD, Wei Y, Church DL, *et al*. Surveillance for plasmid-mediated quinolone resistance determinants in Enterobacteriaceae within the Calgary Health Region, Canada: the emergence of aac(6')-Ib-cr. J Antimicrob Chemother 2008; 61(5): 999-1002.

[166] Hanson ND, Moland ES, Hong SG, *et al*. Surveillance of community-based reservoirs reveals the presence of CTX-M, imported AmpC, and OXA-30 beta-lactamases in urine isolates of Klebsiella pneumoniae and Escherichia coli in a U.S. community. Antimicrob Agents Chemother 2008; 52(10): 3814-16.

[167] Fadel R, Dakdouki GK, Kanafani ZA, *et al*. Clinical and microbiological profile of urinary tract infection at a tertiary-care center in Lebanon. Infect Control Hosp Epidemiol 2004; 25(1): 82-85.

[168] Al-Tawfiq JA, Antony A. Antimicrobial resistance of Klebsiella pneumoniae in a Saudi Arabian hospital: results of a 6-year surveillance study, 1998-2003. J Infect Chemother 2007; 13(4): 230-34.

[169] Youssef MT, Malkawi HI, Shurman AA, *et al*. Molecular typing of multiresistant Klebsiella pneumoniae isolated from children from northern Jordan. J Trop Pediatr 1999; 45(5): 271-7.

[170] Tham J, Odenholt I, Walder M, *et al*. Extended-spectrum beta-lactamase-producing Escherichia coli in patients with travellers' diarrhoea. Scand J Infect Dis 2010; 42(4): 275-80.

[171] Shehabi AA, Masoud H, Maslamani FA. Common antimicrobial resistance patterns, biotypes and serotypes found among Pseudomonas aeruginosa isolates from patient's stools and drinking water sources in Jordan. J Chemother 2005; 17(2): 179-83.

[172] Shehabi AA, Odeh JF, Fayyad M. Characterization of antimicrobial resistance and class 1 integrons found in Escherichia coli isolates from human stools and drinking water sources in Jordan. J Chemother 2006; 18(5): 468-72.

[173] Smith KE, Stenzel SA, Bender JB, *et al*. Outbreaks of enteric infections caused by multiple pathogens associated with calves at a farm day camp. Pediatr Infect Dis J 2004; 23(12): 1098-104.

[174] Cabello FC. Heavy use of prophylactic antibiotics in aquaculture: a growing problem for human and animal health and for the environment. Environ Microbiol 2006; 8(7): 1137-44.

[175] Sidjabat HE, Townsend KM, Hanson ND, *et al*. Identification of bla(CMY-7) and associated plasmid-mediated resistance genes in multidrug-resistant Escherichia coli isolated from dogs at a veterinary teaching hospital in Australia. J Antimicrob Chemother 2006; 57(5): 840-48.

[176] Sidjabat HE, Townsend KM, Lorentzen M, *et al*. Emergence and spread of two distinct clonal groups of multidrug-resistant Escherichia coli in a veterinary teaching hospital in Australia. J Med Microbiol 2006; 55(Pt 8): 1125-34.

[177] Johnson JR, Stell AL, Delavari P. Canine feces as a reservoir of extraintestinal pathogenic Escherichia coli. Infect Immun 2001; 69(3): 1306-14.

[178] Johnson JR, Kuskowski MA, Owens K, *et al*. Phylogenetic origin and virulence genotype in relation to resistance to fluoroquinolones and/or extended-spectrum cephalosporins and cephamycins among Escherichia coli isolates from animals and humans. J Infect Dis 2003 Sep 1; 188(5): 759-68.

[179] Iabadene H, Bakour R, Messai Y, *et al*. Detection of bla CTX-M-14 and aac (3)-II genes in Salmonella enterica serotype Kedougou in Algeria. Med Mal Infect 2009; 39(10): 806-07.

[180] Bouallegue-Godet O, Ben Salem Y, Fabre L, Demartin M, Grimont PAD, Mzoughi R, Weill FX. Nosocomial Outbreak Caused by Salmonella enterica Serotype Livingstone Producing CTX-M-27 Extended-Spectrum beta-Lactamase in a Neonatal Unit in Sousse, Tunisia. J Clin Microbiol 2005; 43(3): pp. 1037-44.

[181] Ahmed SH, Daef EA, Badary MS, *et al*. Nosocomial blood stream infection in intensive care units at Assiut University Hospitals (Upper Egypt) with special reference to extended spectrum beta-lactamase producing organisms. BMC Res Notes 2009; 2: 76.

[182] Ensor VM, Jamal W, Rotimi VO, *et al*. Predominance of CTX-M-15 extended spectrum beta-lactamases in diverse Escherichia coli and Klebsiella pneumoniae from hospital and community patients in Kuwait. Int J Antimicrob Agents 2009; 33(5): 487-89.

[183] Al-Agamy MH, Shibl AM, Tawfik AF. Prevalence and molecular characterization of extended-spectrum beta-lactamase-producing Klebsiella pneumoniae in Riyadh, Saudi Arabia. Ann Saudi Med 2009; 29(4): 253-57.

[184] Talaat M, el-Oun S, Kandeel A, *et al.* Overview of injection practices in two governorates in Egypt. Trop Med Int Health 2003; 8(3): 234-41.

[185] Talaat M, Kandeel A, El-Shoubary W, Bodenschatz C, Khairy I, Oun S, *et al.* Occupational exposure to needlestick injuries and hepatitis B vaccination coverage among health care workers in Egypt. Am J Infect Control 2003; 31(8): 469-74.

[186] Ismail NA, Aboul Ftouh AM, El-Shoubary WH, *et al.* Safe injection practice among health-care workers in Gharbiya Governorate, Egypt. East Mediterr Health J 2007; 13(4): 893-906.

[187] Talaat M, Kandeel A, Rasslan O, *et al.* Evolution of infection control in Egypt: achievements and challenges. Am J Infect Control 2006; 34(4): 193-200.

[188] Versalovic J, Koeuth T, Lupski JR. Distribution of repetitive DNA sequences in eubacteria and application to fingerprinting of bacterial genomes. Nucleic Acids Res 1991 25; 19(24): 6823-31.

[189] Messai Y, Benhassine T, Naim M, *et al.* Prevalence of beta-lactams resistance among Escherichia coli clinical isolates from a hospital in Algiers. Rev Esp Quimioter 2006; 19(2): 144-51.

[190] Welsh J, McClelland M. Fingerprinting genomes using PCR with arbitrary primers. Nucleic Acids Res. 1990 25; 18(24): 7213-18.

[191] Abdallah IM, Araj GF, Matar GM, *et al.* Polymerase chain reaction identification of coagulase-negative Staphylococci and of strain diversity and spread of Staphylococcus epidermidis in a major medical center in Lebanon. Infect Control Hosp Epidemiol 2006; 27(7): 781-83.

[192] Baddour MM, Abuelkheir MM, Fatani AJ, *et al.* Molecular epidemiology of methicillin-resistant Staphylococcus aureus (MRSA) isolates from major hospitals in Riyadh, Saudi Arabia. Can J Microbiol 2007; 53(8): 931-36.

[193] Marsou R, Idrissi L, BenHammida H, *et al.* Relationship of Staphylococcal isolates in a Moroccan hospital by comparing phenotypical and genotypical tests. Pathol Biol (Paris) 2001; 49(2): 109-14.

[194] Balkhy HH, Alsaif S, El-Saed A, *et al.* Neonatal rates and risk factors of device-associated bloodstream infection in a tertiary care center in Saudi Arabia. Am J Infect Control 2010; 38(2): 159-61.

[195] Japoni A, Vazin A, Hamedi M, *et al.* Multidrug-resistant bacteria isolated from intensive-care-unit patient samples. Braz J Infect Dis 2009; 13(2): 118-22.

[196] Borg MA, Cookson BD, Scicluna E. Survey of infection control infrastructure in selected southern and eastern Mediterranean hospitals. Clin Microbiol Infect 2007; 13(3): 344-46.

[197] Abd Elaziz KM, Bakr IM. Assessment of knowledge, attitude and practice of hand washing among health care workers in Ain Shams University hospitals in Cairo. J Prev Med Hyg 2009; 50(1): 19-25.

CHAPTER 12

Antimicrobial Resistance of Gram-Negative Bacteria in Saudi Arabia

Jaffar A. Al-Tawfiq[1][*] and Ziad A. Memish[2]

[1]*Saudi Aramco Medical Services Organization, Dhahran and* [2]*Preventive Medicine Directorate, Saudi Ministry of Health, Riyadh, Saudi Arabia*

Abstract: Much of the focus of today's media is directed on multidrug-resistant gram-positive bacteria. However, resistance within gram-negative bacilli continues to rise, occasionally creating situations in which few or no antibiotics that retain activity are available. Gram-negative bacteria are important causes of urinary tract infections, bloodstream infections, hospital- and healthcare-associated pneumonias, and various intra-abdominal infections. In Saudi Arabia, among Escherichia coli isolates from outpatients, 50% are resistant to ampicillin, 33% are resistant to trimethoprim-sulfamethoxazole (TMP-SMZ), and 14% are resistant to ciprofloxacin. Among isolates from inpatients, 63% of E. coli are resistant to ampicillin, 44% are resistant to TMP-SMZ, and 33% are resistant to ciprofloxacin. Multidrug resistance is detected in 2-28% of outpatient isolates and 7.4-39.6% of inpatient isolates. For *Pseudomonas aeruginosa*, the resistance rates of outpatient and inpatient isolates to piperacillin, ceftazidime, imipenem, and ciprofloxacin are 4.6% and 11.5%, 2.4% and 10%, 2.6% and 5.8%, and 3% and 6%, respectively. Multi-drug resistance is observed in 1—2% of inpatient isolates. Acinetobacter calcoaceticus-baumannii has high rates of resistance to ampicillin (86%), cefoxitin (89%), and nitrofurantoin (89%). The rate of resistance to imipenem is 3%; to ticarcillin-clavulanic acid, 16.5%; to gentamicin, 26%; and to ceftazidime, 38%. Multidrug resistance is observed in 14%-35.8%. Acinetobacter calcoaceticus-baumannii complex were recovered. The organism showed high rates of resistance to ampicillin (86%), cefoxitin (89%), and nitrofurantoin (89%). The rate of resistance to imipenem was 3%; to ticarcillin-clavulanic acid, 16.5%; to gentamicin, 26%; and to ceftazidime, 38%. Multidrug resistance is observed in 14%-35.8%.

Keywords: Trimethoprim-sulfamethoxazole, multidrug-resistant gram-positive bacteria, *Pseudomonas aeruginosa,* Gram-negative bacteria, ampicillin, cefoxitin, nitrofurantoin, ticarcillin-clavulanic acid, gentamicin, ceftazidime, Multidrug resistance.

INTRODUCTION

The focus of today's media is directed on multidrug-resistant gram-positive bacteria such as methicillin-resistant Staphylococcus aureus and vancomycin-resistant Enterococcus. However, resistance within gram-negative bacilli continues to rise, occasionally creating situations in which few or no antibiotics that retain activity are available. Extended-Spectrum B-Lactamase (ESBL)-producing Escherichia coli and Klebsiella sp are emerging threats. Regional and local descriptions of antibiotic resistance add to the global view of antimicrobial resistance [1]. More recently a new antibiotic resistance gene has become widespread in several species of bacteria in India, Pakistan, and the UK. Bacteria with this gene are resistant to nearly all classes of antibiotics. The bacteria appear to have been brought into the UK and other European countries by patients who travelled to India for medical procedures including cosmetic surgery. The gene has the potential to spread worldwide, in part because of the growth in 'medical tourism. The resistance gene, known as New Delhi metallo-ß-lactamase 1 (NDM-1), encodes a protein that breaks down a broad range of antibiotics including carbapenems, regarded as one of the drugs in the last line of defense against multidrug-resistant gram-negative bacteria (a large and diverse group of bacteria that includes pathogens such as *Escherichia coli, Salmonella,* and *Legionella)* [2].

Escherichia coli

Antimicrobial resistance among bacterial pathogens in the developing country is thought to be high and

*****Address correspondence to Jaffar A. Al Tawfiq:** Saudi Aramco Medical Services Organization, Dhahran; Tel: +96638773524; Fax: +96638773790; Email: jaffar.tawfiq@aramco.com

Asad U. Khan and Raffaele Zarrilli (Eds)

rising [3]. Many factors contribute to the emergence of antimicrobial resistance and include increased antimicrobial utilization [4, 5]. In Saudi Arabia, among *E. coli* isolates from outpatients, 50% are resistant to ampicillin, 33% are resistant to trimethoprim-sulfamethoxazole (TMP-SMZ), and 14% are resistant to ciprofloxacin. Among isolates from inpatients, 63% are resistant to ampicillin, 44% are resistant to TMP-SMZ, and 33% are resistant to ciprofloxacin. Multidrug resistance is detected in 2-28% of outpatient isolates and 7.4-39.6% of inpatient isolates [6]. It was reported that there is an increasing rates of resistance to 10 (67%) of 15 antibiotics commonly given to treat infection in outpatients and to 6 (40%) of 15 antibiotics commonly prescribed to infection in inpatients [6]. Ampicillin resistance rate is high and ranges from 55% to 92% among urinary isolates [6-8]. In addition, in a study that compared the resistance rate of *E. coli* from patients and animals revealed that the rate of ampicillin resistance was 70.7% [9]. It seems that ampicillin resistance is associated with resistance to other non-b-lactam antibiotics such as ciprofloxacin, trimethoprim-sulfamethoxazole, and tetracycline [6]. The high rates of resistance to the commonly used oral antibiotics such as ampicillin, tetracycline, and trimethoprim-sulfamethoxazole and quinolone limits the use of these agents to treat infections caused by *E. coli* as out-patient. In Saudi Arabia, the rate of quinolone resistance among *E. coli* is about 13 to *37%* [6, 10-13].

Klebsiella pneumoniae

Klebsiella pneumoniae accounted for 9% of all health care associated bloodstream infections at a general hospital in Saudi Arabia [14]. However, antibiotic resistance of *K. pneumoniae* in Saudi Arabia is limited. Two studies documented the prevalence of antibiotic resistance in this organism over time [15, 16]. The prevalence of ciprofloxacin resistance in *K. pneumoniae* isolates was 4.4% and 9.6% in outpatient and hospital acquired isolates, respectively [15]. In another study, the resistance of *K. pneumoniae* to ciprofloxacin increased from 16% to 27.5% from 2002 to 2005 [17]. Multidrug resistance, defined as resistance to three or more classes of antibiotics, was present in 0.6% and 1.7% of outpatient and hospital-acquired isolates, respectively [15].

Pseudomonas aeruginosa

For *Pseudomonas aeruginosa,* the resistance rates of outpatient and inpatient isolates to piperacillin, ceftazidime, imipenem, and ciprofloxacin are 4.6% and 11.5%, 2.4% and 10%, 2.6% and 5.8%, and 3% and 6%, respectively [18]. Multi-drug resistance is observed in 1-2% of inpatient isolates [18]. In another study, *P. aeruginosa* susceptibility significantly declined after 2007, especially for carbapenem (66% *vs* 26%), ceftazidime (69% *vs* 44%), and ciprofloxacin (67% *vs* 49%) in 2004 and 2009, respectively [19]. One of the interesting observations for *P. aeruginosa* resistance is the difference in the resistance rates to ceftazidime. The resistance rates to this antibiotic vary from as low as 2.4% [18] to as high as 56% [19]. Ceftazidime resistance is due to the selection of *P. aeruginosa* strains with derepression of the chromosomal AmpC b-lactamase gene or efflux pumps. Thus, increased prevalence of ceftazidime-resistant strains is related to increased use of b-lactam antibiotics such as amoxicillin and ceftazidime. This finding correlates with the prescribing habits of each hospital and the selective pressure of certain antibiotics. The resistance rate to imipenem is also variable and was documented in 2.6% and 5.8% of outpatient and inpatient isolates, respectively [18], 9.2% in another study [20]. In a recent study from Riyadh, *P. aeruginosa* susceptibility significantly declined for carbapenem from 66% in 2004 to 26% in 2009 [19].

Acinetobacter calcoaceticus-baumannii

Acinetobacter calcoaceticus-baumannii has high rates of resistance to ampicillin (86%), cefoxitin (89%), and nitrofurantoin (89%). In one study, the rate of resistance to imipenem is 3%; to ticarcillin-clavulanic acid, 16.5%; to gentamicin, 26%; and to ceftazidime, 38% [21]. However, another study showed much higher resistance rates where *A. baumannii* susceptibility was significantly decreased to imipenem (10-55%, meropenem (10-33%), ciprofloxacin (10-22%), and amikacin (6-12%) [19]. In a third study, about 50% of *A. calcoaceticus-baumannii* was resistant to imipenem and 28% were resistant to meropenem [22]. Thus, variation in the resistance rates is probably a reflection of the variation in the antimicrobial prescribing habits.

ESBL PRODUCING ORGANISMS

Pathogens producing Extended-Spectrum Beta-Lactamases (ESBL) are of a major concern throughout the globe and are important causes of multidrug resistant nosocomial and community acquired infections. ESBL enzymes are capable of hydrolyzing and mediating resistance to all penicillins, broad-spectrum cephalosporins, and monobactams. The production of ESBL is the result of mutations in the TEM-1, TEM-2 or SHV-1 genes commonly found in the Enterobacteriaceae family [23]. There are limited data on the on the molecular characterization of ESBL isolates circulating in Saudi Arabia. The prevalence of ESBL-producing bacteria is relatively high in the region and was 31.7% in Kuwait [24], 41% in United Arab Emirates [25] and 55% in Saudi Arabia [26]. In a recent study from Saudi Arabia, 71% of ESBL isolates harbored the CTX-M gene [27]. In that study, a high level (44%) of co-carriage of blaCTX-M and blaSHV genes was observed compared to a rate of 2.27% in an earlier study [26]. In a study of the fecal carriage of ESBL-producing bacteria in the community, ESBL-producing bacteria were found in 12.7% gram negative bacterial isolates [28].

SALMONELLOSIS

Salmonella infection is a major health concern throughout the world with variable patterns of antimicrobial resistance and increasing rates of multiple drug resistant *Salmonella typhi*. However, there is limited data about the resistance pattern of *Salmonella* spp. in Saudi Arabia [29-32]. Because of widespread dissemination of multi-drug resistant strains of *Salmonella spp*, ciprofloxacin became the drug of choice for typhoid fever. However, the emergence of *S. Typhi* with reduced susceptibility to quinolones began to appear in areas with resistance to first-line drugs, thus threatening the efficacy of these agents for treatment of typhoid fever. Reduced susceptibility to fluroquinolone (FQ) results in clinical and microbiological failure with rates of 53.4% and 17.4%, respectively [33]. In Saudi Arabia, the resistance rate of *Salmonella* non-typhi to ciprofloxacin ranges between 0 and 19% [34, 35]. On the second hand, multi-drug resistant *S. typhi* emerged since 1980s and constituted about 20% in one study from Saudi Arabia [35]. However, not all laboratories in Saudi Arabia routinely perform tests for the detection of resistance and reporting of quinolone resistance on *Salmonella spp.*, according to standards of the Clinical and Laboratory Standards Institute.

In conclusion, the development of antimicrobial resistance is a major threat to the recent achievement in the field of infectious diseases. Multiple factors contribute to the development of such resistance. As no new antibiotics with novel mechanisms against many of these gram negative bacilli are expected to be developed in the foreseeable future, there is a clear need for the development of strategies to combat antimicrobial resistance.

REFERENCES

[1]   Al-Tawfiq JA, Stephens G, Memish ZA. Inappropriate antimicrobial use and potential solutions: a Middle Eastern perspective. Expert Rev Anti Infect Ther 2010 Jul; 8(7): 765-74.

[2]   Kumarasamy KK, Toleman MA, Walsh TR, *et al.* Emergence of a new antibiotic resistance mechanism in India, Pakistan, and the UK: a molecular, biological, and epidemiological study. Lancet Infect Dis 2010; 10(9): 597-602.

[3]   Okeke IN, Laxminarayan R, Bhutta Z, *et al.* Antimicrobial in developing countries. Part I: recent trends and current status. Lancet Infect Dis 2005; 5: 481-93.

[4]   Austin DJ, Kristinsson KG, Anderson RM. The relationship between the volume of antimicrobial consumption in human communities and the frequency of resistance. Proc Natl Acad Sci USA 1999; 96(3): 1152-56.

[5]   Steinke D, Davey P. Association between antibiotic resistance and community prescribing: a critical review of bias and confounding in published studies. Clin Infect Dis 2001; 3: S193-S205.

[6]   Al-Tawfiq JA. Increasing antibiotic resistance among isolates of Escherichia coli recovered from inpatients and outpatients in a Saudi Arabian hospital. Infect Control Hosp Epidemiol 2006; 27(7): 748-53.

[7]   Bukharie HA, Saeed IM. Antimicrobial resistance among pathogens causing acute uncomplicated UTIs. Infect Med 2001; 18: 358-62.

[8]   Akbar DH. Urinary tract infection: diabetics and non-diabetic patients. Saudi Med J 2001; 22: 326-29.

[9]   Al-Ghamdi MS, El-Morsy F, Al-Mustafa ZH, *et al.* Antibiotic resistance of Escherichia coli isolated from poultry workers, patients and chicken in the eastern province of Saudi Arabia. Trop Med Int Health 1999; 4: 278-83.

[10]   Akbar DH. Urinary tract infection: diabetics and non-diabetic patients. Saudi Med J 2001; 22: 326-29

[11]   Rafay AM, Nsanze HN. Multi-drug resistance of Escherichia coli from the urinary tract. Saudi Med J 2003; 24:261-264.

[12]   El-Karsh T, Tawfik AF, Al-Shammary F, *et al.* Antimicrobial resistance and prevalence of extended spectrum betalactamase among clinical isolates of gram-negative bacteria in Riyadh. J Chemother 1995; 7: 509-14.

[13]   Kader AA, Nassimuzzaman M. Antimicrobial resistance patterns of gram negative bacteria isolated from urine cultures in Almana General Hospital. Ann Saudi Med 2001; 21: 110-12.

[14]   Al-Tawfiq JA, Abed MS. Prevalence and antimicrobial resistance of health care associated bloodstream infections at a general hospital in Saudi Arabia. Saudi Med J 2009 Sep; 30(9): 1213-18.

[15]   Al-Tawfiq JA, Antony A. Antimicrobial resistance of Klebsiella pneumoniae in a Saudi Arabian hospital: results of a 6-year surveillance study, 1998-2003. J Infect Chemother 2007; 13(4): 230-34.

[16]   Bilal NE, Gedebou M. Clinical and community strains of Klebsiella pneumoniae: multiple and increasing rates of antibiotic resistance in Abha, Saudi Arabia. Br J Biomed Sci 2000; 57: 185-91.

[17]   Akhtar N, Alqurashi AM, Abu Twibah M. *In vitro* ciprofloxacin resistance profiles among gram-negative bacteria isolated from clinical specimens in a teaching hospital. J Pak Med Assoc. 2010; 60(8): 625-27.

[18]   Al-Tawfiq JA. Occurrence and antimicrobial resistance pattern of inpatient and outpatient isolates of Pseudomonas aeruginosa in a Saudi Arabian hospital: 1998-2003. Int J Infect Dis. 2007; 11(2): 109-14.

[19]   Al Johani SM, Akhter J, Balkhy H, *et al.* Prevalence of antimicrobial resistance among gram-negative isolates in an adult intensive care unit at a tertiary care center in Saudi Arabia. Ann Saudi Med 2010; 30: 364-69.

[20]   Al-Jasser AM, Elkhizzi NA. Antimicrobial susceptibility pattern of clinical isolates of Pseudomonas aeruginosa. Saudi Med J 2004; 25: 780-84.

[21]   Al-Tawfiq JA, Mohandhas TX. Prevalence of antimicrobial resistance in Acinetobacter calcoaceticus-baumannii complex in a Saudi Arabian hospital. Infect Control Hosp Epidemiol 2007; 28(7): 870-72.

[22]   Asghar AH, Faidah HS. Frequency and antimicrobial susceptibility of gram-negative bacteria isolated from 2 hospitals in Makkah, Saudi Arabia. Saudi Med J. 2009; 30(8): 1017-23.

[23]   Paterson DL, Bonomo RA. Extended-spectrum beta-lactamases: a clinical update. Clin Microbiol Rev 2005; 18: 657-86.

[24]   Mokaddas EM, Abdulla AA, Shati S, *et al.* The technical aspects and clinical significance of detecting extended-spectrum beta-lactamase-producing Enterobacteriaceae at a tertiary-care hospital in Kuwait. J Chemother 2008; 20: 445-51.

[25]   Al-Zarouni M, Senok A, Rashid F, *et al.* Prevalence and antimicrobial susceptibility pattern of extended-spectrum beta-lactamase-producing Enterobacteriaceae in the United Arab Emirates. Med Princ Pract 2008; 17: 32-36.

[26]   Al-Agamy MH, Shibl AM, Tawfik AF. Prevalence and molecular characterization of extended-spectrum beta-lactamase-producing Klebsiella pneumoniae in Riyadh, Saudi Arabia. Ann Saudi Med 2009; 29: 253-57.

[27]   Bindayna K, Khanfar HS, Senok AC, *et al.* Predominance of CTX-M genotype among extended spectrum beta lactamase isolates in a tertiary hospital in Saudi Arabia. Saudi Med J 2010; 30(8): 859-63.

[28]   Kader AA, Kamath KA. Faecal carriage of extended-spectrum beta-lactamase-producing bacteria in the community. East Mediterr Health J 2009; 15(6): 1365-70.

[29]   Al-Zamil FA, Al-Anazi AR. Serogroups and antimicrobial susceptibility of non-typhoidal salmonellosis in children. Saudi Med J 2001; 22: 129-32.

[30]   Malik GM, Al-Wabel A, El Bagir MM, *et al.* Salmonella Infections in Asir Region, Southern Saudi Arabia: Expatriate Implications. Ann Saudi Med 1993; 13(3): 242-45.

[31]   Peter J, Gosling AIMLS, Mohammed AK. Salmonella Gastroenteritis in Jeddah: A study of 1017 patients over a fourteen-month period. Saudi Med J 1983; 4: 61-66.

[32]   Al-Tawfiq JA. Antimicrobial susceptibility of Salmonella typhi and non-typhi in a hospital in eastern Saudi Arabia. J Chemother 2007; 19(1): 62-65.

[33]   Rupali P, Abraham OC, Jesudason MV, *et al.* Treatment failure in typhoid fever with ciprofloxacin susceptible Salmonella enterica serotype Typhi. Diagn Microbiol Infect Dis 2004; 49(1): 1-3.

[34]   Al-Zamil FA, Al-Anazi AR. Serogroups and antimicrobial susceptibility of non-typhoidal salmonellosis in children. Saudi Med J 2001; 22: 129-32.

[35]   Al-Tawfiq JA. Antimicrobial susceptibility of Salmonella typhi and non-typhi in a hospital in eastern Saudi Arabia. J Chemother 2007; 19(1): 62-65.

β-Lactamases as Major Mechanism of Resistance in Gram-Negative Bacteria

Mariagrazia Perilli[*], Giuseppe Celenza, Cristina Pellegrini and Gianfranco Amicosante

Department of Biomedical Sciences and Technologies, University of L'Aquila, Italy

Abstract: β-lactamases are the major mechanism of resistance against β-lactam antibiotics among Gram-negative bacteria. On the basis of their amino acid sequence, β-lactamases are divided into four classes: A, B, C and D. This classification was first proposed by Ambler. The classes A, C and D include enzymes that hydrolyse their substrates by forming an acyl enzyme through an active site, whereas class B β-lactamases are metallo-enzymes which utilise one or two ions in their active sites. The massive use of expanded-spectrum cephalosporins, since the 1980s, has been conducive for the emergence of extended-spectrum β-lactamases (ESBLs) in the clinical setting, a group of enzymes capable of hydrolysing a wide range of expanded-spectrum β-lactams, including the oxyiminocephalosporins, but they are inactive against cephamicins and carbapenems. The emergence and widespread of ESBLs compromised the usefulness of carbapenems in clinical therapy leading to the emergence and diffusion of carbapenemases and in particular metallo-β-lactamases.

Keywords: β-lactamases, metalloenzymes, ESBL, cephamicins, carbapenems, oxyiminocephalosporins.

INTRODUCTION

The emergence of resistant strains is a recurrent problem from the introduction of antibiotics in clinical practice. Starting from penicillin G, introduced in clinical practice approximately 60 years ago, β-lactam antibiotics - penicillins, cephalosporins, carbapenems and monobactams - respresent more than 60% of all antimicrobials used worldwide. These molecules are preferred because of their versatility, efficacy and safety. All β-lactams are bactericidal agents able to inhibit cell wall synthesis by interfering with the biosynthesis of peptidoglycan, a complex structure that guarantees its survival by efficiently counteracting its own osmotic pressure. The target enzymes are the Penicillin-Binding Proteins (PBPs) which catalyse the formation of the essential peptide cross-links in nascent peptidoglycan. Bacteria utilise several mechanisms to escape the lethal effects of β-lactam antibiotics. In Gram-positive bacteria ,an alteration of PBPs (*i.e.* PBP2' of *Staphylococcus aureus* or PBP 2x of *Streptococcus pneumoniae*) reduced the affinity for β-lactam antibiotics, which are required in a very large amount, often out of the therapeutic range, in order to be effective. In many Gram-negative bacteria the entrance of β-lactams into periplasmic space could be restricted because of the lack or diminished expression of OMPs (Outer Membrane Proteins). Moreover, the major mechanism of β-lactam resistance is the production of β-lactamases, enzymes that catalyse very effciently the irreversible hydrolysis of the amide bond of the β-lactam ring, yielding biologically inactive product(s) [1-3]. β-lactamase production is the cardinal mechanism of resistance in Gram-negative bacteria where they are frequently copiously released into the periplasmic space (until 1 mM of enzyme [4]). Some of these microrganisms may produce constitutive chromosomal β-lactamases, such as class A enzymes in *Klebsiella pneumoniae*, or inducible β-lactamases, such as class C enzymes in *Enterobacter cloacae*, *Enterobacter aerogenes*, *Citrobacter freundii*, *Serratia* spp. and non fermenting rods (*Pseudomonas aeruginosa* and *Acinetobacter* species). Over the last fifty years plasmid-mediated β-lactamases became prevalent among Gram-negative bacteria. As reported by G. Jacoby and K. Bush on their web site (http://www.lahey.org/studies/), the number of identified β-lactamases exceeded 890. The production of β-lactamases is the most important resistance mechanism in *Enterobacteriaceae*, *P. aeruginosa* and

*Address correspondence to Mariagrazia Perilli: Department of Biomedical Sciences and Technologies, University of L'Aquila, Italy; Tel: 9+39-0862-433489; Fax: +39-0862-433433; Email: perilli@univaq.it

Acinetobacter baumannii which are responsible for a variety of infections in hospitalised and community based patients. *Enterobacteriaceae* are important causes of Urinary Tract Infections (UTI), bloodstream infections, hospital acquired pneumonia and various intra-abdominal infections. Within this family, *Escherichia coli* is frequently found in infections in UTIs [5, 6] whereas *Klebsiella* spp. and *Enterobacter* spp. are important causes of pneumonia [7]. Members of the *Enterobacteriaceae* family are frequently are resistant to third-generation cephalosporins because of the production of β-lactamases. Examples are the Extended-Spectrum B-Lactamases (ESBLs), derived from TEM-1, SHV-1, CTX-M- and OXA-types. They are able to hydrolyse broad- and extended-spectrum cephalosporins, monobactams and penicillins [5, 7, 8]. Moreover, *Enterobacteriaceae* may also express AmpC, class A and class B carbapenemases. AmpC β-lactamases hydrolyse third-generation or expanded-spectrum cephalosporins but, unlike ESBLs, they are also active against cephamycins and resistant to inhibition by clavulanate or other β-lactamase inhibitors [9]. *Enterobacter* spp. produce a constitutive chromosomal AmpC β-lactamase the expression of which is induced by continual β-lactam exposure [10]. In *Enterobacteriaceae* carbapenem resistance can arise from: (a) membrane alteration in organisms with AmpC or ESBL enzymes; (b) acquisition of IMP or VIM metallo-β-lactamases; (c) acquisition of the serin-carbapenemases KPC, IMI/NMC, SME or OXA families [11]. Like *E. aerogenes, Pseudomonas* spp. principally *P. aeruginosa* has a chromosomal AmpC β-lactamase that might become derepressed by mutation, conferring resistance to oxyimino-cephalosporins. Beside, resistance in *Pseudomonas* is also attributed to the alteration of permeability that leads to the exclusion of many antibiotics from the cell. The Pseudomonal cells are equipped with pump systems (*i.e.* MexAB-OprM) able to extrude β-lactams, chloramphenicol, fluoroquinolones, macrolides, novobiocin, sulfonamides, tetracycline, and various xenobiotic substances [12]. However, the production of β-lactamases all over the world was ascertained in *P. aeruginosa* less frequently than *Enterobacteriaceae*. Many penicillinases that lack activity against oxyimino-cephalosporins or carbapenems have been reported in *P. aeruginosa*. With the exception of PER-1, extended-spectrum β-lactamases are rare in *P. aeruginosa* [13-16]. Others class A ESBLs, VEB-1 [17, 18] and class D β-lactamases, OXA-types, have been found in isolates of *P. aeruginosa* [18-20]. Since the first identification of IMP-1 in *P. aeruginosa*, in the early 1990s in Japan [21], transferable metallo-β-lactamases (MBLs) like IMP and VIM-types are frequently found in *Pseudomonas* species [22-26]. *Acinetobacter* species have emerged in recent years as one of the major causes of nosocomial infections associated with significant morbidity and mortality. They are also able to survive on dry inanimate surfaces for a prolonged period of time [27]. Multi Drug Resistant (MDR) *A. baumannii* infections often occur in immune-suppressed patients, in patients with serious underlying diseases and in those subjected to invasive procedures and treated with broad-spectrum antibiotics. *A. Baumannii* is frequently implicated in Ventilator-Associated Pneumonia (VAP), urinary tract infections and bacteraemia [28]. In *A. baumannii*, resistance is intrinsic to the species and depends on a not inducible chromosomal AmpC β-lactamase, expressed at low levels. However, AmpC can be over-expressed as a result of the upstream insertion of IS*Aba1* sequences [29]. The most common β-lactamases found in *Acinetobacter* species are OXA-type enzymes [30] as OXA-51-like, OXA-23-like, OXA-24(40)-like OXA-58 [30-33]. The aim of this review is to provide information on biochemical and molecular aspects of the most common serine- and metallo β-lactamases distributed among *Enterobacteriaceae*, *Pseudomonas* and *Acinetobacter* species.

β-LACTAMASES (E.C. 3.5.2.6)

β-lactam antibiotics are the most commonly prescribed drugs, which share the peculiarity of a β-lactam ring (Fig. **1**). β-lactam antibiotics inhibit the growth of sensitive bacteria by inactivating enzymes located in the bacterial cell membrane, which are involved in the third stage of cell wall synthesis. In particular, these compounds interfere with the biosynthesis of the peptidoglycan, an essential element in maintaining the shape and rigidity of the cell wall in both Gram-positive and Gram-negative bacteria [34, 35].

β-lactamases are the commonest cause and the most efficient mechanism of bacterial resistance to β-lactam antimicrobial agents. β-lactamases protect the bacterial cell wall peptidase by hydrolysing the β-lactam bond before the antibiotics reach their specific target enzymes, the Penicillin Binding Proteins (PBPs). These enzymes very efficiently catalyse the irreversible hydrolysis of the amide bond of the β-lactam ring rendering the product biologically inactive (Fig. **2**).

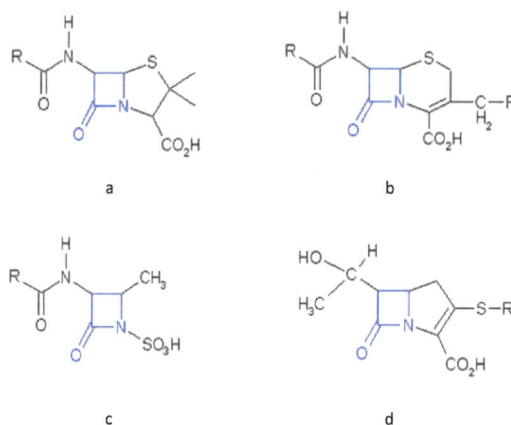

Figure 1: Structure of β-lactam nucleus of principal class of β-lactam antibiotics: **a)** penicillin; **b)** cephalosporin; **c)** monobactam; **d)** carbapenems.

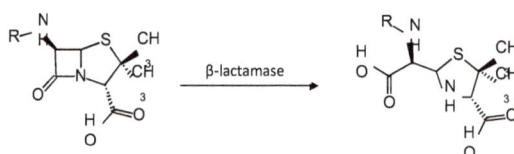

Figure 2: Hydrolysis of β-lactam ring by β-lactamases activity.

To date, over 890 β-lactamase enzymes have been reported (G. Jacoby and K. Bush, http://www.lahey.org/Studies/). Two classification schemes for β-lactamases are currently in use. On the basis of their amino acid sequence, β-lactamases are divided into four classes: A, B, C and D. This classification was firstly proposed by Ambler [36]. The classes A, C and D include enzymes that hydrolyse their substrates by forming a transient or stable acyl enzyme through an active site serine, whereas class B β-lactamases are metallo-enzymes that utilize one or two active site zinc ions. Moreover, a functional classification for β-lactamases, correlated with their molecular structure, was proposed by Bush in 1989 and updated in 1995 and 2010 by the same authors [37-40]. This classification grouped the enzymes on the basis of their ability to hydrolyse specific β-lactams and on their behaviour towards clinically used β-lactamase inhibitors as clavulanic acid, tazobactam and sulbactam. Three functional groups are included in this scheme and each group is divided into subgroups. Group 1 included cephalosporinases belonging to molecular class C active on cefoxitin and usually resistant to clavulanic acid. The new subgroup 1e comprises enzymes with a greater activity against ceftazidime and other oxyimino-β-lactams (*i.e.* GC1, CMY-10, -19, -37 enzymes) [40-43]. Functional group 2 β-lactamases encloses molecular classes A and D and are subdivided in to several subgroups: 2a, 2b, 2be, 2br, 2ber, 2c, 2ce, 2d, 2de, 2df, 2e, and 2f. The biggest group is represented by subgroup 2be that includes ESBLs enzymes. Finally, group 3, subgroups 3a and 3b, includes metallo-β-lactamases. β-lactamases can be chromosomal or plasmid encoded, constitutive or inducible and can be secreted into periplasmic space and into the outer medium in Gram-negative and Gram-positive bacteria respectively. The presence of resistance genes on plasmids and transposons allows the genes to be transferred to related bacteria by conjugation, transduction, or transformation. The capture of new genes by the bacterial cell is largely, but not exclusively, responsible for the development of antibiotic-resistant variant strains of some bacteria. Frequently, β-lactamase genes are carried on genetic elements that utilise site-specific recombination to capture individual antibiotic resistance genes, the integrons. Integrons consist of three peculiar regions: the 5' conserved region (5'CS), the 3' conserved region (3'CS) and a variable region. The 5' CS region includes a receptor site, *attI*, where captured genes are integrated, together with an adjacent sequence coding for a recombinase, *IntI* [44-47].

ACTIVE SITE SERINE β-LACTAMASES

β-lactamases can be also classified on the basis of their catalytic mechanisms in serine and zinc β-lactamases [48]. The serine β-lactamases hydrolyse β-lactams according to the acylation/deacylation pathway. They act by a three-steps mechanism involving the transient formation of an acyl-enzyme (scheme **1**) in which the hydroxyl group of the essential serine residue is esterified by the carbonyl group of the antibiotic moiety [49]. In the following scheme E is the enzyme, C the antibiotic, EC the non covalent Henri-Michaelis complex, EC* the covalent acyl-enzyme and P the inactive degradation product of the antibiotics.

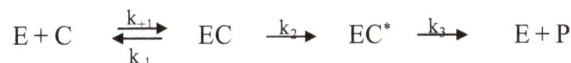

$$E + C \;\; \underset{k_{-1}}{\overset{k_{+1}}{\rightleftharpoons}} \;\; EC \;\; \xrightarrow{k_2} \;\; EC^* \;\; \xrightarrow{k_3} \;\; E + P$$

Scheme 1

According to this scheme, the β-lactam compounds appear to form a similar adduct when reacting with their physiological targets (the DD-peptidases) or with active-site serine β-lactamases. As described in detail by Matagne *et al.* the difference between these two types of enzymes is purely quantitative [50]. The catalytic mechanism of β-lactamases has been studied in detail for the representative enzymes and kinetic data of a plethora of β-lactamases belonging to different classes are available for their interaction with a wide range of β-lactam compounds. Serine β-lactamases are globular proteins which consist of two structural domains, an α and an α/β domain. The active site is situated in a groove between these two domains. Several conserved elements in the active site of serine β-lactamase have been identified which appear to be directly or indirectly involved in the substrate recognition and catalytic processes. Based on sequence aligments Joris *et al.* described almost three structural elements which delimited the active site in all active-site serine penicillin-recognizing enzymes (Table **1**) [51]. Although class A, C and D β-lactamases have similar structures (Fig. **3**) different amino acid residues are involved in the acylation and deacylation steps as well as their catalytic properties can exhibit deep variations. In the class A enzymes, Glu166 residue, which is absent in the other class of enzymes, seems to play a crucial role in the catalytic process.

The first element is the conserved sequence S* - X - X - K with the active serine at the N-terminus of α2 helix (S70 in class A and D β-lactamases, S64 in class C β-lactamases and S62 in the DD peptidase). Downstream one helix-turn was located a lysine residue whose side-chain also points into the active site (residue 73, 67 and 65, respectively). The proximity of the serine and lysine side-chains, which are hydrogen-bonded, suggests the possible involvement of the lysine side-chain amino group in the catalytic process [50, 52]. The second element is the SDN loop of class A β-lactamases corresponding to Y - X - N in class C and D and in some PBPs. It is located on a short loop in the all α domains where it forms one side of the catalytic cavity. The side-chains of the first and third residues point to the active-site cleft, while that of the second residue lies in the protein core. The first residue (Ser or Tyr) is hydroxylated and the third is nearly always an asparagine. In class A β-lactamases, the SDN motif is nearly invariant [53]. The third element (KT(S) G) is on the innermost strand of the β-sheet (α/β domain) and forms the opposite wall of the catalytic cavity. In this element a residue of lysine could be replaced by histidine or arginine residues in a few exceptional cases. A positive charged side-chain, followed by one bearing a hydroxyl group, appears to be universally conserved. The side chain of the lysine residue forms a hydrogen-bond with the hydroxyl group of the serine or tyrosine of the second element [50-56].

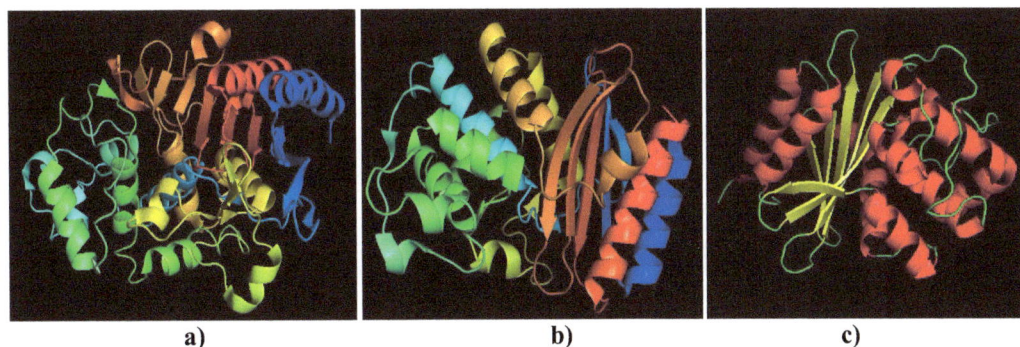

a)   b)   c)

The images sre created by PyMol version 1.3 (available at http://www.pymol.org).

Figure 3: Structures of serine β-lactamases: **a)** class A enzyme: TEM-1 structure **b)** class C enzyme: AmpC structure, **c)** class D enzyme: OXA-24 structure.

Table 1: Structural elements that limit the active site in most serin-β-lactamases.

ENZYME	1st ELEMENT	2nd ELEMENT	3rd ELEMENT
Class A	70Ser-X-X-Lys73	130Ser-Asp-sn(Ser)132	234Lys-Thr-Gly236 234Lys-Ser-Gly236 234Arg-Ser-Gly236
Class C	64Ser-X-X-Lys67	150Tyr-X-Asn152	315Lys-Thr-Gly317
Class D	70Ser-X-X-Lys70	144Tyr-Gly-Asn146	214Lys-Thr-Gly216
DD peptidase	62Ser-X-X-Lys65	159Tyr-Ser-Asn161	298His-Thr-Gly300

Table modified from reference 51.

CATALYTIC MECHANISM OF SERINE β-LACTAMASES

The catalytic mechanism of serine β-lactamases consists in acylation and deacylation steps involving different and specific amino acid residues. The active site of β-lactamases is expected to contain a specific amino acid side-chain which increases the nucleophilicity of the hydroxyl group of Ser-70 by acting as a general base catalyst. Thus, a crucial role in the catalytic mechanism is played by serine active residue. Site-directed mutagenesis experiments demonstrated that the replacement of serine with cysteine at this position can yield active enzyme. Moreover naturally occurring cysteines have never been found in β-lactamases [57, 58]. Crystallographic studies and molecular modelling have shown that the structures of enzymes belonging to A, C and D have the similar "oxyanion holes" including the main chain NH-groups of Ser70 and Ala237 in the class A enzymes, Ser64 and Ser/Ala 318 in the class C and Ser62 and Thr301 in the DD-peptidases [59-61].

The nucleophilic attack of the active site serine γ-O atom on the carbonyl carbon of the β-lactam bond, leads to a negatively charged tetrahedral transition state. The interaction of the β-lactam carbonyl oxygen with the oxyanion hole and by the dipole of the buried helix is necessary in order to stabilise the tetrahedral transition state. The lysine at position 73 has been ascertained in the orientation of the serine proton towards the nitrogen of the leaving group.

MECHANISTIC ASPECTS OF CLASS A β-LACTAMASES

Generally, the mechanism of catalysis is based on the presence of a proton park in the catalytic pocket represented by three residues: Lys73, Ser130 and Glu166. For class A enzymes two distinct residues have been proposed for the role of general base. In one hypothesis, this role is played by the conserved Glu166. This residue in class A β-lactamases is part of a structural element called Ω loop. Crystallographic data have highlighted the presence of a tightly bound water molecule, forming a bridge between the Ser70 hydroxyl group and the Glu166 carboxylate side chain. This water molecule is found at the same position in all class A structures solved by X-ray [59, 62-64]. Although site-directed mutagenesis experiments suggested that Glu166 might play the role of general base in the acylation reaction [65, 66], it seems too far from the Ser70 OH group. Molecular modelling studies [63] have suggested that the conserved water molecule might act as a relay molecule in the transfer of the proton between the Ser70 and Glu166 side chains. Alternatively, the flexibility of the Ω-loop might allow the distance between the two residues to be shortened during the acylation process. Both cases require the presence of a second water molecule, the ε-amino groups of Lys73 and Lys234 and the hydroxyl group of Ser130, which acts as the last proton donor [63]. On the contrary, Mobashery and co-workers [67, 68], suggested that Ser130 can decrease the energy barrier for hydrolysis of substrates by merely hydrogen-bonding to the nitrogen atom of the β-lactam ring in the course of Ser70 acylation. In the second hypothesis [69] formulated on the structural properties of the Glu166Asn mutant of the TEM-1 β-lactamase the authors argued that Glu166 is expendable for acylation and thus proposed an unsymmetrical mechanism, with two different general bases, Lys73 and Glu166, participating in acylation and deacylation respectively.

EXTENDED-SPECTRUM β-LACTAMASES (ESBLs)

Class A enzymes is the largest group of β-lactamases widely distributed among Gram-negative and Gram-positive bacteria. They are largely plasmid encoded and have been found to hydrolyse both penicillins and cephalosporins. Epidemiological studies have shown TEM-1 to be the most common plasmid-mediated β-lactamase in Gram-negative bacteria [5, 8]. In the early 1980s, extended-spectrum antibiotics (*e.g.* ceftazidime, cefotaxime, aztreonam) were introduced in the clinical practice because of their stability to β-lactamases such as TEM-1. Another effective way to threat β-lactamase producing infections was the introduction of β-lactamase inhibitors (*e.g.* clavulanic acid, tazobactam). Both approaches, the use of stable β-lactam antibiotics and β-lactamase inhibitors, determined a strong selective pressure causing numerous mutations in prototype enzymes. The first report of plasmid-encoded β-lactamases capable of hydrolysing the extend-spectrum cephalosporins was published in 1983 [70]. The term "extended-spectrum β-lactamses" was originally applied to the TEM and SHV derivatives (classified as group 2be) that can hydrolyse oxyimino-cephalosporins [5, 8, 40]. These broad-spectrum enzymes retain the activity against penicillins and cephalosporins of subgroup 2b β-lactamases and in addition hydrolyse one or more oxyimino cephalosporins (cefotaxime, ceftazidime, aztreonam). Enzymes belonging to 2be subgroup cannot hydrolyse cephamycins, temocillin or carbapenems efficiently and are inhibited by clavulanic acid. This subgroup includes a large number of enzymes derived from amino acid substitution of TEM-1/2, SHV-1 and CTX-M-types. The CTX-M enzymes hydrolyse cefotaxime more readily than ceftazidime [71]. Many of them hydrolyse cefepime as well. Unlike TEM or SHV ESBLs, CTX-M enzymes are inhibited by tazobactam at least one order of magnitude better than clavulanic acid [5, 8]. A huge number of ESBL variants have been selected by the continuous use of selected antibiotics as cefuroxime or cefotaxime or ceftazidime. As reported by Bush and Jacoby in their authoritative web site (G. Jacoby and K. Bush, http://www.lahey.org/Studies/), at least 92/183 TEM, 43/135 SHV-, 103 CTX-M-, 7 PER-related enzymes exhibit an increased hydrolytic activities against the oxyimino β-lactams [5, 8]. The large majority of these new enzymes belong to the SHV and TEM families. Each variant has from one to five/six amino acid replacements when compared with the parental enzymes. The amino acid residues responsible for the ESBL activity profiles are Val42, Glu104, Arg164, Asp179, Ala237, Gly238, and Glu240 in TEM-types whereas Leu35, Arg205, Gly238 and Glu240 in SHV-type enzymes (Table **2**). A number of residues involved in the extended-spectrum properties of these enzymes were found to be located in close proximity of active site [72]. Even though most of them are not directly involved in the catalytic mechanism, these mutations are able to extend the substrate profile of these enzymes. The hydrophilic side chain of Glu104, in TEM-types, is exposed on the left side of the entrance of the binding site and is hydrogen bonded to Asn132. It may therefore stabilise the catalytically important Ser130 in the conserved SDN loop. The side chain of residue 104 could easily interact with the larger acyl-amido substituents of β-lactams. The change Glu104Lys has been reported among numerous natural TEM mutants. The long lysine side chain could extend out to interact with the carboxylic acid group in the substituents of ceftazidime, aztreonam or ceftibuten. This electrostatic attraction should increase initial binding, possibly decreasing the K_m. However, a TEM-1 mutant produced in laboratory with a change from glutamate to lysine at position 104 (Glu104Lys) showed little impact in K_m for the first two of these β-lactams [73], so that the charge-charge interaction may involve an intermediate rather than the initial Michaelis species. Reduction of the K_m is observed in multiple mutants containing an Arg164Ser change. The arginine residue at position 164 in TEM-1 and other TEM-related enzymes is positioned below the binding site in the omega loop (with Glu166 residue). The guanidinium side chain is strongly linked by electrostatic attraction and hydrogen bonded to conserved Asp179 across the neck of the loop [59, 62]. The common changes found are serine, histidine and cysteine. A reduction in the number of hydrogen bonds or elimination of the electrostatic attraction will weaken the linkage across the neck of the omega loop. This change allows more flexibility in the loop, which in turn opens, increasing the space for bulky β-lactam substituents. The residue Asp179 could interact with Arg164 by electrostatic and hydrogen bonds. Residue 205 in SHV mutants is located on the upper surface of the enzyme near the N-terminal end of helix H9. The exposed amino acid at position 205 is very far (2.2 nm) from the binding site. However, the C-terminal end of this helix forms the upper edge of the binding site. In SHV-type enzymes a radical change is observed whereby the hydrophilic arginine is replaced in SHV-3 and SHV-4 by a hydrophobic leucine.

Glycine at position 238, either in TEM- and SHV variants, is on the inner side of the B3 β-strand and it lies very close to the side chain of residue 69. The common substituents are the following amino acid residues: serine (in some TEM and SHV enzymes), aspartate (in TEM-111), asparagines (TEM-142), arginine (in TEM-178, formerly TEM-AQ [74]. If side chains of both residues 69 and 238 are large, they may displace the B3 β-strand outward so that the lower portion of the binding site becomes slightly expanded. At the end of β-strand B3 is positioned the residue Glu240 that can interact with acylamide substituents of cephalosporins. This side chain would be too far from smaller ligands such as clavulanic acid or sulbactam, and changes here are not seen or expected in inhibitor-resistant variants. Changes observed in the most TEM and SHV natural variants are lysine and arginine. The lysine side chain is able to form an electrostatic bond with the carboxylic acid group on oxyimino substituents. Lys240 is therefore found in variants able to hydrolyse ceftazidime and aztreonam [75, 76]. TEM-24, with lysines at both positions 104 and 240, has the highest V_{max} for ceftazidime [77].

Table 2: Main amino acid substitution in TEM and SHV variants.

Amino Acid Residue in TEM-1	Amino Acid Substitutions in TEM-Variants
Glu104	Lys
Arg164	Ser
	His
	Cys
Gly238	Ser
	Asp
	Asn
	Arg
Glu240	Lys
	Arg
	Val
Amino Acid Residue in SHV-1	**Amino Acid Substitutions in SHV-Variants**
Leu35	Gln
Arg205	Leu
Gly238	Ser
	Ala
Glu240	Lys
	Arg

A residue of valine at position 240 was identified for the first time in a natural TEM-149 ESBL, isolated from *Serratia marcescens* and *Enterobacter aerogenes* in an Italian hospital [78]. Kinetic parameters showed that TEM-149 are able to hydrolyse cefazolin, cefotaxime, ceftazidime, cefepime, aztreonam, and penicillins. Among the oxyimino-cephalosporins, ceftazidime was the best substrate, while cefotaxime was an overall poor substrate (ceftazidime, K_m=19 μM, k_{cat}=8.3 s^{-1}, k_{cat}/K_m=0.44 μM^{-1} s^{-1}; cefotaxime, K_m=43 μM, k_{cat}=0.07 s^{-1}, k_{cat}/K_m=0.0016 μM^{-1} s^{-1}) [78]. Beyond Val240, TEM-149 has the following amino acid substitutions: Lys104, Ser164 and Thr182. The enhanced catalytic efficiencies of TEM-149 for ceftazidime and, slightly, for aztreonam with respect to other TEM-types with the similar aminoacid substitutions (*i.e.* TEM-10) could also be attributed to the presence of a lysine at position 104. The side chain amino group of lysine 104 is able to form an ionic bond with the peculiar side chain of ceftazidime and aztreonam, whereas the acid side chain of the glutamic acid at position 104 induces unfavorable interactions [78]. Thus, Lys104 improves the catalytic activities of ESBLs against ceftazidime and aztreonam and improves them less so against cefotaxime. The arginine at position 164 in TEM variants is located in the omega loop and usually makes a salt bond and a hydrogen bond with Asp179 [78, 79]. The replacement of arginine with the neutral amino acid serine makes the omega loop more flexible because of the elimination of the electrostatic attraction between residues 164 and 179. This allows the accommodation of bulky β-lactam substituents. The combination of mutations found in the TEM-149 enzyme contributes to a better orientation and a better accommodation of ceftazidime and aztreonam in the catalytic site of the enzyme (Fig. **4**).

Fig. **3** shows the molecular modelling of the Michaelis complex of TEM-149 with ceftazidime. The hydroxy group of the serine at position 164 is sufficiently close to the carboxylic oxygens of the aspartate at position 179 to allow the formation of one hydrogen bond. The lysine at position 104 is able to form an ionic bond with the carbonilic oxygens of the oxyimino chain of ceftazidime. The valine at position 240 is placed on the omega loop at the end of the B3 β strand.

In addition, several reports describe the inhibitor-resistant TEM (IRTs) that differ from TEM1/2 by one or more amino acids substitutions (Met69, Trp165, Arg244, Arg275, Asn276) that decrease the affinity for β-lactams and modify the inhibitory activity of suicide substrates such as clavulanic acid [80]. Although, for many years, TEM and SHVwere the predominant ESBL variants, recently a new family of β-lactamases emerged over the world: the CTX-M enzymes. CTX-M enzymes are replacing TEM and SHV variants in many European countries [81] including Italy [82, 83]. It is important to highlight that 103 CTX-M β-lactamases were identified. They divide into five clusters on the basis of their sequence homology, namely CTX-M-1, -M-2, -M-8, -M-9 and -M-25 groups. Groups 1 and 2 evolved by the chromosomal genes of *Kluyvera ascorbata* [84], whereas groups 8 and 9 enzymes evolved from *Kluyvera georgiana* [85]. Once mobilised, *bla*CTX-M genes can be hosted by many elements, but most often by large multi-resistance plasmids. IS*Ecp*1 insertion sequence elements were often involved in the initial mobilization events [86]. CTX-M enzymes are more active against cefotaxime and ceftriaxone than ceftazidime, but point mutations can increase activity against ceftazidime; thus CTX-M-15 and -32 differ from CTX-M-3 and -1, respectively, solely by Asp240Gly substitutions, but are 100-fold more active against ceftazidime [87, 88].

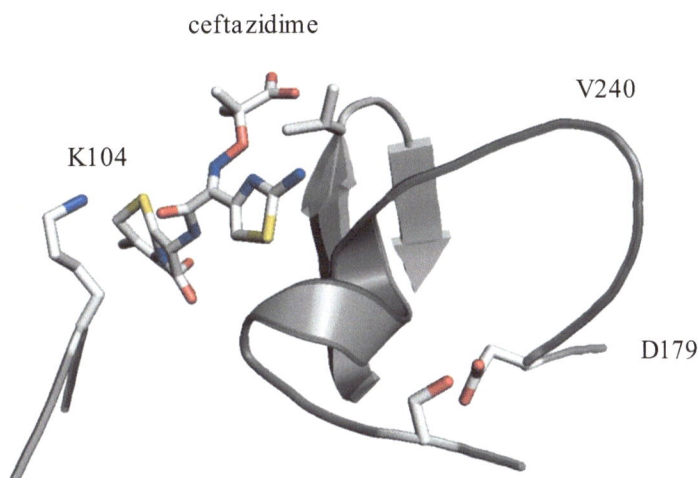

Figure 4: Molecular modeling of the Michaelis complex of TEM-149 with ceftazidime [87].

The Asp240 might be involved in the oxyimino-cephalosporinase activity by fixing cefotaxime in the binding site. In order to investigate the effect of glycine residue at position 240, molecular modelling of the Michaelis complex of CTX-M-44, belonging to CTX-M-2 group, in combination with ceftazidime, cefotaxime and ceftibuten was performed by molecular mechanics calculations [89]. The hypothesis that substitution of the charged and bulky aspartate with the neutral and small glycine residue might favour the accommodation of the C7β substituents of ceftazidime, cefotaxime and ceftibuten by expansion of the binding site. Recent studies on docking between CTX-M-15, belonging to CTX-M-1 group, and cefotaxime reveal that the residues Asn104, Asn132, Gly227, Thr235, Gly236, and Ser237 are responsible for positioning cefotaxime into the active site of the CTX-M-15 [90]. Cephamycins, temocillin and carbapenems are not hydrolysed by CTX-M enzymes, while, as expected, clavulanate, tazobactam and sulbactam showed inhibitory activity. In Italy, CTX-M ESBLs appeared only in 2003 in several *E. coli*, *E. aerogenes* and *C. freundii* isolates with CTX-M-1 enzyme [91, 92]. In 2003, in Italy a second nationwide ESBL survey showed that CTX-M enzymes were widespread [82, 83] in *E. coli* and, in a few cases, in *K. pneumoniae*. All CTX-M found belonged to group 1, with CTX-M-1 and CTX-M-15 predominant and CTX-M-32. Carbapenems are commonly used to treat β-lactamases-producing clinical isolates. Therefore the emergence and widespread of ESBLs compromised the usefulness of carbapenems in clinical terapy leading to the emergence and diffusion of carbapenemases and in particular metallo-β-lactamases.

CLASS A CARBAPENEMASES

Carbapenemases or "carbapenem-hydrolysing enzymes" represent the most versatile family of β-lactamases, with a breadth of spectrum unrivaled by other β-lactam-hydrolysing enzymes. Class A serine carbapenemases of functional group 2f have appeared sporadically in clinical isolates since their first discovery over 20 years ago [93]. These β-lactamases have been detected in *Enterobacter cloacae*, *Serratia marcescens*, and *Klebsiella* spp. as single isolates or in small outbreaks [94]. The three major families of class A serine carbapenemases include NMC/IMI, SME, and KPC enzymes. All these enzymes have the ability to hydrolyse a broad variety of β-lactams, including carbapenems, cephalosporins, penicillins, and aztreonam, and all are inhibited by clavulanate and tazobactam. A fourth member of this class, the GES β-lactamases, was originally identified as an ESBL, however other variants, with low, but detectable imipenem hydrolysis, were discovered. SME-1 (for "*Serratia marcescens* enzyme") was first detected in England from two *S. marcescens* isolates collected in 1982 [95]. The SME-1 β-lactamase, along with the almost identical SME-2 and SME-3, has been found sporadically throughout the United States [96]. The IMI, "imipenem-hydrolysing β-lactamase" and NMC-A, "not metallo-enzyme carbapenemase" enzymes have been detected in rare clinical isolates of *E. cloacae* in the United States, France, and Argentina [94]. NMC-A and IMI-1 have 97% amino acid identity and are related to SME-1, with approximately 70% amino acid identity [97]. In addition to the conserved active site motif of class A β-lactamases, these carbapenemases have conserved cysteine residues at positions 69 and 238 that form a disulfide bridge. The genes for these three β-lactamases are all chromosomally located with the rare exception of bla_{IMI-2} that was found in plasmids from *Enterobacter cloacae* [98]. Biochemical characterisation of purified SME, NMC, and IMI enzymes revealed a broad hydrolytic spectrum that includes penicillins, first generation cephalosporins, aztreonam, and carbapenems. In structure/function studies using site-directed mutagenesis, the ability of the SME-1 enzyme to hydrolyse imipenem could not be attributed to a single amino acid residue [99]. KPC, "*Klebsiella pneumoniae* carbapenemase", enzymes are found on transferable plasmids. Their substrate spectrum includes the aminothiazoleoxime cephalosporins, such as cefotaxime. Although the KPC β-lactamases are predominantly found in *K. pneumoniae*, there are reports of these enzymes in *Enterobacter* spp. and *Salmonella* spp. [100, 101]. KPC enzymes have the closest amino acid identity (about 45%) to SME carbapenemases. In addition, these β-lactamases have the conserved Cys69 and Cys238 residues that form a disulfide bond described for the SME and NMC/IMI enzymes. The GES/IBC family of β-lactamases is an infrequently encountered family that was first described in 2000 with reports of IBC-1 (for "integron-borne cephalosporinase") from an *E.cloacae* isolate in Greece [102] and GES-1 (for "Guyana extended spectrum") in a *K. pneumoniae* isolate from French Guyana [103]. These enzymes differ by only two amino acid substitutions. Their amino acid sequences show that they are distantly related to other class A carbapenemases, with identities of 36%, 35% and 31% with respect to KPC-2, SME-1 and NMC-A [94]. The genes encoding GES enzymes are located in integrons on plasmids. The enzymes have a broad hydrolytic spectrum that included penicillins and extended-spectrum cephalosporins so that they were initially classified as extended-spectrum β-lactamases [102].

CLASS C β-LACTAMASES

AmpC enzymes typically have molecular masses ranging from 34 to 40 kDa and isoelectric points>8.0, although the isoelectric points of plasmid-mediated FOX enzymes are lower (6.7 to 7.2), and AmpC enzyme from *Morganella morganii* has a pI of 6.6. They are active on penicillins and even more active on cephalosporins. They can hydrolyse cephamycins such as cefoxitin and cefotetan; oxyimino cephalosporins such as ceftazidime, cefotaxime, and ceftriaxone; and monobactams such as aztreonam with a rate <1% respect to benzylpenicillin [9, 55]. The rate of hydrolysis for cefepime, cefpirome, and carbapenems is also very low, and the estimated K_m values for cefepime and cefpirome are high, reflecting low enzyme affinity. With preferred cephalosporin substrates, the turnover rate of the *E. cloacae* P99 β-lactamase is diffusion limited rather than catalysis limited, implying that AmpC enzymes have evolved to maximal efficiency. Such data also suggest that AmpC β-lactamase evolved to deal with cephalosporins rather than for some other cellular function, although there is some evidence to suggest that these enzymes play a morphological role. Inhibitors of class A enzymes such as clavulanic acid, sulbactam, and tazobactam have much less effect on AmpC β-lactamases, although some of them are inhibited by tazobactam or sulbactam [104].

AmpC β-lactamases are poorly inhibited by *p*-chloromercuribenzoate and not at all by EDTA. Cloxacillin, oxacillin, and aztreonam, however, are good inhibitors.

Mechanistic Aspects of Class C β-Lactamases

Studies carried on *C. freundii* AmpC suggested the importance of Ser64 and Tyr150 in the catalytic mechanism of class C β-lactamases [105]. Ser64, as Ser70 in class A β-lactamases, allows the nucleophilic attack onto β-lactam carbonyl whereas Tyr150 is considered to be a general basis that increases the nucleophilicity of the active serine residue and water during the acylation and deacylation steps [106, 107]. Mutations of the conserved Lys67 and Tyr150 residues have been found to significantly reduce the activity of the enzyme [108]. Several authors proposed two main reaction mechanisms for these families of enzymes: either a neutral Lys67 or an anionic Tyr150 activating the nucleophilic Ser64 during acylation step. X-ray structures and mutagenesis experiments showed that other active site residues, as Asn152, Lys315, Thr316 and Gly317 are essential to create a dense hydrogen binding network that is commonly considered to be crucial for catalysis [109-110].

CLASS D β-LACTAMASES

Molecular class D β-lactamases correspond almost perfectly to the enzymes classified phenotypically as OXA types for their oxacillinase activity. Oxacillinases are unusual β-lactamases that form a heterogeneous group with respect to their structural or biochemical properties. Historically, the first characterised class D β-lactamases were referred as oxacillinases because they commonly hydrolyse the isoxazolylpenicillin oxacillin faster than classical penicillins [56]. Moreover, further studies on new enzymes belonging to class D, showed for some enzymes a hydrolytic activity against expanded-spectrum cephalosporins, (*i.e.* ceftazidime and cefotaxime), methicillin and aztreonam. The activity of classical β-lactamase inhibitors such as sulbactam, tazobactam and clavulanic acid, is reduced in a number of these enzymes. Among the current variants (more than 160 proteins nowadays identified) about the 40% exhibit low carbapenem-hydrolysing activities with much or absent activity against oxymino-cephalosporins, aztreonam and low sensibility against classical β-lactamase inhibitors [56]. The hydrolytic efficiency of OXA-enzymes against carbapenems, in particular imipenem (but not always meropenem) is much lower (100- to 1000-fold) than MBLs. This property may complicate their recognition.

MECHANISTIC ASPECTS OF CLASS D β-LACTAMASES

Despite the fact that some regions of class D enzymes are structurally very similar to class A enzymes, the binding sites of known class D β-lactamases are more extended with respect to those of class A β-lactamases. This biding site is more hydrophobic than in class A and C β-lactamases [111]. The general mechanism of catalysis is similar to class A and C types even though the detailed catalytic mechanism seems to be quite different in each class. For the acylation step several hypothesis have been proposed based on carbamylated or non carbamylated structure of Lys73 (or Lys70 if using OXA-2 numbering). Lys73 carbamylated may activate Ser70 by deprotonation before the attack to the carbamyl of the β-lactam [112]. The conserved residues Ser118 and Lys73 seem to participate in the proton transfer to the nitrogen atom of β-lactam ring, with the carbamyl group acting as a proton acceptor [113]. If Lys73 is non-carbamylated, the amine side chain of the lysine active Ser70 attacks the β-lactam carbonyl group. Ser118 and Lys73 play crucial roles in proton transfer to the nitrogen group of the β-lactam ring [114, 115]. The last transfer is facilitated by two residues positioned closely to Ser118 (Lys73 and Lys216). In the carbamylated enzyme, the water molecule is not correctly positioned to make possible the attack to the acyl enzyme intermediate. In fact, in class D enzymes, the Lys73 residue acts as a general base and seems to be involved also in the deacylation step [114, 116]. Two possible situations could be distinguished: Lys73 in the unprotonated state and in the carbamylate state. In the unprotonated model the substrate could interact with Arg250 through hydrogen bondings and the catalytic water molecule held in between Lys73 and Trp154 interactions. In the carbamylated Lys73 model a water molecule is kept at the catalytic center due to the strong negative charge of the carbamyl moiety of Lys73. Thus Lys73 plays the role of an acidic residue which deprotonates the catalytic water molecule and subsequently plays the role of a basic residue which protonates the active serine [116]. There is also the possibility that the acylation occurs with carbamylated Lys73 which could be decarbamylated during the formation of acyl enzyme. In this case the deacylation step occurs with a non carbamylate lysine [56].

CLASS B METALLO β-LACTAMASES

MBLs were formally classified as class B according to Ambler [36] classification and group 3 in accordance with Bush-Jacoby-Medeiros [39] functional classification. All MBLs are characterised by their ability to hrdrolysed imipenem and their sensitivity to EDTA or other chelating agents. MBLs are not inhibited by serine β-lactamase inhibitors. Despite the low degree of sequence homology three different subclasses were identified B1, B2 and B3 [117]. On the basis of their hydrolytic activity against imipenem and their spectrum of action *vs* other β-lactams, each subclass is divided into subgroups. The first report of a transferable MBL gene was in 1991 in Japan [118]. Nowadays, twenty-six bla_{IMP} variants were identified worldwide. As demonstrated by Laraki *et al.* [119], despite the broad-spectrum of activity of IMP-1 enzyme, the kinetic parameters are generally lower than those calculated for other subclass B1 enzymes. In 1999 a novel acquired carbapenemase was identified in Italy in a clinical isolate of *P. aeruginosa* at the University Hospital of Verona, VIM-1 metallo-enzyme (Veronese Imipenemase) [120]. VIM-1 shares less than 30% of amino acid identity with IMP-1 metallo enzyme. However, those two enzymes show similar extended spectrum of hydrolysis. Even if the catalytic efficiency of VIM-1 enzyme is comparable with that from other subclass B1 enzymes the high K_m value for almost all substrates with respect to IMP-1 enzyme is noteworthy. Although VIM-1 enzyme exhibits a broad-spectrum activity, it is a better cephalosporinase than penicillinase. In 2002 was reported a novel metallo carbapenemase isolated in a strain of *P. aeruginosa* collected in Sao Paulo, Brazil, SPM-1 (Sao Paulo MBL) [121]. A comparison of SPM-1 amino acidic sequence with other MBLs, shows a low degree of identity, about 30%, with respect to IMP-1 (35.5%), ImiS (32.2%), CphA (32,1%), BCII (30%) and CcrA (27%). However, despite the apparent heterogeneity of the sequence alignment, the phylogenetic analysis demonstrated that SPM-1 is much closer to IMP-1 than to other MBLs [69], thus it has been classified as B1 subclass metallo enzyme. The same year, five multidrug-resistant clinical isolates of *P. aeruginosa* collected in Dusseldorf, Germany, were analyzed, showing the presence of a new MBL designed GIM-1 (German imipenemase) [122]. The most closely related enzymes to GIM-1 are IMP variants, sharing 40% of amino acid identity. The kinetic parameteres of the GIM-1 metallo enzyme are similar to other members of subclass B1 of metallo-β-lactamases. Compared with other MBLs, GIM-1 is not a real good carbapenemase, in fact the catalytic efficiency against imipenem is 10-fold lower than those of IMP-1, VIM-1 and SPM-1 enzymes. Recently, was identified a new metallo-β-lactamase originating from New Delhi, India and called NDM-1. This enzyme is a new subclass of the B1 group and possesses novel amino acids near the active site, suggesting that it has a novel structure [123].

MECHANISTIC ASPECTS OF MBLs

Even if the catalytic mechanisms of action are deeply different, MBLs share with serin β-lactamases the inactivation of the β-lactam antibiotics by cleavage of the amide bond of the β-lactam ring. The chemistry of the reaction in MBLs is the result of the peculiar architecture of the proteins. From an evolutionary stand point, MBLs belong to the zinc metallo-hydrolase family of the β-lactamase fold [124] which includes sixteen groups of enzymes structurally related [125]. These proteins share the same motif αβα, at least in one of their domains (Fig. **5**).

The broad spectrum of activity of MBLs is the result of the high flexibility and adaptability of the active site, in which, a large number of β-lactam substrates can be accommodated, including serin β-lactamase inhibitors like clavulanic acid and sulbactam. It is important to remark that metallo carbapenamases have a low degree of activity against monobactams. Detailed information about the structures of metallo carbapenemases was determined, revealing significant differences in the active site pocket and in a loop involved in substrate binding [126, 127].

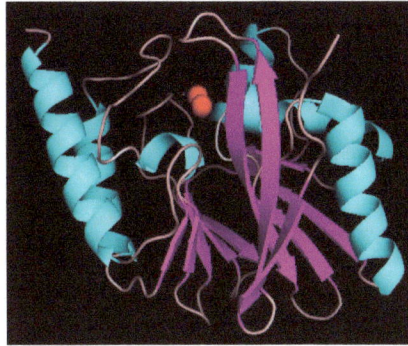

Figure 5: Structure of IMP-1 metallo-β-lactamase The images sre created by PyMol version 1.3 (available at http://www.pymol.org).

The mechanism for the di-zinc form of CcrA from *Bacteroides fragilis* seems to involve the formation of an intermediate (EI). Thus a possible scheme of reaction would involve at least four steps: substrate binding and formation of Michaelis comples (ES), formation of the intermediate (EI) and product release, where the rate constant k_3 that represents the breakdown of the intermediate (EI) into the complex (EP) is the rate limiting step of the reaction. In the proposed mechanism, the Zn1 ion acts as a Lewis acid so that a molecule of water exists as a hydroxide ion, forming an oxyanion hole which polarises the carbonyl group of the β-lactam ring of the substrate. Another similar mechanism was proposed for the monozinc form of BcII enzyme from *Bacillus cereus* [128]. The nucleophilic attack to the carbon of the carbonyl group of the β-lactam ring is performed by the hydroxide ion, but the deprotonation of the hydroxide from Asp90 leads to the formation of a secondary tetrahedral intermediate. The catalytic mechanism of subclass B3 enzymes is essentially similar to that described for subclass B1 enzymes. The oxyanion hole produced by a hydroxide anion bound to Zn1 and stabilised by Zn2 and Asp120 acts as the nucleophile in β-lactam hydrolysis [129]. The mechanism proposed for monozinc subclass B2 enzyme is very different from those proposed for B1 and B3 enzymes in which the nucleophile attack is performed by the hydroxide anion bound to the Zn1 site. Serine-β-lactamase inhibitors as clavulanic acid are unsuccessful to inhibit class B enzymes. As previously mentioned the only molecules known to inhibit all three MBL subclasses are EDTA, o-phenantroline and dipicolinic acid, which indeed have no clinical significance. In fact a clinically useful inhibitor of MBLs should be sufficiently specific to remain inactive against the multitude of human metallo-enzymes.

REFERENCES

[1]   Frère JM. B-lactamases and bacterial resistance to antibiotics. Mol Microbiol 1995; 16(3): 385-95.

[2]   Matagne A, Galleni M, Laraki N, *et al.* B - lactamases , an old but ever renascent problem. Netherlands: A. Van Broekhoven *et al.* (eds.) 2001; 117-29.

[3]   Babic M, Hujer AM, Bonomo RA. What's new in antibiotic resistance? Focus on β-lactamases. Drug Res Updates 2006; 9: 142-56.

[4]   Hechler U, van den Weghe M, Martin HH, *et al.* Overproduced β-lactamase and the outher membrane barrier as resistance factors in Serratia marcescens higly resistant to β-lactamase-stable β-lactam antibiotics. J Gen Microbiol 1989; 135(5): 1275-90.

[5]   Bradford PA. Extended-spectrum β-lactamases in the 21st century: characterization, epidemiology, and detection of this important resistance threat. Clin Microbiol Rev 2001; 14(4): 933-51.

[6]   Caccamo M, Perilli M, Celenza G, *et al.* Occurrence of extended spectrum β-lactamases among isolates of *Enterobacteriaceae* from urinary tract infections in southern Italy. Microb Drug Resist 2006; 12: 257-64.

[7]   Paterson DL. Resistance in Gram-negative bacteria: *Enterobacteriaceae*. Amer J Med 2006; 119(6A): 520-28.

[8]   Paterson DL, Bonomo RA. Extended-spectrum β-lactamases: a clinical update. Clin Microbiol Rev 2005; 18(4): 657-86.

[9]   Jacoby GA. AmpC β-lactamases. Clin Microbiol Rev 2009; 22(1): 161-82.

[10]   Bouza E, Cercenado E. *Klebsiella* and *Enterobacter*: antibiotic resistance and treatment implications. Semin Respir Infect 2002; 17: 215-30.

[11]   Livermore DM. Threat from the pink corner. Ann. Med 2003; 35: 226-34.

[12]   Poole K. Multidrug efflux pumps and antimicrobial resistance in *Pseudomonas aeruginosa* and related organisms. J Mol Microbiol Biotechnol 2001; 3: 255-64.

[13]   Vahaboglu H, Oztürk R, Aygün G, *et al.* Widespread detection of PER-1-type extended-spectrum β-lactamases among nosocomial Acinetobacter and Pseudomonas aeruginosa isolates in Turkey: a nationwide multicenter study. Antimicrob Agents Chemother 1997; 41(10): 2265-69.

[14]   Pagani L, Mantengoli E, Migliavacca R, *et al.* Multifocal detection of multidrug-resistant *Pseudomonas aeruginosa* producine the PER-1 extended-spectrum β-lactamase in Northern Italy. J Clin Microbiol 2004; 42(6): 2523-29.

[15]   Endimiani A, Luzzaro F, Pini B, *et al. Pseudomonas aeruginosa* bloodstream infections: risk factors and treatment outcome related to expression of the PER-1 extended-spectrum β-lactamase. BMC Infect Dis 2006; 6: 52-60

[16]   Empel J, Filczak K, Mròwka A, *et al.* Outbreak of *Pseudomonas aeruginosa* infections with PER-1 extended-spectrum β-lactamase in Warsaw, Poland: further evidence for an international clonal complex. J Clin Microbiol 2007; 45(9): 2829-34.

[17]   Woodford N, Zhang J, Kaufmann ME, *et al.* Detection of *Pseudomonas aeruginosa* isolates producing VEB-type extended-spectrum β-lactamases in the United Kindom. J Antimicrob Chemother 2008; 62(6): 1265-68.

[18]   Mirsalehian A, Feizabadi M, Nakhjavani FA, *et al.* Detection of VEB-1, OXA-10 and PER-1 genotypes in extended-spectrum β-lactamase-producing Pseudomonas aeruginosa strains isolated from burn patients. Burns 2010; 36(1): 70-74.

[19]   Naas T, Nordmann P. OXA-type β-lactamases. Curr Pharm Des 1999; 5: 865-79.

[20]   Poirel L, Girlich D, Naas T, et al. OXA-28, an extended-spectrum variant of OXA-10 β-lactamase from Pseudomonas aeruginosa and its plasmid- and integron-located gene. Antimicrob Agents Chemother 2001; 45: 447-53.

[21]   Watanabe M, Iyobe S, Inoue M, *et al.* Transferable imipenem resistance in *Pseudomonas aeruginosa.* Antimicrob Agents Chemother 1991; 35(1): 147-51.

[22]   Lauretti L, Riccio M, Mazzariol A, *et al.* Cloning and characterization of *bla*$_{VIM}$, a new integron-borne metallo-β-lactamase gene from a *Pseudomonas aeruginosa* clinical isolate. Antimicrob Agents Chemother 1999; 43(7): 1584-90.

[23]   Lee K, Lim J, Yum J, *et al. bla*$_{VIM-2}$ cassette-containing novel integrons in metallo-β-lactamase-producing *Pseudomonas aeruginosa* and *Pseudomonas putida* isolates disseminated in a Korean hospital. Antimicrob Agents Chemother 2002; 46(4):1053-58.

[24]   Walsh TR, Toleman MA, Poirel L, *et al.* Metallo-β-lactamases: the quiet before the storm? Clin Microbiol Rev 2005; 18(2): 306-25.

[25]   Bebrone C. Metallo-β-lactamases (classification, activity, genetic organization, structure, zinc coordination) and their super-family. Biochem Pharmacol 2007; 74(12): 1686-01.

[26]   Pellegrini C, Mercuri PS, Celenza G, *et al.* Identification of *bla*$_{IMP-22}$ in *Pseudomonas spp* in urban wastewater and nosocomial environments: biochemical characterization of a new IMP metallo-enzyme variant and its genetic location. J Antimicrob Chemother 2009; 63(5): 901-08.

[27]   Karageorgopoulos DE, Falagas ME. Current control and treatment of multidrug-resistant *Acinetobacter baumannii* infections. Lancet Infect Dis 2008; 8(12): 751-62.

[28]   Hanlon GW. The emergence of multidrug resistant *Acinetobacter* species: a major concern in the hospital setting. Lett Appl Microbiol 2005; 41(5): 375-78.

[29]   Héritier C, Poirel L, Nordmann P. Cephalosporinase over-expression resulting from isertion of IS*Aba*1 in *Acinetobacter baumannii.* Clin Microbiol Infect 2006; 12(2): 123-30.

[30]   Héritier C, Poirel L, Fournier PE, *et al.* Characterization of the naturally occurring oxacillinase of *Acinetobacter baumannii.* Antimicrob Agents Chemother 2005; 49(10): 4174-79.

[31]   Evans BA, Hamouda A, Towner KJ, *et al.* Novel genetic context of multiple bla OXA-58 genes in Acinetobacter genospecies 3. J Antimicrob Chemother 2010; 65(8): 1586-88

[32]   Merino M, Acosta J, Poza M, *et al.* OXA-24 carbapenemase gene flanked by XerC/XerD-like recombination sites in different plasmids from different Acinetobacter species isolated during a nosocomial outbreak. Antimicrob Agents Chemother 2010; 54(6):2724-27.

[33]   Grosso F, Quinteira S, Peixe L. Emergence of an extreme-drug-resistant (XDR) Acinetobacter baumannii carrying blaOXA-23 in a patient with acute necrohaemorrhagic pancreatitis. J Hosp Infect 2010; 75(1): 82-83.

[34] Frère JM, Nguyen-Distèche M, Coyette J, *et al.* 1992 in The Chemistry of β-lactams; Page MI ed., Blackie, London, pp 148-197.

[35] Ghuysen JM. Serine β-lactamases and penicillin-binding proteins. Annu Rev Microbiol 1991; 45: 37-67.

[36] Ambler RP. The structure of β-lactamases. Philos Trans R Soc Lond B Biol Sci 1980; 289(1036): 321-31.

[37] Bush K. Classification of β-lactamases: groups 1, 2a, 2b, and 2b'. Antimicrob Agents Chemother 1989; 33: 264-70.

[38] Bush K. Classification of β-lactamases: groups 2c, 2d, 2e, 3 and 4. Antimicrob Agents Chemother 1989; 33: 271-76.

[39] Bush K, Jacoby JA, Medeiros AA. A functional classification scheme for β-lactamases and its correlation with molecular structure. Antimicrob Agents Chemother 1995; 39(6): 1211-33.

[40] Bush K, Jacoby GA. Update functional classification of β-lactamases. Antimicrob Agents Chemother 2010; 54(3): 969-76.

[41] Ouellette ML, Bissonnette L, Roy PH. Precise insertion of antibiotic resistance determinants into Tn21-like transposons: nucleotide sequence of the OXA-1 β-lactamase gene. Proc Natl Acad Sci USA 1987; 84: 7378-82.

[42] Doy Y, Paterson DL, Adams-Haduch JM, *et al.* Reduced susceptibility to cefepime among *Escherichia coli* clinical isolates producing novel variants of CMY-2 β-lactamase. Antimicrob agents Chemother 2009; 53: 3159-61.

[43] Lee SH, Jeong SH, Park YM. Characterization of *bla*$_{CMY-10}$ a novel, plasmid-encoded AmpC-type β-lactamase gene in a clinical isolate of Enterobacter aerogenes. J Appl Microbiol 2003; 95: 744-52.

[44] Hall PM, Collis CM. Mobile gene cassettes and integrons: capture and spread genes by site-specific recombination. Mol Microbiol 1995; 15: 593-600.

[45] Rowe-Magnus DA, Guerout AM, Mazel D. Super-integrons. Res Microbiol 1999; 150: 641-51.

[46] Collis CM, Kim MJ, Stokes HW, *et al.* Binding of the purified integron DNA integrase IntI1 to integron- and cassettes-associated recombination sites. Mol Microbiol 1998; 29: 477-90.

[47] Collis CM, Hall RM. Expression of antibiotic resistance genes in the integrated cassettes of integrons. Antimicrob Agents Chemother 1995; 39: 155-62.

[48] Ahmed AM, Shimamoto T. Emergence of a cefepime- and cefpirome-resistant Citrobacter freundii clinical isolate harbouring a novel chromosomally encoded AmpC β-lactamase, CMY-37. Int J Antimicrob Agents 2008; 32: 256-61.

[49] Waley SG. 1992 in The Chemistry of β-lactams; Page MI ed., Blackie, London, pp 198-28.

[50] Matagne A, Lamotte-Brasseur J, Frère JM. Catalytic properties of class A β-lactamases: efficiency and diversity. Biochem J 1998; 330: 581-98.

[51] Joris B, Ledent P, Dideberg O, *et al.* Comparison of sequences of class A β-lactamases and of the secondary structure elements of penicillin-recognizing proteins. Antimicrob Agents Chemother 1991; 35(11): 2294-301.

[52] Herzberg O, Moult J Penicilling-binding and degrading enzymes. Curr Opinion Struct Biol 1991; 1: 946-53.

[53] Jacob F, Joris B, Lepage S, *et al.* Role of the conserved amino acids of the SDN loop (Ser130, Asp131, Asn132) in a class A β-lactamase studied by site-directed mutagenesis. Biochem J 1990; 271: 399-406.

[54] Galleni M, Lamotte Brasseur J, Raquet X, *et al.* The enigmatic catalytic mechanism of active serine β-lactamases. Biochem Pharmacol 1995; 49(9): 1171-78.

[55] Bauvois C. Wouters J Crystal structures of class C β-lactamases: mechanistic implications and perspectives in drug design. In Enzyme-mediated resistance to antibiotics. Mechanisms, Dissemination, and prospects for inhibition. Edited by Robert A. Bonomo and marcelo Tolmasky. ASM Press Washington, D.C. 2007, pp 145-61.

[56] Danel F, Page MGP, Livermore DM. Class D β-lactamases. In Enzyme-mediated resistance to antibiotics. Mechanisms, Dissemination and prospects for inhibition. Edited by Robert A. Bonomo and marcelo Tolmasky. ASM Press Washington, D.C. 2007, pp 163-94.

[57] Sigal IS, Harwood BG, Arentzen R. Thiol-β-lactamase: replacement of the active site serine of RTEM β-lactamase by a cysteine residue. Proc Natl Acad Sci USA 1982; 79: 7157-60.

[58] Jacob F, Joris B, Frère JM. Active site serine mutants of the *Streptomyces albus* G β-lactamase. Biochem J 1991; 277: 647-52.

[59] Herzberg O. Refined crystal structure of β-lactamase from *Staphylococcus aureus* PC1 at 2.0 Å resolution. J Mol Biol 1991; 217: 701-19.

[60] Lobkovsky E, Moews PC, Liu H, *et al.* Evolution of an enzyme activity: crystallographic structure at 2.0 Å resolution of cephalosporinase from the ampC gene of *Enterobacter cloacae* P99 and comparison with a class A penicillinase. Proc Natl Acad Sci USA 1994; 90: 11257-61.

[61]   Kelly JA, Knox JR, Zhao H, *et al.* Crystallographic mapping of β-lactams bound to a D-alanyl-Dalanyl peptidase target enzyme. J Mol Biol 1989; 209: 281-95.

[62]   Knox JR, Moews PC. Beta-lactamase of *Bacillus licheniformis* 749/C. Refinement at 2 Å resolution and analysis of hydration.J Mol Biol 1991; 220: 435-55.

[63]   Jelsch C, Lenfant F, Masson JM, *et al.* B-lactamase TEM-1 of E. coli. Crystal structure determination at 2.5 Å resolution. FEBS Lett 1992; 299(2): 135-42.

[64]   Lamotte-Brasseur J, Dive G, Dideberg O, *et al.* Mechanism of acyl transfer by the class A serine β-lactamase of *Streptomyces albus* G. Biochem J 1991; 279(1): 213-21.

[65]   Leung YC, Robinson CV, Aplin RT, *et al.* Site-directed mutagenesis of β-lactamase I: role of Glu-166. Biochem J 1994; 299(3): 671-78.

[66]   Guillaume G, Vanhove M, Lamotte-Brasseur J, *et al.* Site-directed mutagenesis of glutamate 166 in two β-lactamases. Kinetic and molecular modelling studies. J Biol Chem 1997; 272(9): 5438-44.

[67]   Imtiaz U, Billings E, Knox JR, *et al.* Inactivation of class A 3-lactamases by clavulanic acid: the role of arginine-244 in a proposed nonconcerted sequence of events. J Am Chem Soc 1993; 115: 4435-42.

[68]   Imtiaz U, Billings E, Knox JR, *et al.* A structure-based analysis of the inhibition of class A β-lactamases by sulbactam. Biochemistry 1994; 33(19): 5728-38.

[69]   Strynadka NCJ, Martin R, Jensen SE, *et al.* Structure-based design of a potent transition state analogue for TEM-1 β-lactamase. Nature Struct Biol 1996; 3(8): 688-95.

[70]   Knothe H, Shah P, Kremery V, *et al.* Transferable resistance to cefotaxime, cefoxitin, cefamandole and cefuroxime in clinical isolates of Klebsiella pneumoniae and Serratia marcescens. Infection 1983; 11: 315-17.

[71]   Bonnet R. Growing group of extended-spectrum β-lactamases: the CTX-M enzymes. Antimicrob Agents Chemother 2004; 48(1): 1-14.

[72]   Petrosino J, Cantu III C, Palzkill T. B-lactamases: protein evolution in real time. Trends Microbiol 1998; 6(8): 323-27.

[73]   Sowek JA, Singer SB, Ohringer S, *et al.* Substitution of lysine at position 104 or 240 of TEM β-lactamase enhances the effect of serine 164 substitution of hydrolysis or affinity for cephalosporins and the monobactam aztreonam. Biochemistry 1991; 30: 3179-88.

[74]   Perilli M, Felici A, Franceschini N, *et al.* Characterization of a new TEM-derived ß-lactamase produced in a Serratia marcescens strain. Antimicrob Agents Chemother 1997; 41 (11): 2374-82.

[75]   Huletsky A, Knox JR, Levesque RC. The role of Ser238 and Lys240 in the hydrolysis of third-generation cephalosporins by SHV-type β-lactamases probed by site-directed mutagenesis and three-dimensional modeling. J Biol Chem 1993; 268: 3690-97.

[76]   Cantu III C, Huang W, Palzkill T. Selection and characterization of amino acid substitutions at residues 237-240 of TEM-1 β-lactamase with altered substrate specificity for aztreonam and ceftazidime. J Biol Chem 1996; 37: 22538-45.

[77]   Jacoby GA. Genetics of extended-spectrum b-lactamases. Eur J Clin. MicroBiol Infect. Dis 1994 13(Suppl. 1): 2-11.

[78]   Perilli M, Celenza G, De Santis F, *et al.* E240V substitution increases catalytic efficiency toward ceftazidime in a new natural TEM-type extended spectrum β-lactamase (TEM-149) from *Enterobacter aerogenes* and *Serratia marcescens* clinical isolates. Antimicrob Agents Chemother 2007; 52: 915-19

[79]   Knox, J R. Extended-spectrum and inhibitor-resistant TEM-type β-lactamases: mutations, specificity, and three-dimensional structure. Antimicrob Agents Chemother 1995; 39: 2593-601.

[80]   Chaibi EB, Sirot D, Paul G, *et al.* Inhibitor-resistant TEM β-lactamases: phenotypic, genetic and biochemical characteristics. J Antimicrob Chemother 1999; 43(4): 447-58.

[81]   Livermore DM, Canton R, Gniadkowsky M *et al.* CTM-M: changing the face of ESBLs in Europe. J Antimicrob Chemother 2007; 59: 165-74.

[82]   Luzzaro F, Mezzatesta M, Mugnaioli C, *et al.* Trends in production of extended-spectrum β-lactamases among enterobacteria of medical interest: Report of the second Italian nationwide survey. J Clin Microbiol 2006; 44: 1659-64

[83]   Mugnaioli C., Luzzaro F., De Luca F, *et al.* CTX-M-type extended-spectrum ß-lactamases in Italy: molecular epidemiology of an emerging countrywide problem. Antimicrob Agents Chemother 2006; 50(8): 2700-06.

[84]   Rodriguez MM, Power P, Radice M, *et al.* Chromosome-encoded CTX-M-3 from *Kluyvera ascorbata*: a possible origin of plasmid-borne CTX-M-1-derived cefotaximases. Antimicrob Agents Chemother 2004; 48: 4895-97.

[85]   Olson AB, Silverman M, Boyd DA, *et al.* Identification of a progenitor of the CTX-M-9 group of extended-spectrum β-lactamases from *Kluyvera georgiana* isolated in Guyana. Antimicrob Agents Chemother 2005; 49: 2112-15.

[86]   Poirel L, Decousser JW, Nordmann P. Insertion sequence IS*Ecp1B* is involved in expression and mobilization of a *bla*CTX-M β-lactamase gene. Antimicrob Agents Chemother 2003; 47: 2938-45.

[87]   Poirel L, Gniadkowski M, Nordmann P. Biochemical analysis of the ceftazidime-hydrolysing extended-spectrum β-lactamase CTX-M-15 and of its structurally related b-lactamase CTX-M-3. J Antimicrob Chemother 2002; 50: 1031-34.

[88]   Cartelle M, del Mar TM, Molina F, *et al.* High-level resistance to ceftazidime conferred by a novel enzyme, CTX-M-32, derived from CTX-M-1 through a single Asp240-Gly substitution. Antimicrob Agents Chemother 2004; 48: 2308-13.

[89]   Celenza G, Luzi C, Aschi M. Natural D240G Toho-1 mutant conferring resistance to ceftazidime: biochemical characterization of CTX-M-43. J Antimicrob Chemother 2008; 62(5): 991-97.

[90]   Shakil S, Khan AU. Interaction of CTX-M-15 enzyme with cefotaxime: a molecular modelling and docking study. Bioinformation 2010; 4(10): 468-72.

[91]   Sanguinetti M, Posteraro B, Spanu T, *et al.* Characterization of clinical isolates of Enterobacteriaceae from Italy by the BD Phoenix extended-spectrum b-lactamase detection method. J Clin Microbiol 2003; 41: 1463-68.

[92]   Pagani L, Dell'Amico E, Migliavacca R, *et al.* Multiple CTX-M-type extended-spectrum b-lactamases in nosocomial isolates of *Enterobacteriaceae* from a hospital in northern Italy. J Clin Microbiol 2003; 41: 4264-69

[93]   Medeiros AA, Hare RS. B-lactamase-mediated resistance to penems and carbapenems amongst *Enterobacteriaceae*, abstr. 116. 26th Intersci. Conf. Antimicrob Agents Chemother American Society for Microbiology, Washington, DC. 1986.

[94]   Queenan AM, Bush K. Carbapenemases: the versatile β-lactamases. Clin Microbiol Rev 2007; 20(3): 440-58.

[95]   Yang Y, Wu P, Livermore DM. Biochemical characterization of a β-lactamase that hydrolyzes penems and carbapenems from two *Serratia marcescens* isolates. Antimicrob Agents Chemother 1990; 34: 755-58.

[96]   Queenan AM, Shang W, Schreckenberger P, *et al.* SME-3, a novel member of the *Serratia marcescens* SME family of carbapenem-hydrolyzing β-lactamases. Antimicrob Agents Chemother 2006; 50: 3485-87.

[97]   Rasmussen BA, Bush K, Keeney D, *et al.* Characterization of IMI-1 β-lactamase, a class A carbapenem-hydrolyzing enzyme from *Enterobacter cloacae*. Antimicrob Agents Chemother 1996; 40: 2080-86.

[98]   Yu YS, Du XX, Zhou ZH, *et al.* First isolation of *bla*IMI-2 in an *Enterobacter cloacae* clinical isolate from China. Antimicrob Agents Chemother 2006; 50: 1610-11.

[99]   Majiduddin FK, Palzkill T. Amino acid residues that contribute to substrate specificity of class A β-lactamase SME-1. Antimicrob Agents Chemother 2005; 49: 3421-27.

[100] Hossain A, Ferraro MJ, Pino RM, *et al.* Plasmid-mediated carbapenem-hydrolyzing enzyme KPC-2 in an *Enterobacter* spp.Antimicrob Agents Chemother 2004; 48: 4438-40.

[101] Miriagou V, Tzouvelekis LS, Rossiter S, *et al.* Imipenem resistance in a *Salmonella* clinical strain due to plasmid-mediated class A carbapenemase KPC-2. Antimicrob Agents Chemother 2003; 47: 1297-300.

[102] Giakkoupi P, Tzouvelekis LS, Tsakris A, *et al.* IBC-1, a novel integron-associated class A β-lactamase with extended-spectrum properties produced by an Enterobacter cloacae clinical strain. Antimicrob Agents Chemother 2000; 44: 2247-53.

[103] Poirel L, Le Thomas I, Naas T, *et al.* Biochemical sequence analyses of GES-1, a novel class A extended-spectrum β-lactamase, and the class 1 integron In52 from *Klebsiella pneumoniae*. Antimicrob Agents Chemother 2000; 44: 622-32.

[104] Monnaie D, Frère JM. Interaction of clavulanate with class C β-lactamases. FEBS Lett 1993; 334: 269-71.

[105] Usher KC, Blaszczak LC, Weston GS, *et al.* Three dimensional structure of AmpC β-lactamase from E. coli bound to a transition-state analogue: possible implications for the oxyanion hypothesis and for inhibition design. Biochemistry 1998; 37: 16082-92.

[106] Dubus A, Ledent P, Lamotte-Brasseur J, *et al.* The roles of residues Tyr150, Glu272 and His314 in class C β-lactamases. Proteins 1996; 25(4): 473-85.

[107] Diaz N, Suàrez D, Sordo TL. Molecular dynamics simulations of class C β-lactamase from *Citrobacter freundii*: insights into the base catalyst for acylation. Biochemistry 2006; 45(2): 439-51.

[108] Goldberg SD, Iannuccilli W, Nguyen T, *et al.* Identification of residues critical for catalysis in a class C β-lactamase by combinatorial scanning mutagenesis. Protein Sci 2003; 12: 1633-45.

[109] Monnaie D, Dubus A, Cooke D, *et al.* Role of residue Lys315 in the mechanism of action of the Enterobacter cloacae 908R β-lactamase. Biochemistry 1994; 33: 5193-201.

[110] Zhang Z, Yu Y, Musser JM, *et al.* Amico acid sequence determinants of extended-spectrum cephalosporin hydrolysis by the class C P99 β-lactamase. J Biol Chem 2001; 276: 46568-74.

[11] Monaghan C, Holland S, Dale JW. The interaction of antraquinone dyes with the plasmid-mediated OXA-2 β-lactamase. Biochem J 1982; 205: 413-17.

[112] Sunt T, Nukaga M, Mayama K, *et al.* Crystallization and preliminary X-ray study of OXA-1, a class D β-lactamase. Acta Crystallogr D Biol Crystallogr 2001; 57: 1912-14.

[113] Maveyraud L, Golemi-Kotra D, Ishiwata A, *et al.* High resolution X-ray structure of an acyl enzyme species for the class D OXA-10 β-lactamase. J Am Chem Soc 2002; 124: 2461-65.

[114] Paetzel M, Danel F, Castro L, *et al.* Crystal structure of the class D β-lactamase OXA-10. Nat Struct Biol 2000; 7: 918-25.

[115] Pernot L, Frenois F, Rybkine T, *et al.* Crystal structures of the class D β-lactamase OXA-13 in the native form and in complex with meropenem. J Mol Biol 2001; 310: 859-74.

[116] Hata M, Fujii Y, Tanaka Y, *et al.* Substrate deacylation mechanisms of serine β-lactamases. Biol Pharm Bull 2006; 29(1): 2151-59.

[117] Garau G, García-Sáez I, Bebrone C, *et al.* Update of the standard numbering scheme for class B β-lactamases. Antimicrob Agents Chemother 2004; 48(7): 2347-49.

[118] Osano E, Arakawa Y, Wacharotayankun R, *et al.* Molecular characterization of an enterobacterial metallo β-lactamase found in a clinical isolate of *Serratia marcescens* that shows imipenem resistance. Antimicrob Agents Chemother 1994; 38(1): 71-78.

[119] Laraki N, Franceschini N, Rossolini G, *et al.* Biochemical characterization of the *Pseudomonas aeruginosa* 101/1477 metallo-β-lactamase IMP-1 produced by *Escherichia coli*. Antimicrob Agents Chemother 1999; 43(4): 902-06.

[120] Lauretti L, Riccio M, Mazzariol A, *et al.* Cloning and characterization of bla_{VIM}, a new integron-borne metallo-β-lactamase gene from a *Pseudomonas aeruginosa* clinical isolate. Antimicrob Agents Chemother 1999; 43(7): 1584-90.

[121] Toleman M, Simm A, Murphy T, *et al.* Molecular characterization of SPM-1, a novel metallo-β-lactamase isolated in Latin America: report from the SENTRY Antimicrobial Surveillance Programme. J Antimicrob Chemother 2002; 50(5): 673-79.

[122] Castanheira M, Toleman M, Jones R, *et al.* Molecular characterization of a β-lactamase gene, bla_{GIM-1}, encoding a new subclass of metallo-β-lactamase. Antimicrob Agents Chemother 2004; 48(12): 4654-61.

[123] Yong D, Toleman MA, Giske CG, *et al.* Characterization of a new metallo-β-lactamase gene, blaNDM-1, and a novel erythromycin esterase gene carried on a unique genetic structure in *Klebsiella pneumoniae* sequence type 14 from India. Antimicrob Agents Chemother 2009; 53(12): 5046-54.

[124] Neuwald A, Liu J, Lipman D, *et al.* Extracting protein alignment models from the sequence database. Nucleic Acids Res 1997; 25(9): 1665-77.

[125] Daiyasu H, Osaka K, Ishino Y, *et al.* Expansion of the zinc metallo-hydrolase family of the β-lactamase fold. FEBS Lett. 2001; 503(1): 1-6.

[126] Damblon C, Jensen M, Ababou A, *et al.* The inhibitor thiomandelic acid binds to both metal ions in metallo-β-lactamase and induces positive cooperativity in metal binding. J Biol Chem 2003; 278(31): 29240-51.

[127] Garau G, Bebrone C, Anne C, *et al.* A metallo-β-lactamase enzyme in action: crystal structures of the monozinc carbapenemase cpha and its complex with biapenem. J Mol. Biol 2005; 345(4):785-95.

[128] Bounaga S, Laws A, Galleni M, *et al.* The mechanism of catalysis and the inhibition of the *Bacillus* cereus zinc-dependent β-lactamase. Biochem J 1998; 331 (Pt 3): 703-11.

[129] Spencer J, Read J, Sessions R, *et al.* Antibiotic recognition by binuclear metallo-β-lactamases revealed by x-ray crystallography. J Am Chem Soc 2005; 127(41): 14439-44.

Index

A

Aminoglycosides 157
Antimicrobials for treatment of mrsa 136-137

C

Classification of beta-lactamases.. 37
Carbapenem resistance 39-42
Commercial methods for esbl detection 121
Campylobacter 152-153

D

Detection of drug resistance 107-109
DNA sequencing 109

E

Enterobacteriaceae..76-83
ESBL-diversity 117-118

F

Flow cytometric assay 109

G

Genetic basis of methicillin resistance 131-132

H

Heterogenously resistant mrsa...135-136
High prevalence of tb and drug resistant tuberculosis 91-93
HIV-TB co- morbidity... 93

I

Induction of mrps 12-14

M

Molecular mechanisms of drug resistance..103-106
Mechanisms of antimicrobial resistance..63-64
Mechanism responsible for antimicrobial drug resistance in *acinetobacter baumannii*.....142-145
Mechanisms of antibiotic resistance in *campylobacter* 153-155
MDR enterobacteriacae 56
MRSA..48-50
Management of drug resistance in tuberculosis.. 110

O

Oxacillin susceptible mrsa (os-mrsa).. 136

P

Prevalence of antimicrobial resistance in *salmonella*... 157
Prevalence of antimicrobial resistance in *e. coli*...160-161
Pharmacogenetics of mrps..19-22

Poor implementation of dots..94

R

Resistance phenotypes and detection 57-58
Resistance mechanisms and phenotypes 59-60

S

Spread of antimicrobial resistance in *salmonella* 159-160
Social issues 95-96

T

The omega loop 119
Topology of mrps 4-12
Transfer of antimicrobial resistance determinants in campylobacter 155-156
Types of drug resistance 101-102

V

Virulence factors of ca-mrsa... 134-135
VRE 53

W

Worldwide scenario of drug resistant tb 102-103

www.ingramcontent.com/pod-product-compliance
Lightning Source LLC
Chambersburg PA
CBHW050835220326

41598CB00006B/371